Temporomandibular Joint Disorders - New Perspectives in Diagnosis and Treatment

Edited by Dragana Gabrić, Marko Vuletić and Ivica Pelivan

Published in London, United Kingdom

Temporomandibular Joint Disorders - New Perspectives in Diagnosis and Treatment
http://dx.doi.org/10.5772/intechopen.1009041
Edited by Dragana Gabrić, Marko Vuletić and Ivica Pelivan

Contributors
Aisha Faraz, Ajit Sinha, Ashok Prasanna, Atilade Waheed Adegbiji, Bilal Hasan, Chandrsekaran Krithika, Chitathoor Sridhar, Denise Trochesset, Elahe Aleebrahim-Dehkordi, Elvin Gunel, Hima John, Huseyin Kurtulmus, Jiss Mary George, Madiha Khan, Mahmoud Bahrami Dashtaki, Mohamed Arafa, Mohamed M. Ghoneim, Noopur Srivastava, Oyebanji Anthony Olajuyin, Pooja Chaudhuri, Pranav Parasher, S. Nachiappan, Sarah Allal, Segun Mathew Agboola, Sina Ahmadi, Sonam Khurana, Sufyan Ahmed, Taha Fayad, Tharanikumar Sivakumar, Toye Gabriel Olajide, U. Elaveyini

First published in London, United Kingdom, 2026 by IntechOpen
IntechOpen is the global imprint of INTECHOPEN LIMITED, registered in England and Wales, registration number: 11086078, 167-169 Great Portland Street, London, W1W 5PF, United Kingdom

For EU product safety concerns: IN TECH d.o.o., Prolaz Marije Krucifikse Kozulić 3, 51000 Rijeka, Croatia, info@intechopen.com or visit our website at intechopen.com.

British Library Cataloguing-in-Publication Data
A catalogue record for this book is available from the British Library

Temporomandibular Joint Disorders - New Perspectives in Diagnosis and Treatment
Edited by Dragana Gabrić, Marko Vuletić and Ivica Pelivan
p. cm.
Print ISBN 978-1-83634-686-9
Online ISBN 978-1-83634-685-2
eBook (PDF) ISBN 978-1-83634-687-6

Meet the editors

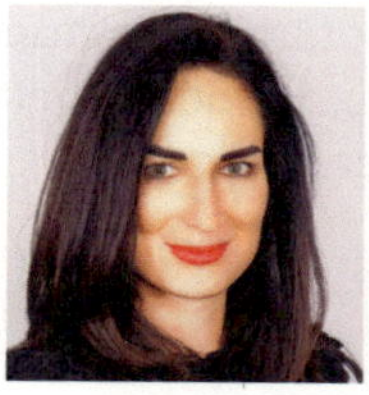

Dragana Gabrić, DMD, Ph.D., is a Full Professor, Scientific Advisor, and Specialist in Oral Surgery at the Department of Oral Surgery, School of Dental Medicine, University of Zagreb. She currently serves as the Head of the Clinical Department of Oral Surgery at the University Dental Clinic, University Hospital Center Zagreb, and is the Head of the Reference Center for Dental Implantology of the Ministry of Health of the Republic of Croatia. Professor Gabrić is the author and coauthor of many cited scientific and professional papers and reviews, as well as 36 book chapters. She has been an invited speaker at numerous international scientific and professional conferences and universities, and holds one registered patent. Her professional affiliations include membership in the Croatian Chamber of Dental Medicine, the Croatian Society of Oral Surgeons, the Croatian Association for Dental Implantology, and the Croatian Medical Association. Additionally, she is a member of the Laser and Health Academy, the Croatian Association for Minimally Invasive Dental Medicine, and the Croatian Society for Maxillofacial, Plastic and Reconstructive Surgery of the Face and Neck.

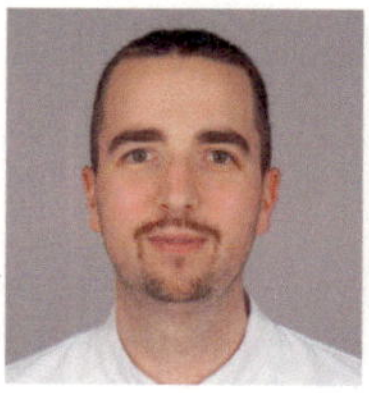

Marko Vuletić is an Assistant Professor at the Department of Oral Surgery, School of Dental Medicine, University of Zagreb. He earned his Ph.D. in 2017 and became a specialist in Oral Surgery in 2019. Since 2020, he has been working as an oral surgeon at the Clinical Department of Oral Surgery at the Clinic of Dentistry, University Hospital Centre Zagreb. He actively participates in clinical teaching of students and residents, postgraduate teaching in dental implantology, and continuing education courses in dental medicine. He continuously improves his scientific and professional skills and has participated in numerous national and international scientific and professional conferences. He has also been an invited lecturer at congresses and has conducted many workshops in Croatia and abroad. He is the author and co-author of more than 100 scientific, professional, and review papers, as well as book chapters and conference papers published in national and international journals.

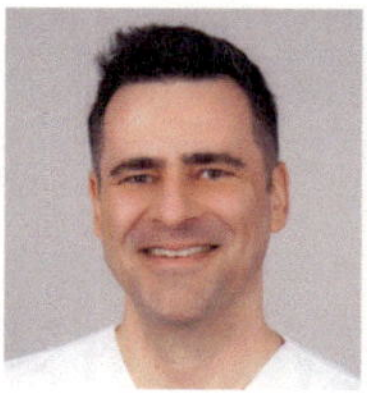

Ivica Pelivan is an Associate Professor in the Department of Removable Prosthodontics at the School of Dental Medicine, University of Zagreb, where he has been employed since 2004. He obtained his Ph.D. in 2010 and became a specialist in prosthodontics the same year. He serves as a lecturer for continuing education courses and as an invited speaker at international congresses, and is both an author and a co-author of various scientific and professional papers. His involvement includes clinical teaching for students and residents, as well as postgraduate education in dental implantology and prosthodontics. He also leads continuing education courses in dental medicine. Pelivan has participated in a wide range of national and international scientific and professional congresses and conferences. These events frequently invite him to lecture, and he has conducted numerous workshops both in Croatia and internationally. He has authored and co-authored numerous scientific, professional, and review papers, as well as book chapters and conference papers, published in both national and international journals. He is a member of several professional organizations, including the Croatian Chamber of Dental Medicine, Croatian Prosthodontics, Croatian Association for Dental Implantology, Croatian Medical Association, Croatian Endodontics Society, European Endodontic Society, and the European Association for Osseointegration.

Contents

Preface

Temporomandibular joint disorders (TMDs) represent a heterogeneous group of conditions that affect the temporomandibular joint, masticatory muscles, and associated structures, often presenting with pain, functional limitation, and a wide spectrum of overlapping symptoms. Despite their high prevalence and significant impact on quality of life, TMDs remain challenging to diagnose and manage due to their multifactorial etiology, variable clinical presentation, and frequent association with otologic, neurologic, musculoskeletal, and psychosocial factors.

Over the past decades, advances in imaging, biomechanics, regenerative medicine, pain science, and minimally invasive interventions have significantly expanded our understanding of temporomandibular joint pathology. At the same time, clinical practice has evolved toward a more conservative, patient-centered, and multidisciplinary approach. This edited volume, *Temporomandibular Joint Disorders – New Perspectives in Diagnosis and Treatment*, aims to reflect these developments by presenting contemporary insights into both fundamental concepts and emerging strategies in the field of TMDs.

The chapters included in this book explore a broad range of topics, beginning with updated perspectives on anatomy, pathophysiology, and differential diagnosis of temporomandibular disorders. Special attention is given to conditions that mimic or coexist with TMDs, highlighting the importance of accurate diagnosis and interdisciplinary collaboration. The volume further addresses conservative and minimally invasive treatment modalities, including physiotherapy, pharmacological management, intra-articular therapies, and neuromodulation techniques, emphasizing evidence-based decision-making and individualized care.

In addition, the book discusses surgical management strategies for advanced or refractory cases, outlining contemporary protocols, indications, and outcomes while stressing the importance of careful patient selection. Emerging fields such as regenerative medicine, platelet-rich plasma therapies, and artificial intelligence-assisted diagnostics are also examined, offering a glimpse into future directions in both research and clinical practice.

This volume is intended for oral and maxillofacial surgeons, dentists, orthodontists, otolaryngologists, physiotherapists, pain specialists, and researchers with an interest in temporomandibular joint disorders. By bringing together contributions from experts across disciplines, we hope this book will serve as a practical reference, an educational resource, and a catalyst for further collaboration and innovation in the diagnosis and treatment of TMDs.

The editors would like to express their sincere appreciation to all contributing authors for their expertise and dedication, as well as to the IntechOpen editorial team for their professional support throughout the development of this volume.

Dragana Gabrić, DDM, PhD
Full Professor,
Specialist in Oral Surgery,
Department of Oral Surgery,
School of Dental Medicine,
University of Zagreb,
Zagreb, Croatia

Head
Clinical Department of Oral Surgery,
University Hospital Centre Zagreb,
Zagreb, Croatia

Ministry of Health Reference Center for Dental Implantology, Head
Croatia

Marko Vuletić, DMD, PhD
Assistant Professor,
Specialist in Oral Surgery,
Department of Oral Surgery,
School of Dental Medicine,
University of Zagreb,
Zagreb, Croatia

University Hospital Centre Zagreb,
Zagreb, Croatia

Ivica Pelivan, DMD, PhD
Associate Professor,
Specialist in Prosthodontics,
Department of Removable Prosthodontics,
School of Dental Medicine,
University of Zagreb,
Zagreb, Croatia

Section 1

Temporomandibular Joint Disorders – New Perspectives in Diagnosis

Chapter 1

Temporomandibular Joint Dysfunction: Clinical Evaluation and Physiotherapeutic Approaches

Pooja Chaudhuri

Abstract

Temporomandibular joint disorders (TMDs) refer to a range of conditions that impact the temporomandibular joint, masticatory musculature, and related structures. They are the significant cause of orofacial pain and functional limitations, impacting quality of life and daily function. A thorough comprehension of temporomandibular joint anatomy and biomechanics is crucial to achieve accurate diagnosis and effective physiotherapeutic management. This paper provides a comprehensive overview of TMDs, including their anatomical and biomechanical foundations, current diagnostic and evaluation techniques, and emerging physiotherapy interventions. This narrative review was conducted to explore recent developments for evaluation, diagnosis, and management of temporomandibular joint disorders (TMDs), with a focus on conservative and physiotherapy-based interventions. The TMJ is a complex synovial joint with unique biomechanical features that allow for both hinging and gliding motions. Dysfunction in this joint often results from musculoskeletal imbalances, trauma, or parafunctional habits. Evaluation of TMD includes clinical assessment (e.g., range of motion, joint sounds, palpation), validated outcome measures (e.g., JFLS, OHIP-TMD), and imaging. Physiotherapy interventions—such as manual therapy, muscle energy techniques (MET), soft tissue mobilization, neuromuscular re-education, and patient-specific exercise programs—have shown significant improvements in pain reduction and functional outcomes. New perspectives include tele-rehabilitation and integration of digital tools for objective assessment and monitoring. Early and accurate diagnosis combined with a multidisciplinary physiotherapy approach is crucial for effective TMD management. Continued research and clinical innovation are essential to refine physiotherapeutic protocols and incorporate technology-driven care tailored to individual patient needs.

Keywords: temporomandibular joint disorders, TMD, physiotherapy, biomechanics, manual therapy, muscle energy technique, DC/TMD, soft tissue mobilization

1. Introduction

Temporomandibular joint (TMJ) is a distinctive synovial joint that links the mandible to the temporal bone of the skull. It is formed by the articulation of the condylar process of the mandible with the mandibular fossa and articular eminence of the temporal bone. Although it is typically classified as a synovial hinge joint, the

TMJ is considered anatomically unique. Unlike most synovial joints, which are lined with hyaline cartilage, the TMJ is covered by fibrocartilage, which contributes to its specialized function and structure [1, 2]. This unique feature allows the joint to withstand repeated stress and complex movements required for functions, such as chewing, speaking, and yawning [3, 4].

2. Design and function

The temporomandibular joint (TMJ) is a form of diarthrodial joint, specifically classified as a ginglymoarthrodial joint, which allows both hinging and gliding movements [5]. It features a synovial cavity, an articular cartilage, and a fibrous capsule that encases the joint. Within this cavity, synovial fluid provides lubrication, and several ligaments offer structural support. Anatomically, the TMJ is formed by the articulation between the mandibular condyle and the mandibular fossa of the temporal bone [6].

3. Anatomy

The temporomandibular joint (TMJ) (**Figure 1**) is a type of compound synovial joint with a modified ovoid bicondylar structure. It is formed through the articulation of the mandibular head, the articular disc located within the joint, and the articular eminence of the temporal bone [1–3].

The upper part of the temporomandibular joint (TMJ) is formed by the squamous part of the temporal bone, specifically known as the glenoid fossa, which accommodates the mandibular condyle [1]. Located behind this fossa is the posterior articular ridge, and next to it lies a bony projection referred to as the postglenoid process. This postglenoid region also helps form the superior boundary of the external auditory canal [7].

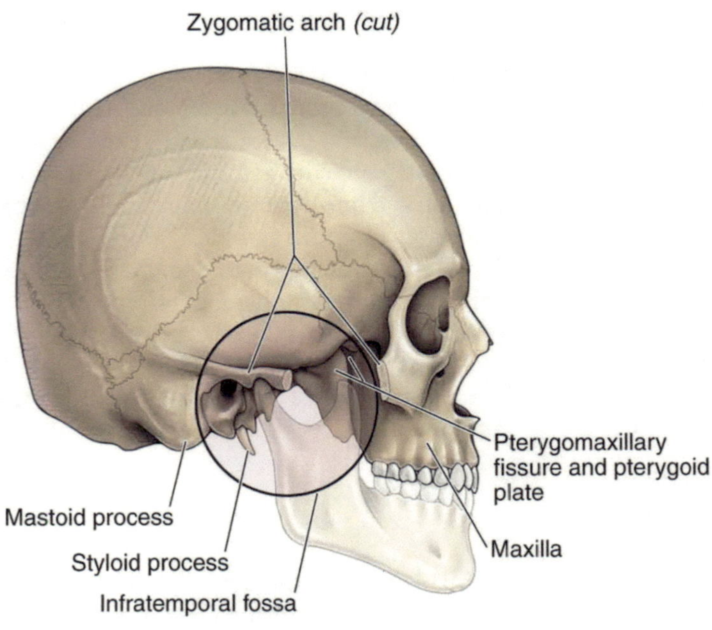

Figure 1.
The temporomandibular joint.

Anterior surface of glenoid fossa in temporal bone comprises the articular eminence, which creates a medial bone projection toward the posterior border of the zygomatic bone. The slightly inclined preglenoid plane leads into this eminence, which lies anterior to the glenoid fossa and forms part of the cranial base. This anatomical configuration supports and guides the dynamic movements of both the mandibular condyle and the articular disc during jaw motion [3, 5]. On the lateral aspect of the articular eminence, adjacent to the root of the zygomatic process, a bony prominence known as the articular tubercle is present [1].

The mediolateral part of glenoid fossa is larger when compared to the anteroposterior part. The lower articular region of the glenoid fossa corresponds to the upper portion of the mandible. It is formed by the mandibular condyle, which typically measures around 15–20 mm in its transverse dimension and approximately 8–10 mm in the anteroposterior direction [3, 4].

The articular disc that is situated between the mandibular condyle and the glenoid fossa is typically biconcave or oval in configuration. This fibrocartilaginous structure measures approximately 2 mm in thickness anteriorly and about 3 mm posteriorly, while the central region is comparatively thinner [3, 5]. The anterior segment of the disc is composed superiorly of fibroelastic fascia and inferiorly of fibrous connective tissue. Superiorly, the disc articulates with the postglenoid process, serving to stabilize its position and prevent forward displacement during mouth opening. Inferiorly, it restricts excessive rotational movement of the disc in relation to the mandibular condyle [5, 7].

The anterior part of the articular disc connects with the joint capsule, articular eminence, condyle, and the upper part of the lateral pterygoid muscle [1].

The posterior part of the articular disc connects to the bilateral retro-disc tissue, glenoid fossa, temporal bone, and condyle [3].

Laterally and medially, the cartilaginous disc is anchored to the mandibular condyle, while its margins show partial continuity with the fibrous capsule that encloses the joint [3, 4].

Multiple ligaments regulate the mechanical forces acting on the temporomandibular joint (TMJ) and contribute to its proprioceptive feedback. Sensory input arises not only from the joint capsule but also from the masticatory muscles, cutaneous receptors, and receptors located within the periodontal ligament [1, 3]. The strain detected by the articular ligaments is particularly significant for maintaining proper TMJ function [5].

3.1 Sphenomandibular ligament (SML)

The sphenomandibular ligament is considered a remnant of Meckel's cartilage. It originates from the spine of the sphenoid bone, which also gives rise to the pterygospinous ligament, and extends toward the mandible, where it blends with the medial wall of the TMJ capsule [7]. Passing through the petrotympanic fissure, it maintains connections with the malleus and contributes fibers to the anterior ligament of the malleus. The ligament descends further to insert into the lingula of the mandible, thereby linking the sphenoid, middle ear, and mandible. Along its course, it is crossed by the mylohyoid nerve and associated vessels, and it also establishes continuity with the pterygomandibular fascia. Anatomically, it lies superior and lateral to the lateral pterygoid muscle, internal maxillary artery, auriculotemporal nerve, inferior alveolar nerve, and middle meningeal artery. Functionally, the SML helps limit excessive forward translation of the mandibular condyle, particularly once the mouth has opened beyond approximately 10 degrees [1, 7].

3.2 Stylomandibular ligament (STML)

The stylomandibular ligament extends from the styloid process of the temporal bone to the posterior border of the mandible, typically near the angle. It is regarded as a condensation of the deep cervical fascia, particularly the parotid fascia [7, 8]. Functionally, it restricts excessive mandibular protrusion. From an embryological perspective, it develops from Reichert's cartilage, which originates from the first and second branchial arches and also contributes to the formation of the stapes in the middle ear. Along its course, the ligament lies over the medial surface of the medial pterygoid muscle [5].

3.3 Pterygomandibular ligament (PTML)

The pterygomandibular ligament, also referred to as the pterygomandibular raphe, represents a localized thickening of the buccopharyngeal fascia. It extends from the hamulus of the medial pterygoid plate of the sphenoid bone to the posterior region of the retromolar trigone of the mandible. The ligament serves as an anatomical boundary between two muscles: anteriorly, it provides attachment for the buccinator, while posteriorly, it connects with the superior pharyngeal constrictor. Developmentally, it arises from mesenchymal tissue associated with the first and second branchial arches. Functionally, the PTML contributes to controlling mandibular motion by restricting excessive movements [7, 8].

3.4 Pinto ligament (discomalleolar or malleolomandibular ligament)

Embryologically, this ligament originates from the tympanic portion of the temporal region. It is composed of two distinct segments. The first lies within the middle ear, where it connects to the malleus and is related to the anterior ligament of the malleus. The second segment extends beyond the tympanic cavity, reaching the posterosuperior portion of the TMJ capsule, where it associates with the retrodiscal tissues by traversing the petrotympanic fissure. Functionally, the ligament serves dual roles: within the TMJ, it provides protection to the synovial membrane by buffering stresses from adjacent structures, while in the middle ear, it is thought to participate in maintaining or modulating pressure equilibrium [3, 9].

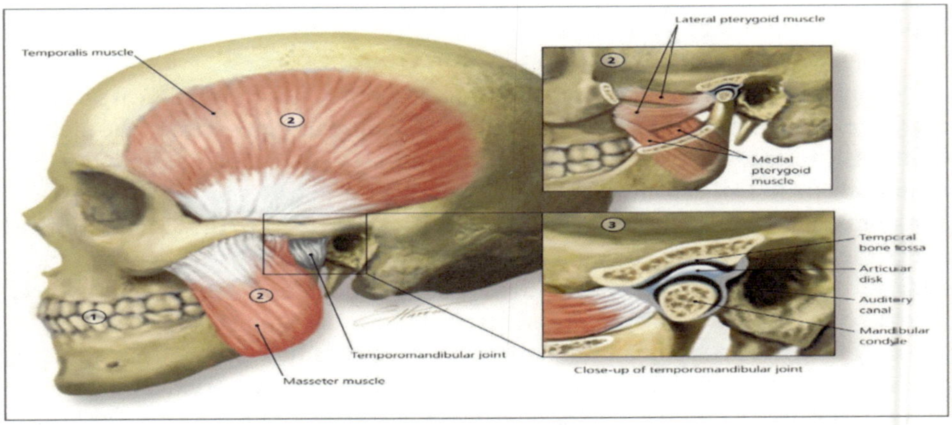

Figure 2.
Anatomy and Structure of TMJ joint.

- The collateral ligament comprises two symmetrical fiber bundles that arise from the intermediate zone of the articular disc and insert into the medial and lateral poles of the mandibular condyle. Its primary role is to firmly secure the disc to the condyle, ensuring coordinated movement between these structures [5, 7].

TMJ is closely related to various muscles that function to move and protect the joint itself. Muscles primarily responsible for *jaw closure* include the masseter, temporalis, and the lateral (external) pterygoid. Conversely, *jaw opening* is facilitated by the medial (internal) pterygoid, digastric, mylohyoid, and geniohyoid muscles (**Figure 2**).

4. Function

During mouth opening, the temporomandibular joint exhibits a coordinated sequence of movements involving both the discomandibular and discotemporal compartments. Initially, a rotational movement occurs within the discomandibular space, followed by translational motion in the discotemporal space [1, 3]. Lateral movement of the condyle is achieved through a combination of rotation and anterior sliding on one side, accompanied by anteromedial translation and rotation of the contralateral condyle. Posterior displacement of one condyle may also occur simultaneously with anterior gliding of the opposite condyle. Protrusive motion, whether bilateral or unilateral, is produced through anterior sliding of the condyles [3, 4].

The versatility of TMJ kinematics allows for a wide range of essential functions, including:

1. Mastication (chewing)
2. Sucking
3. Swallowing
4. Speech and phonation
5. Facial expressions
6. Respiration
7. Protrusion, retrusion, and lateral movements of the mandible
8. Mouth opening
9. Regulation of middle ear pressure [1, 4, 5].

5. Blood supply and lymphatics

The *arterial supply* of the temporomandibular joint (TMJ) is primarily provided by the superficial temporal and maxillary arteries, along with contributions from the masseteric artery. Additional vascular input arises from several branches of the external carotid system, including the posterior auricular, ascending pharyngeal, and ascending palatine arteries [7, 9].

Venous drainage occurs predominantly via the pterygoid venous plexus located in the retrodiscal region. This plexus communicates with multiple venous pathways, including the internal maxillary, sphenopalatine, middle meningeal, deep temporal, masseteric, and inferior alveolar veins [7].

The *lymphatic drainage* of the TMJ is less clearly defined, as lymph node involvement may vary in pathological conditions. In general, the lymphatics associated with the joint are linked to the submandibular triangle, where regional lymph nodes play a role in drainage [8, 9].

6. Nerves

The temporomandibular joint (TMJ) contains a variety of *proprioceptive receptors*, particularly within the articular disc. These include Golgi-Mazzoni and Ruffini corpuscles, as well as both myelinated and unmyelinated nerve fibers that contribute to sensory feedback [1, 4].

Regarding *capsular innervation*, the anterolateral portion of the joint capsule is supplied by the masseteric nerve, a branch of the mandibular division (V3) of the trigeminal nerve. The lateral capsule, in contrast, receives its innervation primarily from the auriculotemporal nerve, another branch of the mandibular nerve (cranial nerve V) [1, 4].

7. Muscular relations of the TMJ

The temporomandibular joint (TMJ) maintains direct contact with four key masticatory muscles: the *masseter, temporalis, lateral (external) pterygoid, and medial (internal) pterygoid*.

- *Masseter muscle*: This muscle, through its perimysium, attaches anteriorly to the articular disc. It originates from the zygomatic arch, with multiple muscular layers, and inserts into the lateral surface of the mandibular ramus and the coronoid process. Functionally, it elevates the mandible. Its innervation is provided by the masseteric branch of the mandibular nerve (V3) [3, 5, 8, 10].

- *Temporalis muscle*: Arising from the temporal fossa and the medial aspect of the zygomatic process, the temporalis inserts onto the coronoid process of the mandible. Occasionally, its anterior fibers may connect with the articular disc. Like the masseter, its main action is mandibular elevation, and it is supplied by the deep temporal branches of the mandibular nerve (V3) [3, 5, 8].

- *Lateral (external) pterygoid muscle*: This muscle has two distinct heads.

    o The *superior head* originates from the outer surface of the greater wing of the sphenoid bone and inserts anteromedially into the TMJ capsule or the anteromedial aspect of the condylar neck, contacting the disc anteriorly.

    o The *inferior head* arises from the lateral plate of the pterygoid process of the sphenoid and attaches to the pterygoid fovea on the condylar neck. Bilateral contraction produces mandibular protrusion, while unilateral contraction causes contralateral deviation. The muscle advances the condyle during mouth opening and assists in pulling the disc anteromedially during closure. Both heads are active in the early phases of opening and closing [3, 5, 8].

- *Medial (internal) pterygoid muscle*: Originating from the pterygoid fossa, the pyramidal process of the palatine bone, and the maxillary tuberosity, this muscle inserts onto the medial surface of the mandibular angle and ramus. It elevates and protrudes the mandible and, like the lateral pterygoid, is innervated by branches of the mandibular nerve (V3) [3, 5, 8].

Classically, these four muscles are identified as the *primary masticatory muscles*. However, the *suprahyoid and infrahyoid muscles* also contribute significantly to mandibular motion.

- *Suprahyoid muscles*: This group includes the digastric, mylohyoid, stylohyoid, and geniohyoid, which assist in mouth opening by stabilizing or depressing the mandible when the hyoid bone is fixed.

- *Infrahyoid muscles*: Comprising the sternohyoid, omohyoid, sternothyroid, and thyrohyoid, these muscles stabilize or reposition the hyoid bone, enabling efficient mandibular and tongue movements.

8. Mandibular kinematics and muscular coordination

Mandibular movements all along both functional and parafunctional activities involve intricate neuromuscular coordination, influenced by both central and peripheral nervous system inputs [1, 3]. The temporomandibular joint (TMJ) facilitates approximately 2000 movements each day [8].

8.1 Jaw opening

The primary muscles involved in jaw opening are the digastric, mylohyoid, and geniohyoid. During slow mouth opening and at maximum mandibular opening, the temporalis muscle remains largely inactive, although slight activity may be observed in the medial pterygoid [3, 5].

8.2 Jaw closure

During mandibular closure without tooth contact, the temporalis muscle shows minimal or no activity. In this case, elevation of the mandible is primarily achieved through the action of the masseter and medial pterygoid muscles [3, 5, 11].

8.3 Retrusion

Controlled mandibular retrusion during closure is mainly achieved by the posterior fibers of the temporalis, assisted by the synergistic activity of the suprahyoid and infrahyoid muscle groups [1, 5, 12].

8.4 Protrusion

Forward displacement of the mandible in the absence of occlusal contact occurs through bilateral activation of the lateral and medial pterygoid muscles, with additional contribution from the masseter [3, 4, 11].

8.5 Lateral movements

When the mandible shifts laterally without tooth contact, the motion is driven mainly by the medial and posterior fibers of the temporalis on the same side, in combination with contralateral activation of the lateral and medial pterygoids, along with the anterior temporalis fibers. The suprahyoid muscles remain active during this action, maintaining the mandible in a slightly depressed and protruded position [4, 8, 11].

9. Mandibular kinematics

Functionally, movements of mandible are mostly complicated, involving six degrees of freedom that combine both rotational and translational components. These movements are made possible through the interaction of four articular surfaces—two lower and two upper joints [1, 3]. Although the temporomandibular joints (TMJs) do not operate independently of each other, classifying mandibular movements in isolation is essential for understanding their biomechanics [8].

10. Types of movements

Jaw movements have been widely studied, especially where the upper and lower teeth meet. The first person to describe these movements in three dimensions was Ulf Posselt [13].

Typically, condylar rotation and the translation of the condyle-disc complex occur simultaneously. On average, for every 1 mm, the jaw moves forward or backward, and the condyle rotates about 2 degrees during opening or closing [14].

11. Mandibular rotational movements

The mandible (lower jaw) exhibits rotational movements around fixed points known as axes during opening and closing. These movements occur within the temporomandibular joint (TMJ), specifically within the inferior joint compartment, situated between the condyle and the articular disc, and rotation occurs along three principal planes—horizontal, vertical, and sagittal—each defined by a specific axis [5].

11.1 Horizontal axis (hinge axis)

The horizontal axis facilitates the opening and closing of the mouth, akin to a door hinge. This movement is termed "hinge movement" and is considered the purest form of rotational motion in the mandible. When the condyles occupy their highest position within the articular fossae and mouth opening occurs solely through rotation without translation, the movement takes place around an axis referred to as the *terminal hinge axis* [15].

11.2 Vertical (frontal) axis

The vertical axis runs perpendicular to horizontal axis and is involved in lateral (side-to-side) movements of the mandible. This axis allows for movements, such as chewing and grinding, where the mandible shifts from side to side [5].

11.3 Sagittal axis

The sagittal axis is oriented from front to back and is associated with forward and backward movements of the mandible. This axis plays a role in actions, such as protrusion and retrusion of the jaw [5, 16].

12. Translational motion

Translation describes the type of motion in which all points of an object move simultaneously at the same speed and in the same direction. Within the masticatory system, translation is observed during mandibular protrusion. In normal function, mandibular movements involve both *rotation and translation* occurring together; as the mandible rotates around one or more axes, those axes themselves continually shift in spatial orientation [1, 5].

Mandibular kinematics, however, extend beyond simple rotation and translation. Lateral or eccentric bodily displacements, combined with these fundamental movements, highlight the mandible's behavior as a dynamic, free-floating structure. Its motion is finely regulated by coordinated pairs of synergistic and antagonistic muscles, which generate graded forces through multiple vectors. This intricate muscular and articular interaction produces highly complex, three-dimensional mandibular movements—an adaptive mechanism made possible by the unique dual-joint design of the TMJ, unmatched by any other joint system in the body [3–5].

Earlier studies examined mandibular movements based on geometric principles using mechanical devices. Posselt, for example, created the gnatho-tensiometer, an instrument capable of recording border movements across all three planes and producing what is known as the Posselt diagram [13]. Advances in technology have since enabled improved position tracking methods, allowing for the detailed analysis of mandibular kinematics with high spatial and temporal resolution [17, 18].

13. Relationship of temporomandibular joint with occlusion

Mandibular movements are influenced not only by the morphology of bones, muscles, and ligaments but also by the occlusal relationships of the teeth [3]. According to the *Glossary of Prosthodontic Terms*, occlusion is described as the static contact between the masticatory surfaces of maxillary and mandibular teeth [19]. However, when analyzed functionally, occlusion is better understood as the biological and dynamic interaction of the masticatory system that governs dental relationships [15].

Occlusion encompasses a broad spectrum of concepts [20]. The biomechanics of occlusal contact, particularly between teeth with varying cusp inclinations, represents a highly complex system [21]. From a clinical perspective, alterations in the TMJ—such as intracapsular exudate or changes within joint tissues—are often associated with occlusal dynamics [4, 22].

14. Temporomandibular joint disorders

Temporomandibular disorders (TMD) are a group of conditions characterized by craniofacial pain arising from the temporomandibular joint (TMJ), masticatory muscles, or the neural structures of the head and neck [3]. They represent the most common source of nondental orofacial pain [22]. Epidemiological studies indicate that TMD affects approximately 10–15% of adults, although only about 5% seek clinical intervention [23]. The incidence typically peaks between 20 and 40 years of age, with women being affected nearly twice as often as men, contributing to significant economic costs through reduced productivity and work absence. Symptom presentation varies from mild discomfort to severe pain, often accompanied by restricted mandibular function. The broad spectrum of TMD is reflected in its classification (**Table 1**), with common subtypes, including myofascial pain disorder, disc displacement disorders, osteoarthritis, and autoimmune-related TMJ involvement [22, 26, 27].

TMDs are increasingly recognized as a heterogeneous group of painful neuromusculoskeletal conditions involving the masticatory system and associated tissues [28]. Reported prevalence rates range from 5–31%, with onset spanning from childhood through adulthood [29]. Beyond physical symptoms, TMD significantly compromises quality of life by affecting daily activities, psychological well-being, and social functioning [30].

Given this clinical burden, there is a pressing need for effective and accessible management strategies. Although formal rehabilitation-based clinical practice guidelines specific to TMD are currently lacking, valuable peer-reviewed resources exist for orthopedic physical therapists and other conservative practitioners, guiding evaluation and management [30]. However, as research in this field continues to evolve, updated frameworks are required. Consequently, the purpose of this two-part series is to present an evidence-informed, supplementary framework to aid clinicians in the conservative assessment and treatment of TMD [31].

14.1 Etiology

The causes of temporomandibular disorders (TMD) are multidimensional, arising from the interaction of biological, psychological, and social influences rather than a single factor [32, 33]. Conditions that are frequently linked to TMD include chronic headache syndromes, fibromyalgia, autoimmune diseases, sleep-related breathing disorders, and psychiatric disturbances [31]. Evidence from a large prospective cohort involving more than 6000 individuals revealed that people with depression had over twice the likelihood of developing TMD (rate ratio = 2.1; 95% CI, 1.5–3; $P < .001$), while those with anxiety experienced a notable increase in the risk of myofascial pain (rate ratio = 1.8; 95% CI, 1.2–2.6; $P < .001$) [34]. Behavioral risk factors also contribute, as smoking has been shown to elevate the risk of TMD, particularly among women below the age of 30 years [35, 36].

Articular disorders (intra-articular)
Congenital or developmental disorders
Condylar hyperplasia
First and second branchial arch disorders
Idiopathic condylar resorption
Degenerative joint disorders
Inflammatory: capsulitis, synovitis, polyarthritides (rheumatoid arthritis, psoriatic arthritis, ankylosing spondylitis, Reiter syndrome, gout)
Noninflammatory: osteoarthritis
Disk derangement disorders
Displacement with reduction
Displacement without reduction (closed lock)
Perforation
Infection
Neoplasia
Temporomandibular hypermobility
Dislocation
Joint laxity
Subluxation
Temporomandibular hypomobility
Ankylosis: true ankylosis (bony or fibrous) or pseudoankylosis
Postradiation fibrosis
Trismus
Trauma
Contusion
Fracture
Intracapsular hemorrhage
Masticatory muscle disorders (extra-articular)
Local myalgia
Myofascial pain disorder
Myofibrotic contracture
Myositis
Myospasm
Neoplasia

Information from References [24, 25].

Table 1.
Classification of temporomandibular joint disorders.

14.2 Classification

Temporomandibular disorders (TMD) are broadly classified as either *intra-articular*, referring to conditions that occur within the joint, or extra-articular, which involve the surrounding musculature [37]. Among these, musculoskeletal disorders represent the most frequent etiology, accounting for more than half of all TMD cases [38]. Within the intra-articular group, the most prevalent pathology is articular disk displacement, characterized by an altered condyle-disk relationship [22]. To provide greater clarity and diagnostic consistency, the International Research Diagnostic Criteria for Temporomandibular Dysfunction (RDC/TMD) Consortium Network introduced a revised classification system in 2013, which is summarized in **Table 1** [39].

14.3 Differential diagnosis

Clinicians should maintain a high index of suspicion for temporomandibular disorders (TMD) when evaluating patients who report pain localized to the temporomandibular joint region. A wide range of conditions can present with symptoms resembling TMD, making differential diagnosis essential. Examples include dental pathology, such as caries or abscess, oral mucosal lesions (herpes simplex, herpes zoster, aphthous ulcers, and lichen planus), muscle-related problems due to overuse (clenching, bruxism, excessive chewing, or spasm), and trauma or dislocation of the joint. Other disorders that may simulate TMD include maxillary sinusitis, salivary gland disease, trigeminal or postherpetic neuralgia, glossopharyngeal neuralgia, giant cell arteritis, primary headache syndromes, and malignancy-related pain [40, 41]. Additionally, TMD-like manifestations may be observed in patients with autoimmune conditions, particularly systemic lupus erythematosus, Sjögren syndrome, and rheumatoid arthritis [42]. A detailed overview of these differential diagnoses with their clinical presentations is summarized in **Table 2** [2, 24].

Condition	Location	Pain characteristics	Aggravating factors	Typical findings
Dental conditions				
Caries	Affected tooth	Intermittent to continuous dull pain	Hot or cold stimuli	Visible decay
Cracked tooth	Affected tooth	Intermittent dull or sharp pain	Biting, eating	Often difficult to visualize crack
Dry socket	Affected tooth	Continuous, deep, sharp pain	Hot or cold stimuli	Loss of clot, exposed bone
Giant cell arteritis	Temporal region	Sudden onset of continuous dull pain	Visual disturbance, loss of vision	Scalp tenderness, absence of temporal artery pulse
Migraine headache	Temporal region, behind the eye, cutaneous allodynia	Acute throbbing, occasionally with aura	Activity, nausea, phonophobia, photophobia	Often normal, aversion during ophthalmoscopic examination, normal cranial nerve findings
Neuropathic conditions				
Glossopharyngeal neuralgia	Most often ear, occasionally neck or tongue	Paroxysmal attacks of electrical or sharp pain	Coughing, swallowing, touching the ear	Pain with light touch

Condition	Location	Pain characteristics	Aggravating factors	Typical findings
Postherpetic neuralgia	Site of dermatomal nerve and its distribution	Continuous, burning, sharp pain	Eating, light touch	Hyperalgesia
Trigeminal neuralgia	Unilateral trigeminal nerve	Paroxysmal attacks of sharp pain	Cold or hot stimuli, eating, light touch, washing	Pain with light touch
Salivary stone	Submandibular or parotid region	Intermittent dull pain	Eating	Tenderness at gland, palpable stone, no salivary flow
Sinusitis	Maxillary sinus, intraoral upper quadrant	Continuous dull ache	Headache, nasal discharge, recent upper respiratory infection	Tenderness over maxillary sinus or upper posterior teeth

Information from references [13, 14].

Table 2.
Conditions that may mimic temporomandibular disorders.

15. Clinical examination of temperomandibular joint

Classical clinical features of temporomandibular joint (TMJ) disorder include orofacial pains, joint noises (such as clicking or popping), and restricted jaw movement, particularly limited mouth opening. This limitation may occur suddenly, presenting as jaw locking, or it may develop gradually over time [43, 44].

15.1 Pain

In the temporomandibular joint (TMJ) region, pain is typically localized and rarely radiates to distant areas. It is important to ask the patient whether activities such as chewing, yawning, swallowing, or speaking influence the pain. If discomfort is associated with any of these actions, a TMJ disorder is likely. However, in rare cases, conditions affecting the parotid gland or the cervical spine might cause odynophagia.

A comprehensive assessment of pain characteristics is essential in patients with suspected temporomandibular disorders (TMD). Sharp, localized, and intense pain is more suggestive of an arthrogenic origin, whereas a dull, diffuse, and less intense ache typically reflects a muscular source. The presence of a painful click is often indicative of intra-articular meniscal subluxation, while progressively worsening spontaneous pain over several weeks may signal arthritis. Conversely, persistent, low-grade pain localized to the masticatory muscles—particularly when aggravated toward the end of the day—is frequently associated with myalgia [24].

15.2 Pain referred from the temporomandibular joint

Pain arising from temporomandibular joint (TMJ) structures can originate either from the masticatory muscles or the joint itself. Within the joint, the most frequent sources are the intracapsular tissues situated posterior to the condyle, including the posterior segment of the meniscus, its capsular attachments, the joint capsule, and the retromeniscal fat pad. TMJ-related pain is commonly accompanied by headache, otalgia, or postauricular discomfort, and in certain cases, may even be referred to the maxillary region.

15.3 Pain referred to the temporomandibular joint area

At times, pain perceived in the temporomandibular joint (TMJ) region may be referred from the cervical spine. In such cases, it is important to conduct a preliminary cervical assessment to rule out neck-related contributions before attributing symptoms solely to the TMJ. Additionally, various other structures can contribute to pain in the TMJ region, which may be categorized as either neurological or non-neurological in origin.

15.4 Neurological disorders

15.4.1 Atypical facial neuralgia

This condition may present unilaterally or bilaterally and is frequently of uncertain etiology. The clinical picture is often characterized by a burning sensation, paresthesia (a feeling of pins and needles), and persistent pain that fluctuates in intensity over time. In some cases, it may develop following dental procedures [45, 46].

15.4.2 Trigeminal nerve neuritis

This condition is mostly seen in individuals aged from 45 to 60 years, with a greater prevalence among females and a predilection for the right side. Affected patients usually describe unilateral, sharp, shooting pain that radiates from the ear toward the temporal region and maxilla, and occasionally extends to the forehead or pharynx. Due to the obscure nature of the pain, it is sometimes misattributed, leading to unnecessary dental extractions.

Although sensory loss is rare, distinct trigger points are often present. Even light stimulation of these points can provoke referred pain. After each episode, there is usually a brief refractory phase, lasting up to 30 seconds, during which no further pain can be provoked despite additional stimuli. Episodes of pain are brief, typically lasting only a few seconds, and may occur sporadically—daily, weekly, or even monthly—either as isolated incidents or in groups.

15.4.3 Herpes zoster oticus infection

This condition can produce dysesthesia preceding the development of typical vesicular eruptions, and unlike other neuropathic pain disorders, true trigger points are absent. Approximately 15% of facial palsies of peripheral origin are attributed to herpes zoster infection.

15.4.4 Peripheral facial palsy of unknown origin (Bell's palsy)

This can be due to cranial neuritis. It primarily affects individuals in 20- to 50-year age group. Although typically not aching, some patients may experience pain around the ear at onset. The condition results in facial muscle palsy, marked by drooping of the mouth on the affected side. Additional symptoms may include reduced pain sensation, altered taste, decreased tear production, and increased salivation [47].

15.4.5 Peripheral neuropathy

This condition is commonly associated with diabetes, temporal arteritis, and or Raynaud's phenomenon. It typically presents with a burning sensation and reduced sensation in areas, such as the eye or lips.

15.4.6 Non-neurological conditions

Otitis externa, parotitis, and otitis externa.

These conditions can produce pain radiating to the TMJ region. In otitis, discomfort often worsens with pressure applied to the tragus, whereas in parotitis (particularly epidemic parotitis), pain intensifies with palpation of the parotid gland. They are more frequently observed in children and are typically accompanied by fever.

15.4.7 Paranasal sinusitis

This condition often produces a persistent, pounding pain that is most noticeable around the orbital region and may extend toward the cheek and teeth. In the case of dental infections or abscesses, patients typically experience pain in the cheek that is elicited by percussion and tends to worsen after consuming sweet foods. A dental abscess is further characterized by localized gingival swelling.

15.4.8 Cluster headache (Horton's neuralgia)

This condition occurs more frequently in men and typically presents on one side of the face. It is mostly accompanied by excessive tearing, nasal congestion, and redness of the face on the affected side. The hallmark feature is the sudden onset of severe, unilateral headache centered in or around the eye. These attacks develop within 5–10 minutes, persist for 45 minutes to a few hours, and tend to recur in cluster patterns [48].

15.4.9 Temporal arteritis

Temporal arteritis, a manifestation of giant-cell arteritis and an autoimmune disorder, typically occurs in men above the age of 50. It most often presents on one side and is commonly linked with polymyalgia rheumatica. Clinically, it produces a throbbing pain around the temporal arteries, with the overlying skin appearing red, tender, and warm [49]. Laboratory findings usually reveal an elevated erythrocyte sedimentation rate (ESR).

15.4.10 Leaking cerebral aneurysm

This condition presents abruptly with a sudden, severe headache, often accompanied by nausea, vomiting, light sensitivity, and neck stiffness. When the aneurysm is located at the posterior communicating artery, it may produce pain along the first branch of the trigeminal nerve. It is regarded as the most frequent cause of what is termed ophthalmoplegic migraine [50].

16. History

During the assessment, the examiner should inquire about the onset, character, location, intensity, and duration of pain, and identify factors that aggravate or alleviate symptoms [51]. In addition to the pain history, several other relevant aspects should be explored with the patient:

- *Is there joint clicking?* When the meniscus is anteriorly subluxated, the normal alignment between the condyle and meniscus is disrupted, often producing a clicking sound during mouth opening.

- *Is jaw movement restricted, either in range or due to locking?* If the mouth-opening range is reduced, it is important to determine whether the limitation developed suddenly or gradually. Sudden locking requires assessment of whether the patient can still open or close the mouth. Inability to open often indicates meniscus displacement, typically unilateral, with at least 1 cm of opening usually preserved. Inability to close suggests a luxation of the mandibular condyle. Rapidly developing severe limitation may result from hysteria or tetanus, in which case, mouth opening is entirely impossible. Gradual onset of restricted movement is most commonly associated with TMJ arthrosis.

- *Any crepitus?* Crepitus occurs when joint surfaces move over an irregular area, often due to advanced joint *changes*. It is commonly observed in osteoarthrosis.

- *Does the patient experience clenching or teeth grinding?* This habit is most often observed at night, particularly in individuals under stress. Patients may be unaware of it, so input from family members or close contacts may be necessary.

- *Are there symptoms such as tinnitus, vertigo, or hearing difficulties?* Vertigo can arise from altered vestibular signals linked to TMJ dysfunction. Additional symptoms may include mild hearing loss, a feeling of fullness in the ear, and tinnitus. Have there been changes in sensibility? These can indicate peripheral neuropathy. It frequently affects the lips, cornea, and conjunctiva. In atypical facial neuralgia severe diminished facial sensibility is often found. Trigeminal neuritis is seldom accompanied by disturbed sensibility.

17. Observation

17.1 Observe

Look for local swelling, facial asymmetry, chin deviation, and tooth wear.

17.2 Causes of swelling

Bacterial or inflammatory arthritis (commonly rheumatoid, rarely psoriatic or gout-related).

In children, swelling may be due to parotid gland inflammation.

17.3 Bell's palsy signs

Drooping of the mouth on the same (ipsilateral) side as the affected area
Smoothing out facial wrinkles on the same side.

17.4 Childhood TMJ inflammation

Can disrupt mandibular growth centers.
May lead to asymmetrical development of the lower face.

17.5 Advanced arthrosis

Can result in facial and cranial asymmetry.
May cause narrowing of the external auditory canal.

17.6 Synovitis effects

Jaw deviation toward the affected side (ipsilateral) on opening.
Deviation toward the opposite side (contralateral) on closing.

17.7 Tooth wear

Abnormal wear may indicate bruxism (teeth grinding).

17.8 Malocclusion and missing teeth

May contribute to TMJ disorders.
There is a *bilateral relationship* between the dental structure and TMJ health:

- Changes in dental alignment can affect the TMJ.
- TMJ dysfunction can lead to altered dental occlusion.

18. Functional examination

18.1 Active movement

The effects of all five active jaw movements are assessed in relation to pain, range of motion, deviation, joint sounds, and crepitus [52, 53].

18.1.1 Opening of the mouth

Since it is not feasible to quantify temporomandibular joint (TMJ) mobility in angular degrees, evaluation is usually performed by measuring the interincisal distance at maximum mouth opening. In adults, this value typically averages 36–38 mm, although it may range between 30 and 67 mm depending on factors, such as age and sex [13, 14]. A simple and rapid clinical screening method involves asking the patient to insert their own knuckles vertically between the upper and lower incisors, which provides a practical estimate of opening capacity (**Figures 3** and **4**).

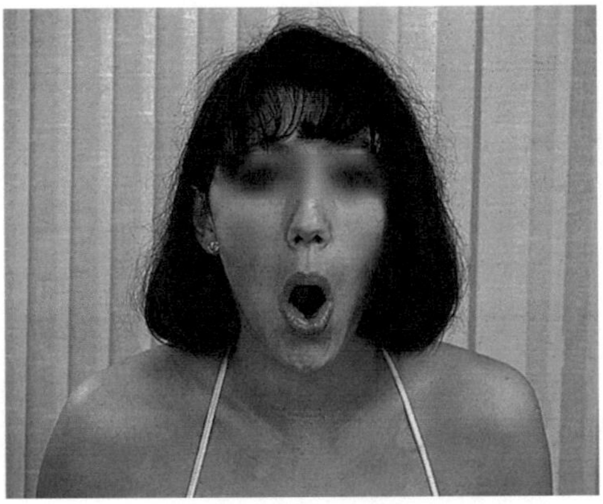

Figure 3.
Opening of the mouth (Active).

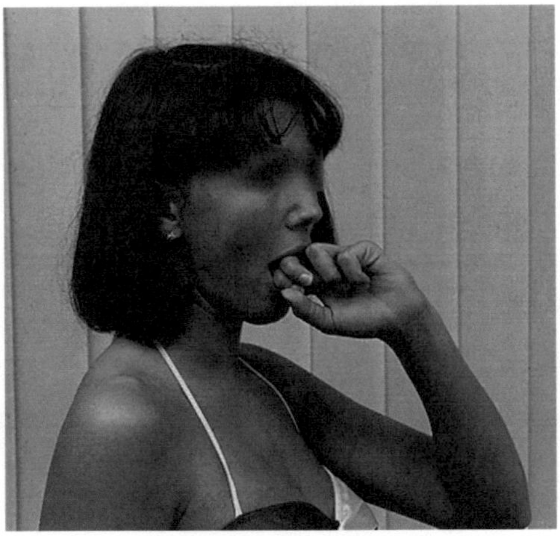

Figure 4.
Assessing the ROM.

18.1.2 Closing of the mouth

Patient is instructed to close their mouth (**Figure 5**).

18.1.3 Deviation of the mandible to the left and right

When the mandible deviates to one side, it rotates around a vertical axis passing through the ipsilateral mandibular ramus, while at the same time, the contralateral mandibular condyle translates anteriorly (**Figure 6**) [54].

18.1.4 Forward protrusion of Chin

This movement is carried out primarily by the lateral and medial pterygoid, masseter, geniohyoid, and digastric muscles. Any disturbance in this function is generally attributed to an intra-articular dysfunction rather than muscular impairment (**Figure 7**) [54].

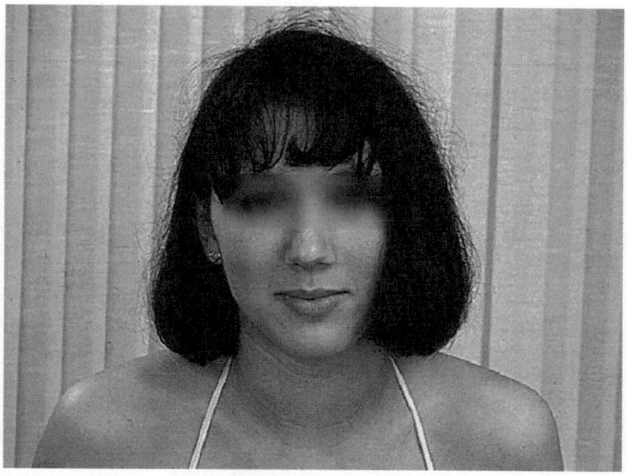

Figure 5.
Closing of the mouth (Active).

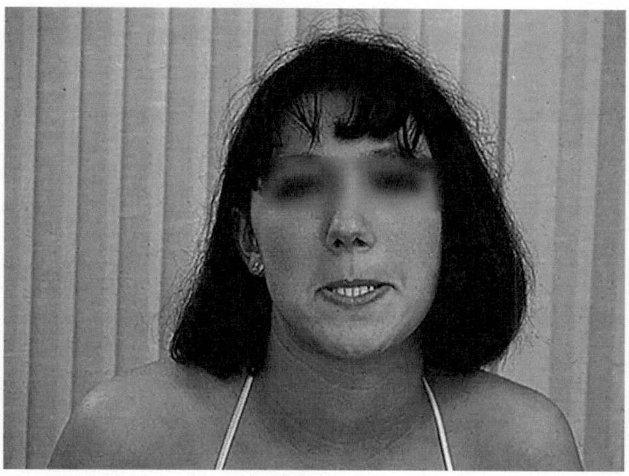

Figure 6.
Deviation of mandible (Active).

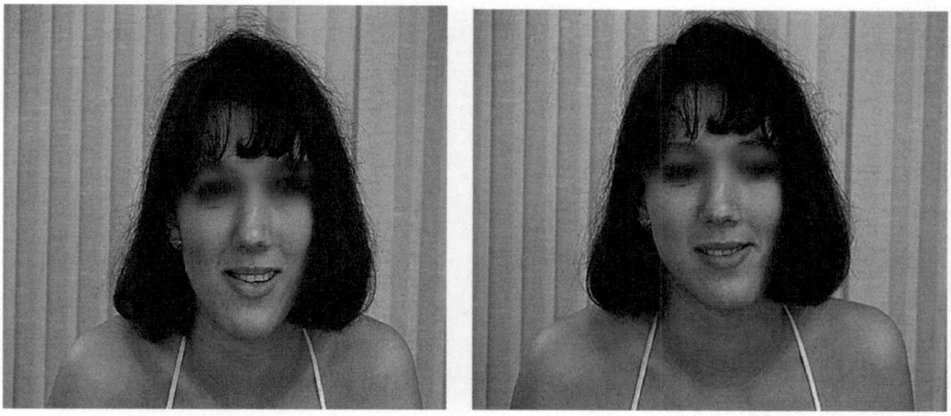

Figure 7.
Forward protrusion of chin (Active).

19. Resisted isometric movements

19.1 Resisted opening of the mouth

To assess the strength of the lateral pterygoid, the examiner supports the patient's chin with one hand while placing the other on the vertex of the head. With the mouth slightly opened (about 1 cm), the patient is instructed to open further against firm resistance applied by the examiner, thereby preventing mandibular movement (**Figure 8**) [54].

19.2 Resisted closing of the mouth

To evaluate the strength of the mouth-closing muscles, a rubber pad approximately 1-cm thick is positioned between the teeth. The patient is instructed to bite down with maximal effort, which engages the masseter, temporalis, and medial pterygoid muscles (**Figure 9**) [54].

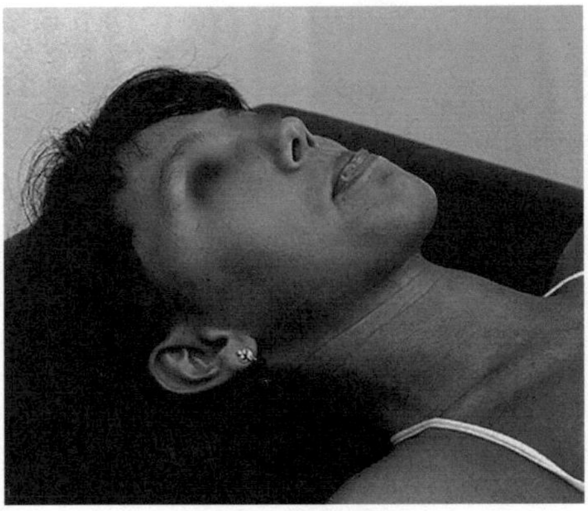

Figure 8.
Resisted opening of mouth.

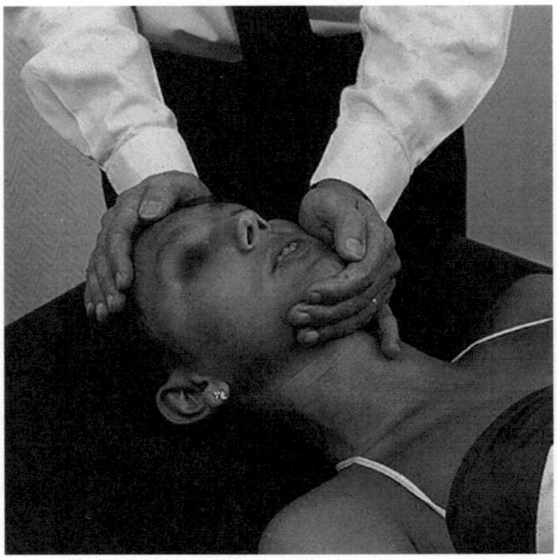

Figure 9.
Resisted closing of mouth.

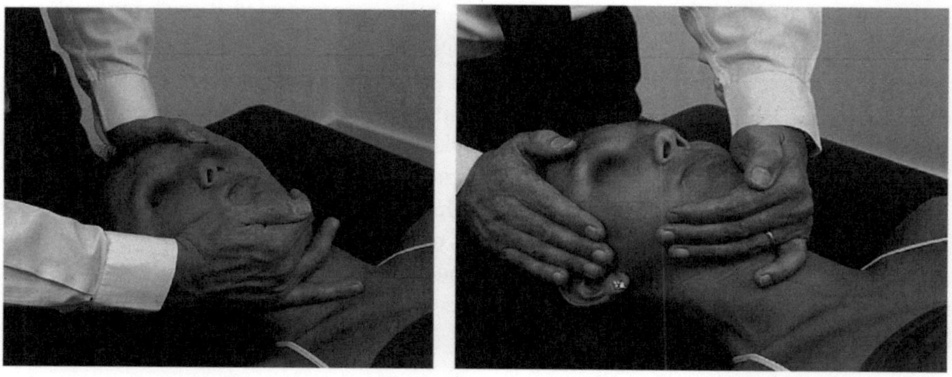

Figure 10.
Resisted deviation of the mandible to the left.

19.3 Resisted deviation of mandible to right and left

To evaluate the function of the lateral pterygoid, the examiner steadies the patient's head by placing one hand on the temporal region and the other on the chin. The patient is instructed to move the jaw sideways against the applied resistance. When the chin is pushed to one side, the opposite lateral pterygoid muscle is primarily engaged (**Figure 10**) [54].

20. Palpation

Palpation of the temporomandibular joint (TMJ) is carried out during active opening, closing, and lateral deviations of the mandible. During mouth opening, the joint is best examined by placing a finger just below the zygomatic arch, anterior to the condyle, whereas during closing, the finger can be positioned either anterior

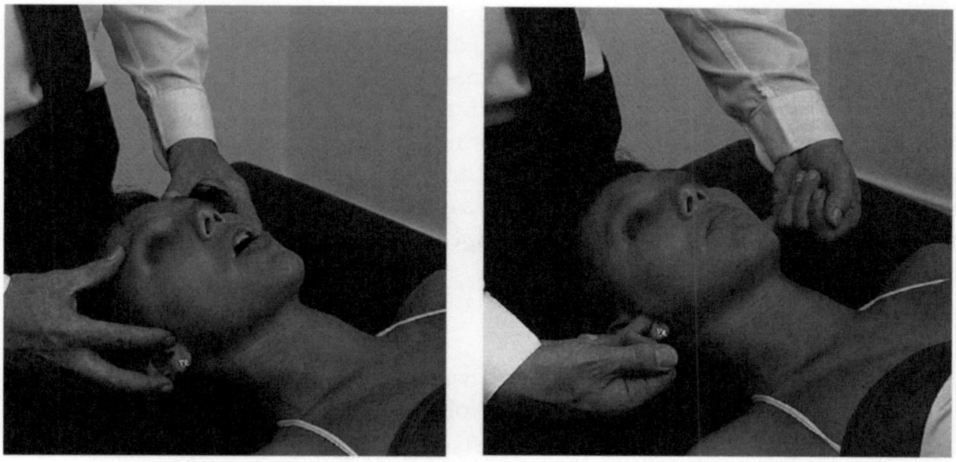

(a) (b)

Figure 11.
Palpation of the TMJ (a) Anterior to tragus; (b) in the external auditory meatus.

to the tragus or within the external auditory meatus to apply gentle anterior pressure against the posterior joint surface. Normally, a concavity is felt as the condyle translates forward, but in cases of significant effusion, a bulging sensation may be detected. While palpating, the examiner should note abnormal joint noises, crepitation, or restrictions in anteroposterior condylar movement. The coronoid process can also be appreciated by placing the fingers beneath the zygomatic arch during mandibular opening and closing, where it is felt through the overlying masseter. Palpation should also include assessment of tenderness over the joint capsule, peri-dental bone, and masticatory muscles. The masseter can be examined both during mouth opening and with teeth clenched, while the temporalis is best assessed by palpation during clenching **(Figure 11)** [55].

21. Technical investigations

The erythrocyte sedimentation rate (ESR) is often elevated in systemic inflammatory conditions and infections, serving as a useful but nonspecific marker. Conventional radiographs contribute little in the diagnosis of temporomandibular disorders, aside from detecting degenerative changes, such as arthrosis [13]. Computed tomography (CT) offers a more detailed assessment of the bony components of the joint and provides accurate information about the position and integrity of the meniscus [14, 15]. In contrast, magnetic resonance imaging (MRI) has become the preferred modality in recent years for evaluating soft-tissue abnormalities, particularly in cases of suspected internal derangement.

22. Special tests

22.1 Chvostek's sign

The purpose of this test is to check for irritability or hyperexcitability of the facial nerve, which may occur due to compression or inflammation. To perform the test, the examiner gently taps over the glandula parotis, situated just in front of the ear, where the branches of the facial nerve emerge. A positive Chvostek's sign is indicated by involuntary twitching or contraction of facial muscles toward the same side of the face, particularly around the mouth, eye, or nose. This response suggests facial nerve irritation or heightened neuromuscular excitability, and while it is more commonly associated with conditions such as hypocalcemia, it may also be relevant in TMJ assessments when nerve involvement is suspected (**Figure 12**).

22.2 Cotton roll test or bite test

The cotton roll test helps distinguish between muscular and joint-related TMJ pain. The patient bites on a piece of cotton roll placed unilaterally between the teeth. If pain decreases on the same side, it suggests a muscle problem. If pain decreases on the opposite side, it indicates a joint (intra-articular) issue, such as disc displacement (**Figure 13**) [56, 57].

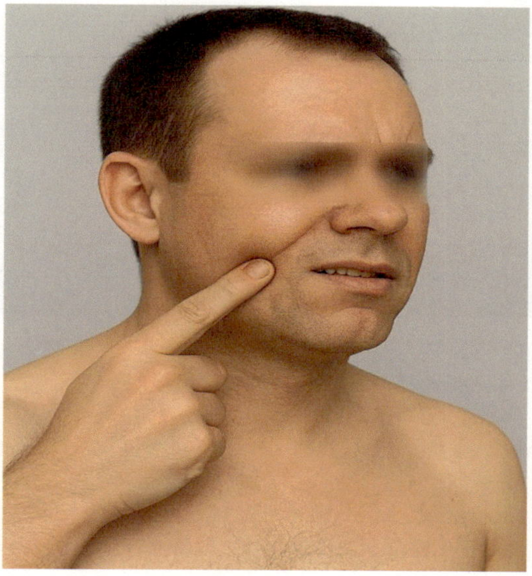

Figure 12.
Chvostek's sign.

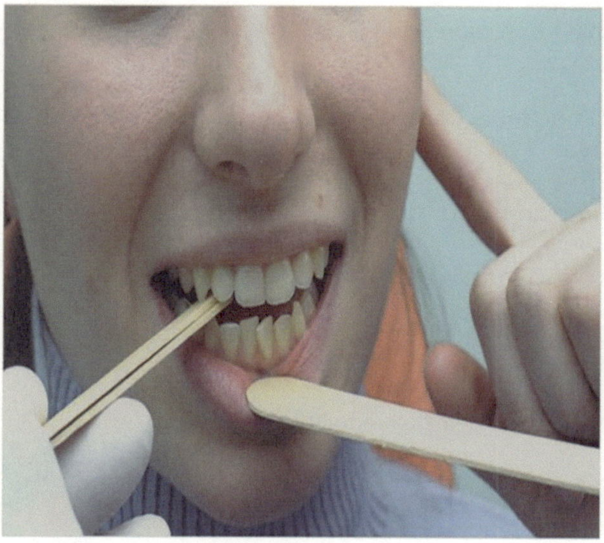

Figure 13.
Cotton roll test.

22.3 Joint auscultation test or stethoscope test

This test detects abnormal joint sounds in the TMJ during movement. For this, a stethoscope is placed directly over the TMJ region while the patient is instructed to slowly open and close the mouth. Any abnormal acoustic phenomena during mandibular movements are carefully noted, as they may indicate internal derangements or degenerative changes (**Figure 14**) [58–60].

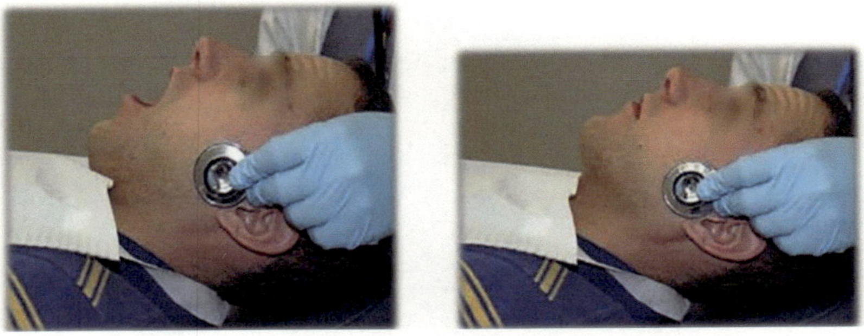

Figure 14.
Joint auscultation test or stethoscope test.

23. Outcome measures for TMDs

Self-report outcome measures (SROMs) are essential tools for evaluating the impact of temporomandibular disorders [61]. Many reliable and valid questionnaires are available, like:

23.1 Functional assessment

- Jaw Functional Limitation Scale (JFLS-8 & JFLS-20)—Measures functional limitations of jaw
- Mandibular Functional Impairment Questionnaire (MFIQ)—Assesses mandibular dysfunction.

23.2 Oral health and quality of life (QoL)

Oral Health Impact Profile (OHIP):

- OHIP-TMD, OHIP-22, and OHIP-14—Region-specific QoL tools tailored for TMD populations.
- OHIP-49—Broad oral health-related QoL measure.

23.2.1 Sleep quality

Pittsburgh Sleep Quality Index (PSQI)—Reliable for evaluating sleep disturbances in TMD populations.

23.2.2 General health QoL

Short Form Health Survey (SF-36)—A general QoL measure, valid in modified form for TMD assessment.

24. Physiotherapy management

Physiotherapy plays a crucial role in managing temporomandibular disorders (TMDs) as it targets the musculoskeletal and neuromuscular imbalances responsible for the symptoms. The main objectives of physiotherapy are to reduce pain, enhance jaw mobility, and improve the patient's overall quality of life. Interventions are tailored to each individual, depending on their clinical findings and specific requirements.

24.1 Manual therapy techniques

Physiotherapists use various manual therapy techniques to target the TMJ and surrounding structures:

- *Joint Mobilization*: Gentle movements of the TMJ to improve mobility and reduce pain by addressing joint restrictions and misalignments.

- *Joint Manipulation*: In cases requiring more forceful intervention, manipulation techniques may be applied to restore normal joint function.

- *Soft tissue mobilization*: Gentle direct pressure is applied to the masticatory muscles surrounding the TMJ to help reduce muscle tension and promote relaxation and enhance relaxation.

    a. *Myofascial release (MFR)*: Gentle, sustained pressure applied to fascial restrictions around the jaw, neck, and face. It helps to improve tissue mobility and reduce pain. Often applied to the *masseter and temporalis* muscles (**Figure 15**).

    b. *Cross-fiber friction massage*: Breaks down adhesions and promotes healing. Often used on *chronic tight areas* (**Figure 16**).

    c. *Intra-oral soft tissue mobilization*: It involves accessing the *medial and lateral pterygoid* and inner masseter through the oral cavity using gloves. It releases deep muscle tension contributing to TMJ dysfunction (**Figure 17**).

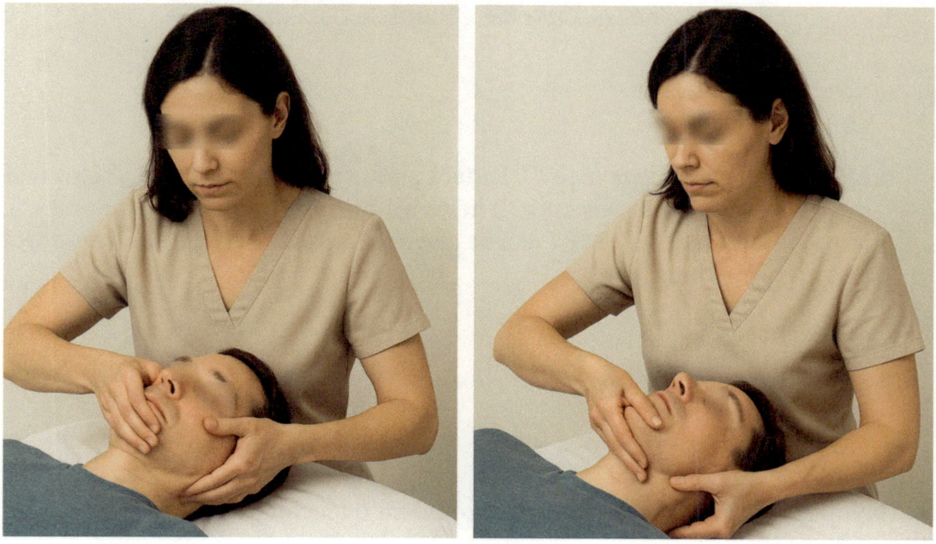

Figure 15.
Myofascial release for TMJ disorders.

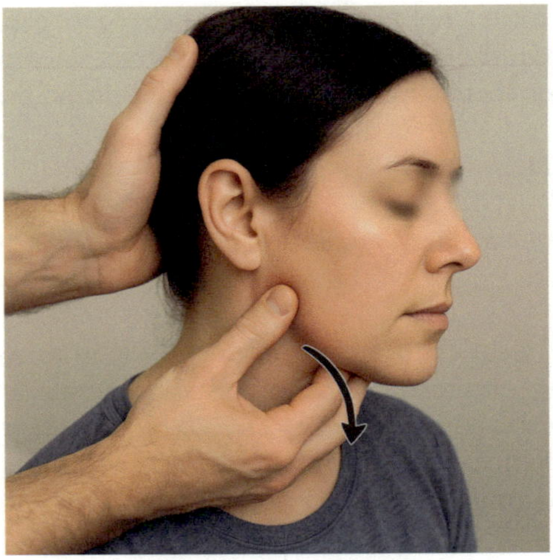

Figure 16.
Cross-fiber friction massage.

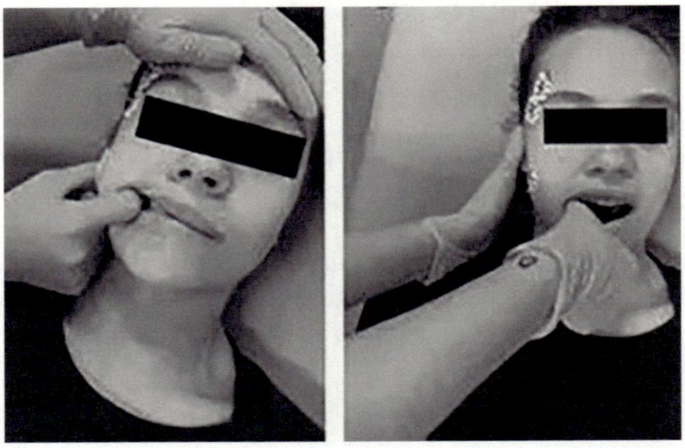

Figure 17.
Intra-oral soft tissue mobilization.

d. *Muscle energy technique (MET)*: Patient performs isometric contractions while the therapist applies resistance. It helps lengthen shortened muscles and improve joint mobility. MET can be given to masseter, temporalis, suprahyoid, and pterygoid muscles.

1. Masseter muscle MET

   Position: Patient supine, jaw slightly open.

   Procedure:

- Therapist resists gentle jaw-closing movement (clenching)
- Hold 5–7 seconds

DOI: http://dx.doi.org/10.5772/intechopen.1012775

- Relax and gently stretch open the mouth
- Repeat 3–5 times

2. Temporalis muscle MET

   Position: Fingers at temporal fossa.

   Procedure:

   - Patient clenches teeth gently against resistance
   - Hold 5 seconds
   - Relax and stretch jaw open

3. Suprahyoid MET for opening restriction

   Procedure:

   - Patient opens mouth slightly
   - Therapist applies downward and backward resistance
   - Hold → relax → stretch into opening

   Treatment Protocol:
   Sessions: 2–3 times per week depending on severity
   Repetitions: 3–5 per muscle per session

e. *Trigger point therapy*: Pressure is applied to areas of muscle hypersensitivity to relieve referred pain and reduce muscle tightness.

24.2 Therapeutic exercises

Rehabilitative exercises are fundamental in restoring jaw function. These may include:

- *Range of motion exercises*: Improve jaw flexibility and mobility.
- *Strengthening and isometric exercises*: Enhance the strength and endurance of masticatory muscles.
- *Postural exercises*: Correct postural imbalances that may contribute to TMJ dysfunction, especially involving the head, neck, and shoulders.

24.3 Physical modalities

Several modalities are used to complement manual therapy and exercise:

- *Therapeutic ultrasound*: Delivers deep heat to tissues using high-frequency sound waves, promoting blood flow, tissue repair, and pain reduction.

- *Laser therapy*: Low-Level Laser Therapy (LLLT), which is also known as cold laser therapy, is a non-invasive modality that stimulates cellular activity to aid healing and reduce inflammation.

- *TENS*: It blocks pain signals. TENS uses electrical impulses and stimulates endorphin release by placing electrodes over the TMJ region.

24.4 Patient education and self-care

Patient education is essential for treatment success. Physiotherapists instruct patients on home exercises, posture correction, and self-management strategies. Consistent participation in self-care plays a vital role in long-term outcomes.

24.5 Collaborative approach

For patients with dentures, physiotherapists may work in collaboration with dentists or prosthodontists. Poor denture fit can impact TMJ health, and physiotherapy can help patients adjust to new dentures, reduce muscle tension, and restore jaw mobility.

24.6 Limitations and considerations

Based on individual factors, which include the type of temporomandibular joint disorder, its comorbidities, and response of patient to a particular treatment, the effectiveness of physiotherapy interventions will vary. Some cases involve complex interactions between joint, muscular, and psychosocial components, which may not be fully resolved by physiotherapy alone. Moreover, treatment outcomes depend heavily on patient compliance and realistic expectations.

While current evidence supports the benefits of certain physiotherapy techniques in TMD management, more high-quality, long-term research is needed to solidify their efficacy.

24.7 Future directions

Emerging trends in TMD physiotherapy show promising potential:

- *Tele-rehabilitation and mobile apps*: Improve access to care in rural or low-access areas.

- *VRT (Virtual Reality) and biofeedback*: Enhance patient engagement and adherence to therapy.

- *Advanced diagnostics*: High-resolution imaging and personalized diagnostics may improve treatment precision.

- *Mindfulness and cognitive behavioral strategies*: Address psychological aspects of TMD and promote holistic care.

- *Genetic and biomarker research*: May lead to personalized, targeted interventions in the future.

Appendix

Home exercise program

Chin tucks [62]

- In a standing or seated position with your back and neck straight.
- Gently pull your chin backward, as if making a "double chin."
- Keep your head facing forward without tilting up or down.
- Hold the position for up to 5 seconds.
- Repeat the movement 8–10 times (**Figure A1**)

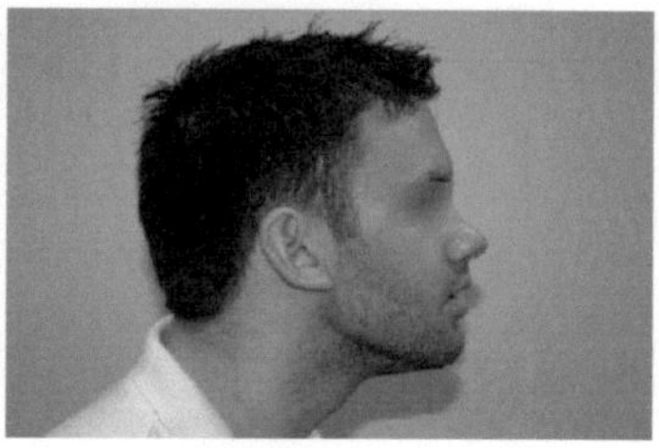

Figure A1.

Relaxed jaw

- Gently rest your tongue on the roof of your mouth.
- Let your teeth separate slightly and allow your jaw muscles to relax (**Figure A2**).

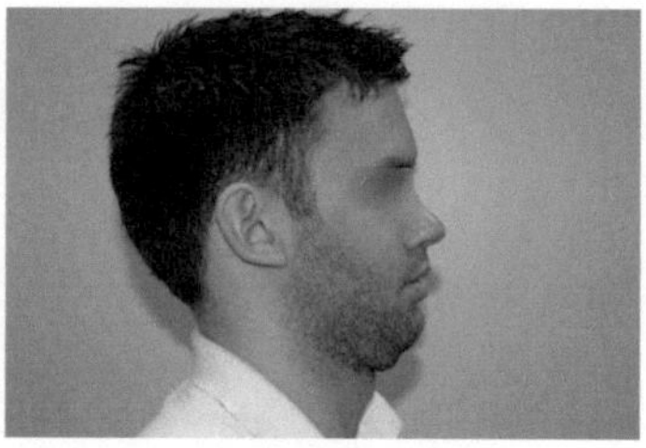

Figure A2.

Goldfish exercise

- Rest your tongue gently on the roof of your mouth.
- Place one index finger over your TMJ area and the other on your chin.
- Slowly lower your jaw and then bring it back up with gentle guidancefrom your finger:

  a. open halfway.

  b. open fully

- Use a mirror to check that your jaw moves straight without deviation.
- Repeat the movement 6–8 times, about 4–6 times per day (**Figure A3**).

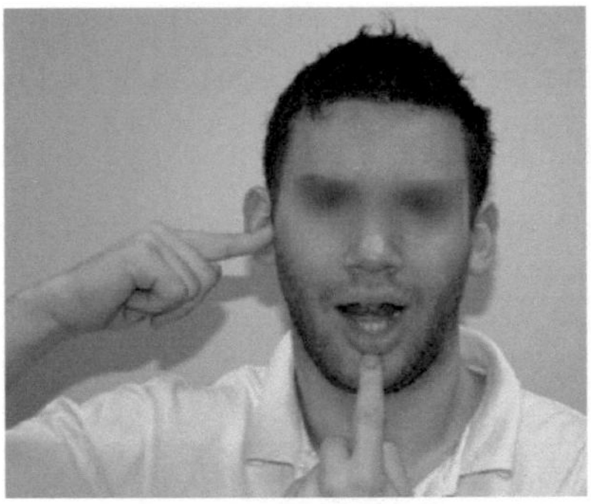

Figure A3.

Unsupported goldfish

- Place the tongue gently against the roof of the mouth.
- Position one index finger over each TMJ.
- Slowly open and close the mouth through:

    a. partial opening.

    b. full opening

- Perform the movement in front of a mirror to ensure the jaw tracksin a straight line without deviation.
- Repeat 6–8 times, 4–6 times daily (**Figures A4** and **A5**)

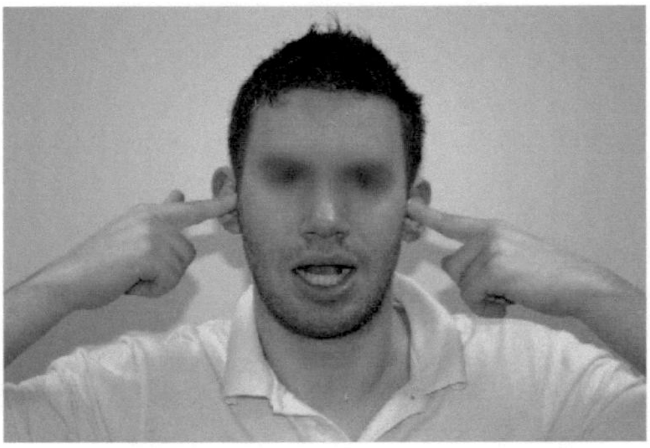

Figure A4.

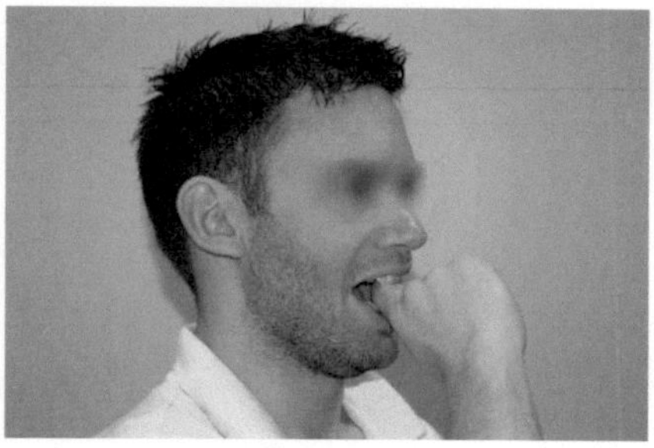

Figure A5.

Stabilization exercises

- Position the jaw in a neutral posture, either with the mouth partiallyopen or at a comfortable distance of one knuckle width apart.
- Apply gentle, steady pressure using your thumb while maintainingthe jaw's alignment.
- Perform the exercise slowly, avoiding any sudden or forceful movements (**Figures A6, A7** and **A8**).

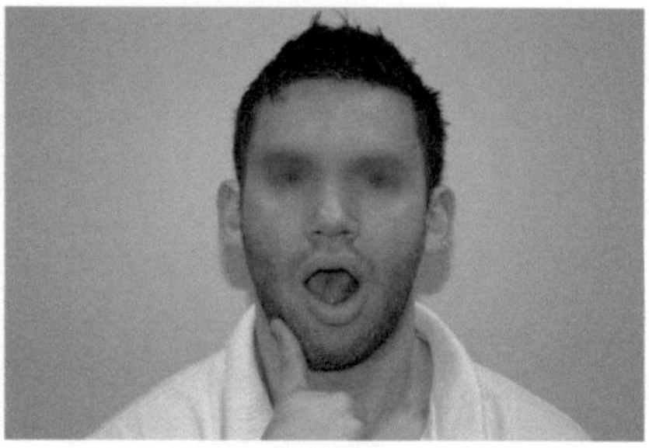

Figure A6.

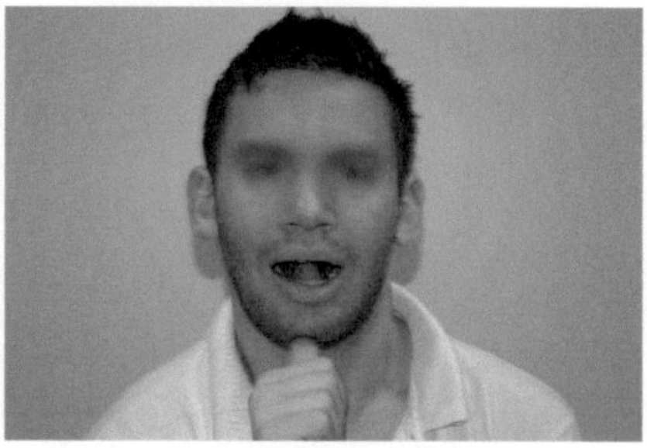

Figure A7.

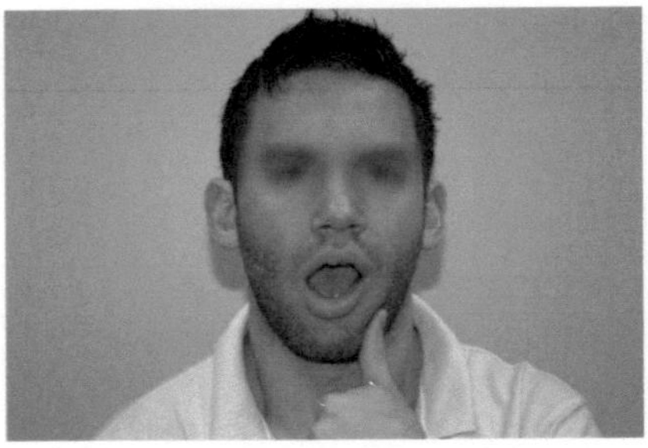

Figure A8.

Author details

Pooja Chaudhuri
Department of Physiotherapy, School of Allied Medical Sciences, University of Science and Technology, Ribhoi, Meghalaya, India

*Address all correspondence to: drpoojachaudhuri1@gmail.com

References

[1] Standring S. Gray's Anatomy: The Anatomical Basis of Clinical Practice. 41st ed. London: Elsevier; 2015

[2] Standring S. Gray's Anatomy: The Anatomical Basis of Clinical Practice. 42nd ed. London: Elsevier; 2021

[3] Okeson JP. Management of Temporomandibular Disorders and Occlusion. 8th ed. Elsevier; 2019

[4] Tanaka E, Detamore MS, Tanimoto K. Lubrication of the temporomandibular joint. Cells, Tissues, Organs. 2008;**187**(1):1-11

[5] Wright EF. Manual of Temporomandibular Disorders. 4th ed. Wiley-Blackwell; 2019

[6] Gray H. Gray's Anatomy: The Anatomical Basis of Clinical Practice. 42nd ed. London: Elsevier; 2021

[7] Sicher H, DuBrul EL. Oral Anatomy. 6th ed. Mosby; 1975

[8] Zarb GA, Carlsson GE. Temporomandibular Joint Function and Dysfunction. Munksgaard; 1990

[9] Rees LA. The structure and function of the mandibular joint. British Dental Journal. 1954;**96**(6):125-133

[10] Burch JG. The cranial attachment of the mandibular joint meniscus. Journal of the American Dental Association (1939). 1966;**73**(6):1314-1320

[11] Posselt U. Physiology of Occlusion and Rehabilitation. 2nd ed. Blackwell Scientific Publications; 1968

[12] Ando E, Shigeta Y, Ogawa T. Kinematic analysis of limitation of mouth opening of temporomandibular disorders by rotation and translation of the condyle [Article in Japanese]. Nihon Hotetsu Shika Gakkai Zasshi. Apr 2005;**49**(2):231-241. DOI: 10.2186/jjps.49.231

[13] Posselt U. Physiology of Occlusion and Rehabilitation. 2nd ed. Blackwell Scientific Publications; 1968

[14] Lundeen HC, Gibbs CH, editors. Advances in Occlusion. Postgraduate Dental Handbook Series. Vol. 14. Boston: J. Wright-PSG; 1982. ISBN: 0884161684

[15] Dawson PE. Functional Occlusion: From TMJ to Smile Design. Mosby; 2007

[16] Lundeen HC, Gibbs CH. Advances in occlusion: Rotation and translation of the mandible. Dental Clinics of North America. 1992;**36**(3):593-607

[17] The American Academy of Prosthodontics. Glossary of Prosthodontic Terms. 9th ed. Journal of Prosthetic Dentistry. 2017;**117**(5S):e1-e105. DOI: 10.1016/j.prosdent.2016.12.001

[18] Dawson PE. Functional occlusion: From TMJ to Smile Design. St. Louis (MO): Mosby; 2007

[19] The American Academy of Prosthodontics. Glossary of prosthodontic terms. 9th ed. The Journal of Prosthetic Dentistry. 2017;**117**(5S):e1-e105

[20] Dawson PE. Functional Occlusion: From TMJ to Smile Design. Mosby; 2007

[21] McNeill C. Science and Practice of Occlusion. Quintessence Publishing; 1997

[22] Schiffman E, Ohrbach R. Executive summary of the diagnostic criteria for temporomandibular disorders (DC/TMD) for clinical and research applications. Journal of the American Dental Association (1939). 2016;**147**(6):438-445

[23] Slade GD, Bair E, Greenspan JD, et al. Signs and symptoms of first-onset TMD and sociodemographic predictors: The OPPERA prospective cohort study. The Journal of Pain. 2013;**14**(12 Suppl):T20-T32

[24] Okeson JP. Management of Temporomandibular Disorders and Occlusion. 7th ed. St. Louis: Elsevier; 2013

[25] Scbiffman E, Obrbacb R, Trueloye E, et al. Diagnostic criteria for temporomandibular disorders (DC/TMD) for clinical and research applications: Recommendations of the international RDC/TMD consortium network and orofacial pain special interest group. Journal of Oral & Facial Pain and Headache. 2014;**28**(1):6-27

[26] Dworkin SF, LeResche L. Research diagnostic criteria for temporomandibular disorders: Review, criteria, examinations and specifications, critique. Journal of Craniomandibular Disorders. 1992;**6**(4):301-355

[27] Qamar Z, Alghamdi AMS, Haydarah NKB, et al. Impact of temporomandibular disorders on oral health-related quality of life: A systematic review and meta-analysis. Journal of Oral Rehabilitation. 2023;**50**(8):706-714. DOI: 10.1111/joor.13472

[28] de Leeuw R, Klasser GD. Orofacial Pain: Guidelines for Assessment, Diagnosis, and Management. 6th ed. Chicago (IL): Quintessence Publishing Co, Inc.; 2018

[29] Cairns BE. Pathophysiology of TMD pain—Basic mechanisms and their implications for pharmacotherapy. Journal of Oral Rehabilitation. 2010;**37**(6):391-410

[30] Durham J, Newton-John TRO, Zakrzewska JM. Temporomandibular disorders. BMJ. 2015;**350**:h1154

[31] Klasser GD, Greene CS. The changing field of temporomandibular disorders: what dentists need to know. Journal of the Canadian Dental Association. 2009;**75**(1):49-53

[32] Manfredini D, Piccotti F, Ferrato G, Guarda-Nardini L. Age peaks of different RDC/TMD diagnoses in a patient population. Journal of Dentistry. 2010;**38**(5):392-399

[33] Fillingim RB, Ohrbach R, Greenspan JD, et al. Psychological factors associated with development of TMD: The OPPERA prospective cohort study. The Journal of Pain. 2013;**14**(12 Suppl):T75-T90

[34] Maixner W, Fillingim R, Sigurdsson A, Kincaid S, Silva S. Sensitivity of patients with painful temporomandibular disorders to experimentally evoked pain. Pain. 1998;**76**(1-2):71-81

[35] Sanders AE, Slade GD, Bair E, et al. General health status and incidence of first-onset temporomandibular disorder: The OPPERA prospective cohort study. The Journal of Pain. 2013;**14**(12 Suppl):T51-T62

[36] Chisnoiu AM, Picos AM, Popa S, et al. Factors involved in the etiology of temporomandibular disorders—A literature review. Clujul Med. 2015;**88**(4):473-478. DOI: 10.15386/cjmed-485

[37] Klasser GD, Greene CS. The changing field of temporomandibular disorders: What dentists need to know. Journal of the Canadian Dental Association. 2009;**75**(1):49-53

[38] Guarda-Nardini L, Manfredini D, Ferronato G. Temporomandibular joint osteoarthritis: An open-label trial of 76 patients treated with arthrocentesis plus hyaluronic acid injections. International Journal of Oral and Maxillofacial Surgery. 2007;**36**(7):610-615

[39] Ohrbach R, Dworkin SF. The evolution of TMD diagnosis: Past, present, future. Journal of Dental Research. 2016;**95**(10):1093-1101

[40] Zakrzewska JM, Hamlyn PJ. Facial pain. In: Oxford Textbook of Neuroscience and Anaesthesia. Oxford University Press; 2013

[41] Fromm GH, Terrence CF, Maroon JC. Trigeminal neuralgia: Current concepts regarding etiology and pathogenesis. Archives of Neurology. 1984;**41**:1204-1207

[42] Mumenthaler M. Giant-cell arteritis: Cranial arteritis, polymyalgia rheumatica. Journal of Neurology. 1978;**218**:219-236. DOI: 10.1007/BF00312878

[43] Rocabado M. Arthrokinematics of the temporomandibular joint. Dental Clinics of North America. 1983;**27**(**3**):573-594

[44] Hodges JM. Managing temporomandibular joint syndrome. Laryngoscope. 1990;**100**:60-66

[45] Adour KK. Current concepts in neurology: Diagnosis and management of facial paralysis. New England Journal of Medicine. 1982;**307**:348-351

[46] Adour KK, Wingerd J. Idiopathic facial paralysis (Bell's palsy): Factor affecting severity and outcome in 446 patients. Neurology. 1974;**24**:1112-1116

[47] Adour KK, Byl FM, Hilsinger RL Jr, Kahn ZM, Sheldon MI. The true nature of Bell's palsy: Analysis of 1000 consecutive patients. Laryngoscope. 1978;**88**:787-801

[48] Kudrow L. Cluster Headache: Mechanisms and Management. London: Oxford University Press; 1980

[49] Mumenthaler M. Giant-cell arteritis: Cranial arteritis, polymyalgia rheumatica. Journal of Neurology. 1978;**218**:219-236

[50] Minervini G, Franco R, Marrapodi MM, et al. Correlation between temporomandibular disorders (TMD) and posture evaluated through the diagnostic criteria for temporomandibular disorders (DC/TMD): A systematic review with meta-analysis. Journal of Clinical Medicine. 2023;**12**(7):2652. DOI: 10.3390/jcm12072652

[51] Minervini G, Franco R, Marrapodi MM, et al. Economic inequalities and temporomandibular disorders: A systematic review with meta-analysis. Journal of Oral Rehabilitation. 2023;**50**(8):715-723. DOI: 10.1111/joor.13491

[52] Mezitis M, Rallis G, Zachariades N. The normal range of mouth opening. Journal of Oral and Maxillofacial Surgery. 1989;**47**:1028-1029

[53] Claes J. Het temporomandibulair pijndysfunctiesyndroom in otorhinolaryngologie. Acta Otorhinolaryngol. 1981;**35**(2):170-183

[54] Okeson JP. Management of Temporomandibular Disorders and Occlusion. 7th ed. St. Louis, MO: Mosby; 2013

[55] Meyer RA. The temporomandibular joint examination. In: Walker HK, Hall WD, Hurst JW, editors. Clinical Methods: The History, Physical, and Laboratory Examinations. 3rd ed. Butterworths; 1990

[56] McPhee SJ, Hammer GD. Pathophysiology of Disease: An Introduction to Clinical Medicine. 8th ed. McGraw-Hill Education; 2020

[57] Royal Surrey Hospital. TMJ Information [Internet]. Guildford: Royal Surrey County Hospital; [cited 2026 Jan 21]. Available from: https://www.royalberkshire.nhs.uk/media/42kcqthn/physiotherapy-management-of-temporomandibular-joint-pain_dec23.pdf?

[58] Walker HK, Hall WD, Hurst JW, editors. Clinical Methods: The History, Physical, and Laboratory Examinations. 3rd ed. Butterworths; 1990. (See chapter on the temporomandibular joint examination, which describes auscultation of crepitus, clicking, and grinding in TMJ motion.) NCBI

[59] Huddellston-Slater JJR, van Selms MKA, Lobbezoo F, Naeije M. The clinical assessment of TMJ sounds by means of auscultation, palpation or both. Journal of Oral Rehabilitation. 2002;**29**(9). DeepDyve

[60] Dagar SR, Turakiya V, Pakhan AJ, Jaggi N, Kalra A, Vaidya V. Modified stethoscope for auscultation of temporomandibular joint sounds. Journal of International Oral Health. 2014;**6**(2):40-44

[61] Garrigós-Pedrón M, Elizagaray-García I, Domínguez-Gordillo AA, et al. Temporomandibular disorders: Improving outcomes using a multidisciplinary approach. Journal of Multidisciplinary Healthcare. 2019;**12**:733-747. DOI: 10.2147/JMDH.S178507

[62] Royal Surrey County Hospital NHS Foundation Trust. Physiotherapy Management of Temporomandibular Joint (TMJ) Pain [Internet]. Guildford (UK): Royal Surrey County Hospital NHS Foundation Trust; 2021

Chapter 2

MR Imaging in Temporomandibular Joint Disorders: From Diagnostic Fundamentals to Advanced Applications

Sonam Khurana, Pranav Parasher and Denise Trochesset

Abstract

Temporomandibular joint (TMJ) disorders include a broad range of developmental, inflammatory, and neoplastic conditions that can interfere with joint function and affect quality of life. Magnetic resonance imaging (MRI) is the reference standard for TMJ evaluation because it provides detailed multiplanar visualization of osseous and soft-tissue structures without ionizing radiation. This review summarizes MRI assessment of TMJ anatomy, normal variations, and internal derangements, including disc displacement, pseudodisc formation, adhesions, marrow changes, and joint effusion. MRI features of inflammatory arthropathies, cystic and tumor-like lesions, and primary or metastatic malignancies are described with attention to diagnostic relevance. Imaging protocols and sequence selection are explained in relation to accurate depiction of disc and condyle relationships and adjacent soft tissues. Recent developments in MRI, including ultrashort echo time imaging, zero echo time imaging, real-time cine evaluation, diffusion-based techniques, and quantitative T2 mapping, are reviewed for their ability to detect early biochemical changes and improve diagnostic precision. The combined anatomic, pathologic, and technical information provides a comprehensive overview of current and emerging applications of MRI in TMJ disorders.

Keywords: temporomandibular joint, magnetic resonance imaging, internal derangement, arthropathy, cystic lesions, tumor, advanced imaging

1. Introduction

Temporomandibular joint (TMJ) disorders are a major cause of orofacial pain and dysfunction, affecting up to one-third of the population [1–3]. Women are more frequently affected, particularly between the second and fourth decades of life, although only a minority of patients seek clinical care [1–7]. Internal derangement, defined by an abnormal positional relationship between the articular disc and condyle, is the most common subtype of temporomandibular disorders (TMD). Additional etiologies include inflammatory arthritis, developmental abnormalities, cystic lesions, and neoplasms [4].

Accurate diagnosis requires detailed visualization of osseous and soft-tissue joint structures. Magnetic resonance imaging (MRI) is the reference standard because it provides high-contrast, multiplanar evaluation of the disc, capsule, synovium, and adjacent musculature without ionizing radiation [8]. MRI is highly sensitive for detecting disc displacement, joint effusion, marrow alterations, and inflammatory changes not evident on radiography or computed tomography [9]. Advances in MRI hardware and pulse sequences have improved spatial resolution and efficiency, enabling assessment of joint motion and tissue composition through dynamic and quantitative techniques [10–14]. Emerging ultrashort and zero echo time (UTE and ZTE) sequences further enhance depiction of osseous structures while maintaining a radiation-free workflow [15].

This review summarizes MRI evaluation of TMJ anatomy, internal derangements, arthropathies, cystic and tumor-like lesions, and malignancies, and outlines recent technological developments relevant to clinical practice.

2. Anatomy

2.1 Normal anatomy

The TMJ is a synovial articulation permitting both hinge and gliding movements between the mandibular condyle and the temporal bone. The principal components of TMJ include the articular disc, bony articular surfaces, fibrous capsule, and associated ligaments [1–3]. The disc is a fibrocartilaginous, biconcave structure dividing the joint into inferior and superior compartments, which contribute to rotation and translation, respectively [1–5]. Initial opening results from condylar rotation within the lower compartment, producing an interincisal distance of approximately 25 mm, followed by anterior translation within the upper compartment to achieve maximal opening of about 50 mm [16–18]. The joint also allows lateral excursions of roughly 10 mm, protrusion of about 9 mm, and limited retrusion of approximately 1 mm [17].

The disc is composed of anterior, intermediate, and posterior regions, with thicker peripheral bands [19]. In physiologic alignment, it remains interposed between the condyle and temporal bone in both closed- and open-mouth positions. In the closed-mouth position, the anterior band lies anterior to the condylar head, while the posterior band and bilaminar zone rest superiorly, typically between the 11- and 12-o'clock positions. With opening, the intermediate zone moves between the condyle and articular eminence (**Figure 1**) [5, 20, 21]. The anterior portion attaches to the capsule, the superior head of the lateral pterygoid muscle (LPM), and the condylar head, whereas the posterior attachment comprises the bilaminar zone. This zone includes a superior elastic layer attached to the postglenoid process and an inferior collagenous layer attached to the posterior condylar neck, with intervening loose connective tissue containing vessels, nerves, and elastic fibers that facilitate disc return during closure (**Figure 2**) [1, 4, 9].

On coronal imaging, the disc appears crescent-shaped and is anchored medially and laterally by collateral ligaments [1, 4]. Both articular surfaces are covered with

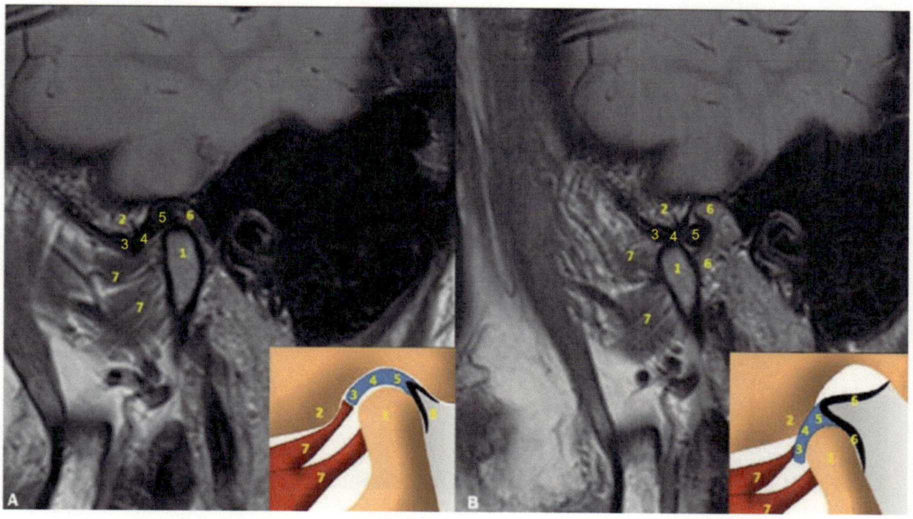

Figure 1.
TMJ Anatomy. Sagittal PD-weighted images and schematic drawings demonstrating the anatomy of the TMJ in closed-mouth and open-mouth positions (A and B, Respectively). 1, Mandibular condyle; 2, Articular eminence of the temporal bone; 3, Articular disc (anterior band); 4, articular disc (intermediate band); 5, articular disc (posterior band); 6, bilaminar zone; 7, superior and inferior bellies of the lateral pterygoid muscle. Source: Ref. [7] https://pmc.ncbi.nlm.nih.gov/articles/PMC10165975/. License: https://creativecommons.org/licenses/.

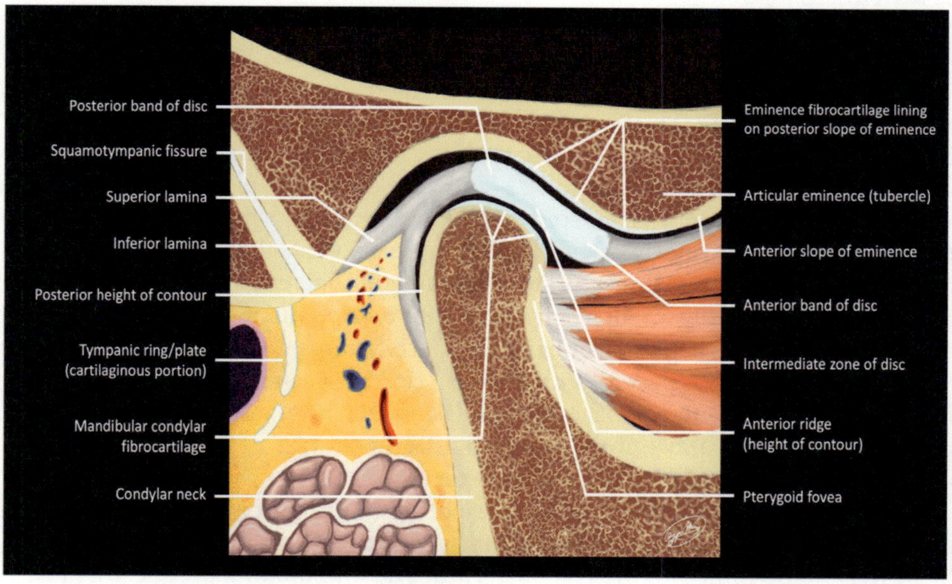

Figure 2.
Sagittal oblique illustration demonstrating the osseous structures of the TMJ.

fibrocartilage, providing greater durability under occlusal loading and enhanced reparative capacity compared with hyaline cartilage (**Figure 3**) [22, 23]. Mandibular motion is primarily driven by the masseter, temporalis, and medial and lateral pterygoids. The lateral pterygoid is especially important; its superior head inserts on the disc–condyle complex to stabilize the mandible during opening, while the inferior head attaches to the condylar neck and facilitates anterior translation [1, 2, 4, 9, 22].

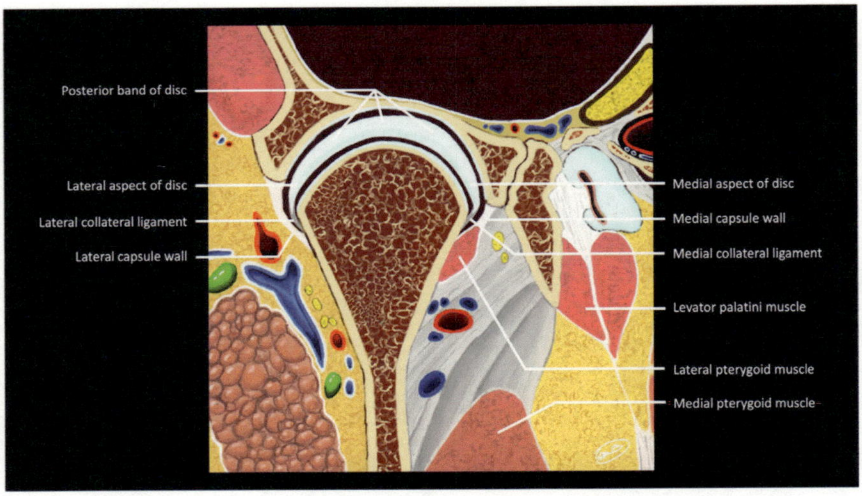

Figure 3.
Coronal oblique illustration demonstrating the osseous structures of the TMJ.

These anatomic features form the basis for understanding their characteristic appearances on conventional and advanced MRI sequences.

2.2 MRI anatomy

On MRI, marrow fat within the mandibular condyle shows high signal intensity on T1-weighted sequences, whereas cortical bone and the articular disc appear uniformly low in signal on both T1- and T2-weighted images because of low proton density and short T2 relaxation times [24]. The disc typically has a biconcave shape with homogeneously low to intermediate signal on T1- and T2-weighted sequences [25, 26]. Under normal conditions, the posterior band demonstrates central hyperintensity on all sequences due to transversely oriented collagen fibers, while the anterior band and the intermediate zone remain hypointense because of their compact, linearly organized collagen. Vertically oriented compact fibers create a distinct vertical low-signal line at the junction of the posterior band and the bilaminar zone [27]. MRI sequences, however, may not always provide a clear distinction between the posterior band and the posterior attachment, since the posterior band contains loosely arranged collagen fibers that extend into those of the posterior attachment [28, 29]. This overlap can complicate evaluation of partial disc displacement.

Thin horizontal low-signal lines representing the superior and inferior surfaces of the posterior band may also mimic anterior extensions of the laminae of the posterior attachment [26]. The posterior band and bilaminar zone are most accurately assessed in the open-mouth position. During opening, distension of the venous plexus within the bilaminar zone produces high T2 signal (**Figure 4**) and the enhancement seen following gadolinium administration [4, 30]. TMJ bone marrow signal changes with age as hematopoietic marrow is gradually replaced by fatty marrow. In infancy, marrow shows T1 signal similar to muscle and appears hyperintense relative to muscle on fluid-sensitive sequences. With maturation, fatty marrow becomes predominant and produces signal characteristics that are isointense to fat on all sequences [25].

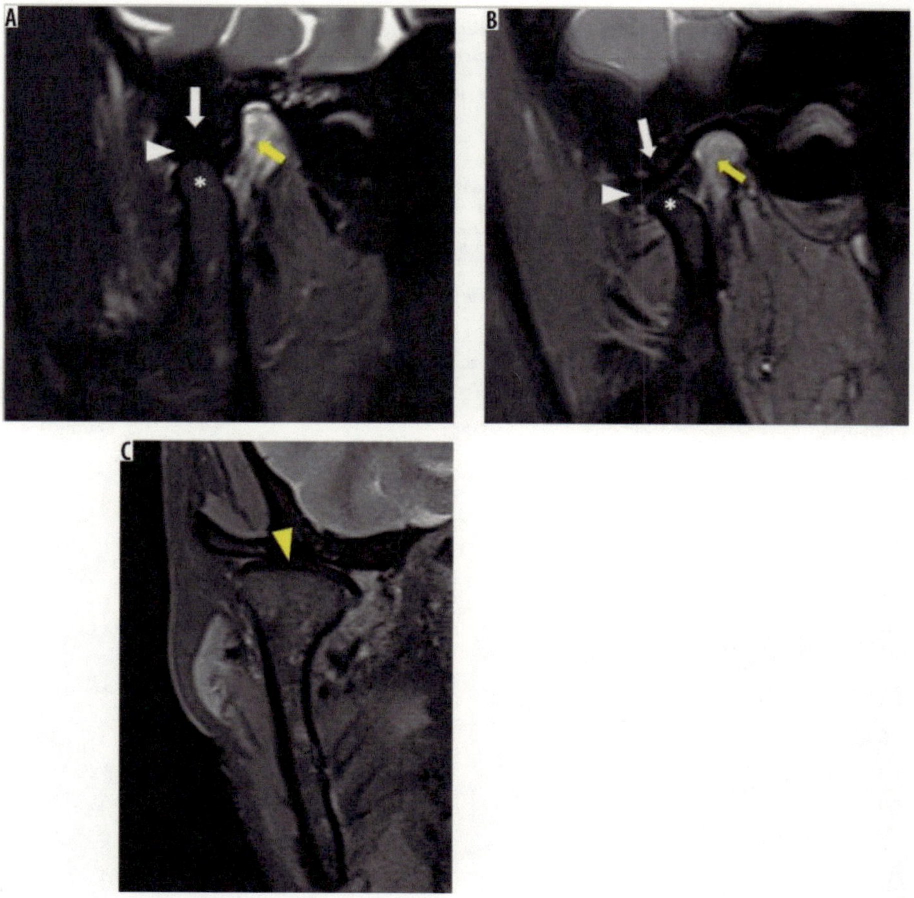

Figure 4.
Normal anatomy of temporomandibular joint (open mouth). Sagittal oblique T2W-FS (A) and proton density fat saturation (PD-FS) (B) images show normal anterior translation of condylar head (asterisk) below the articular eminence (white arrow) with disc interposing between them (white arrowhead). Retrodiscal tissue (yellow arrow) appears normal high signal and is better assessed on T2W images. Coronal oblique PD-FS (C) shows normal disc signal and position (yellow arrowhead). The signal of the disc is better assessed on PD images. Source: Ref. [26] https://pmc.ncbi.nlm.nih.gov/articles/PMC7016362/. License: http://creativecommons.org/licenses/by-nc-nd/4.0/.

3. MRI protocol

MRI is the most reliable technique for evaluating intra-articular TMJ pathology, with reported diagnostic accuracy of approximately 95% for disc position and morphology and 93% for osseous changes [31]. A comprehensive protocol typically includes static and dynamic acquisitions using proton density (PD)–weighted, T1-weighted, and T2-weighted sequences with section thicknesses of 3 mm or less (**Table 1**).

Axial T1-weighted images are generally acquired first and serve as reference images for subsequent plane selection (**Figure 5**). Axial and coronal T1-weighted images assess condylar contour, marrow signal, and the masticator space, with coronal views particularly useful for detecting medial or lateral disc displacement.

Plane/Orientation	Sequence	Slice thickness	TR (ms)	TE (ms)	Mouth position
Axial (localizer)	T1	2 mm, 0 skip	500	Minimal (5-30)	Closed
Coronal (bilateral)	T1	3 mm, 0.5 skip	500	Minimal (5-30)	Closed
Sagittal oblique (bilateral)	T1	3 mm, 0.5 skip	500	Minimal (5-30)	Closed and open
Sagittal oblique (bilateral)	PD	3 mm	3500	85	Closed and open
Sagittal oblique (bilateral)	T2	3 mm	3500	85	Closed and open
Sagittal oblique (bilateral)	Dynamic cine (SSFSE PD)	3 mm	1180–2000	64	During opening/closing

Table 1.
MRI protocol for TMJ evaluation.

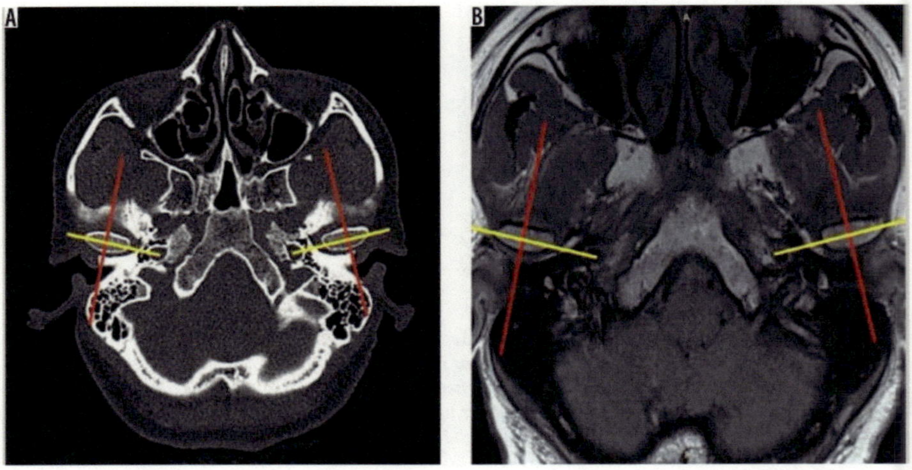

Figure 5.
Planning technique. Axial computed tomography and magnetic resonance images are used to plan coronal oblique images along the horizontal long axis of the head of the mandibular condyle (yellow lines). Sagittal oblique images are obtained perpendicular to this plane (red lines). Source: Ref. [26] https://pmc.ncbi.nlm.nih.gov/articles/PMC7016362/. License: http://creativecommons.org/licenses/by-nc-nd/4.0/.

Oblique sagittal (parasagittal) images, angled approximately 30° from the midsagittal plane and perpendicular to the condylar long axis, are obtained bilaterally in both closed- and open-mouth positions. PD, T1, and T2-weighted acquisitions are performed in the oblique sagittal plane (closed and open mouth). Fat-suppressed, fluid-sensitive sagittal oblique sequences improve sensitivity for inflammatory arthropathies [32].

Contrast-enhanced imaging is not routinely required but may be used when infection, tumor, or inflammatory arthropathy is suspected [2, 3]. When indicated, fat-suppressed gadolinium-enhanced T1-weighted imaging in multiple planes aids in evaluating synovitis and the posterior attachment [1]. For osseous assessment, three-dimensional T1-weighted fast spoiled gradient-echo sequences at 3.0 T depict condylar erosions as focal interruptions of the cortical hypointense line [11, 33, 34]. High-resolution bilateral surface coils with a small field of view optimize signal-to-noise ratio and enable simultaneous imaging of both joints.

Dynamic evaluation uses rapid sequential acquisitions, most commonly single-shot fast spin echo (SSFSE) PD-weighted sequences obtained during gradual mouth opening and closing. Cine reconstruction allows assessment of disc–condyle motion. Mechanical opening devices, such as the Burnett device, may assist with incremental opening but do not reproduce physiologic movement because lateral pterygoid contraction is not engaged. Alternative functional approaches, including balanced steady-state free precession imaging at 3 T, have also been described [25].

4. MRI features of anatomical variants and TMJ pathology

4.1 Foramen tympanicum

Incomplete ossification of the tympanic plate can result in a persistent foramen tympanicum (foramen of Huschke). The tympanic plate begins as a U-shaped cartilaginous structure at birth and normally ossifies by about 5 years of age, although a small residual opening measuring 3–4 mm may occasionally remain. The foramen is located along the anteroinferior wall of the external auditory canal, posteromedial to the TMJ. Patients with a persistent foramen may present with salivary otorrhea during mastication, a visible defect or polyp in the anterior canal wall, or even herniation of TMJ soft tissues into the external auditory canal during movement. It may also lead to intraoperative communication during TMJ arthroscopy or serve as a pathway for spread of infection, inflammation, or tumor between the TMJ and auditory canal. On MRI, retrodiscal tissue may protrude through the defect (**Figure 6**). Evaluation should include closed- and open-mouth imaging with thin sections (approximately 3 mm) to assess the degree of herniation [35].

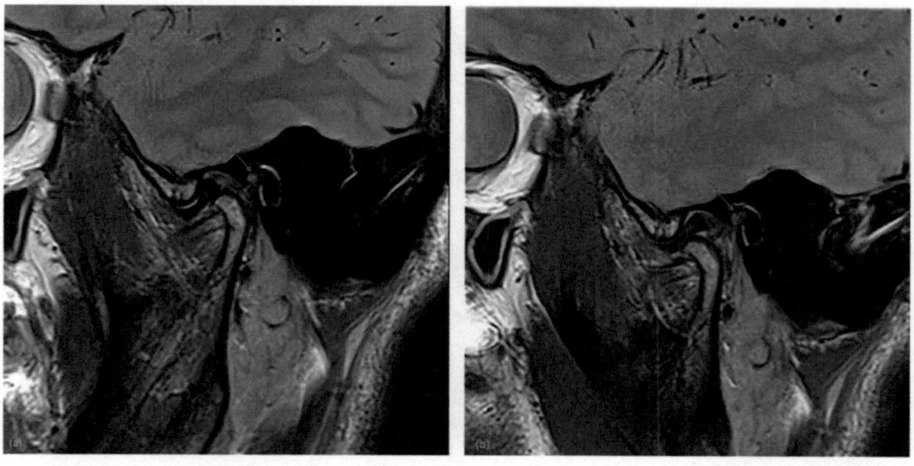

Figure 6.
Proton density weighted magnetic resonance images demonstrating temporomandibular joint herniation through the left foramen tympanicum. (a) Sagittal closed mouth and (b) Sagittal open mouth images demonstrate a similar degree of temporomandibular joint herniation. Source: Ref. [35] https://pubmed.ncbi.nlm.nih.gov/29988923/. License: http://creativecommons.org/licenses/by-nc-nd/4.0/.

4.2 Internal derangement

Internal derangement is defined as an abnormal positional relationship between the mandibular condyle and the articular disc [9]. Disc displacement occurs in 16–31% of asymptomatic individuals and is more frequent in patients with TMJ symptoms [36]. When the disc repositions during mouth opening, an audible or palpable click may be present. In more advanced cases, the disc remains displaced in both closed- and open-mouth positions, leading to restricted opening and absence of clicking. The condition is more common in women, with peak incidence between 20 and 40 years of age [37]. Proposed etiologies include trauma, malocclusion, bruxism, psychological stress, and developmental skeletal abnormalities [38].

Disc displacement may be anterior, anterolateral, anteromedial, lateral, medial, or posterior. Anterior displacement is most common, accounting for approximately half of cases, followed by anterolateral displacement in about one-third. Posterior displacement is rare (<1%) and often presents as acute open-lock with inability to close the mouth [1, 3, 4, 23, 31]. Sagittal imaging is optimal for assessing anterior and posterior displacement, whereas coronal imaging is more sensitive for medial and lateral patterns. Mediolateral abnormalities such as the "floating disc" sign may be noted when the disc is present but the condyle is not visualized on the same slice [20]. Anterior displacement is diagnosed when the junction of the posterior band and bilaminar zone lies anterior to the 11-o'clock position relative to the condyle. Displacement is further classified as reducible or non-reducible based on whether normal disc–condyle alignment is restored on mouth opening [1, 3, 4].

4.2.1 Disc displacement with reduction

In anterior disc displacement with reduction (ADDwR), the disc is positioned anterior to the condyle in the closed-mouth position but resumes a normal position during mouth opening (**Figures** 7 and **8**) [2, 4, 9, 31]. MRI accordingly demonstrates anterior displacement on closed-mouth views with normalization on open-mouth views. Associated features may include a rounded or biconvex disc, abnormal disc orientation [37], and early T2 hyperintensity within the bilaminar zone. With progressive degeneration, signal intensity on both T1- and T2-weighted sequences decreases [38]. Quantitatively, displacement is present when the posterior band lies anterior to the normal 11-o'clock position relative to the vertical condylar axis [19].

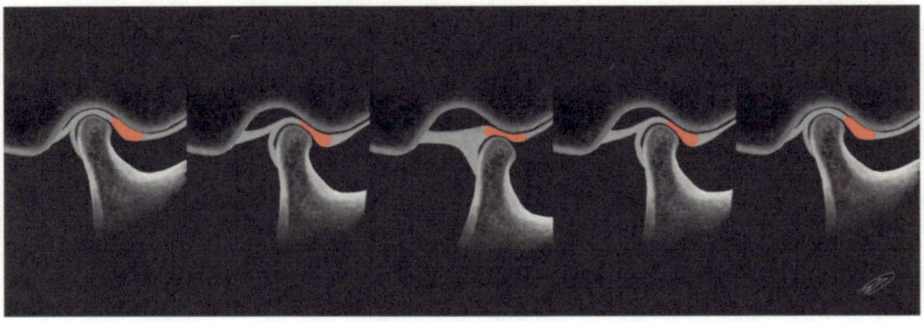

Figure 7.
Diagrammatic representation of disc displacement with reduction.

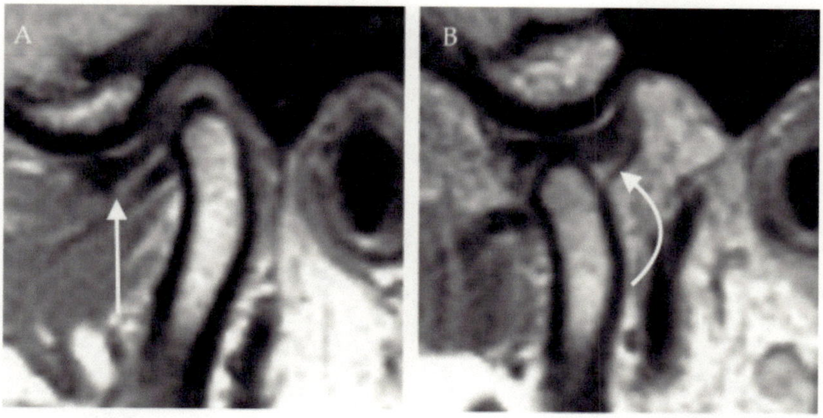

Figure 8.
Anterior disc displacement with reduction. Proton density sagittal image of the TMJ in closed mouth (A) position shows anterior displacement of the articular disc with otherwise normal bow-tie appearance (straight arrow). The mandibular condyle is situated in an anatomic location within the mandibular fossa. On open mouth images (B), normal condylar rotation and anterior translation are noted. Note the recapture of the articular disc, which is now in the normal position (curved arrow). The bow-tie appearance of the articular disc is preserved. Source: Ref. [3] https://pubmed.ncbi.nlm.nih.gov/35454054/. License: https://creativecommons.org/licenses/by/4.0/.

4.2.2 Disc displacement without reduction

In anterior disc displacement without reduction (ADDwoR), the disc remains displaced in both closed- and open-mouth positions, preventing normal condylar translation (**Figures 9** and **10**). This fixed displacement corresponds clinically to "closed lock." MRI demonstrates persistent anterior disc displacement and loss of coordinated disc–condyle motion [2, 4, 9]. Displacement may be complete, involving the full mediolateral extent of the disc, or partial, affecting only a segment. Partial displacement is more frequently encountered in ADDwR and may present as rotational displacement, in which the lateral disc portion is displaced anteriorly while the medial portion maintains normal alignment [31, 39].

4.2.3 Disc morphology and signal alterations

In early disease, the disc retains its normal biconcave shape. With progression, structural alterations develop, including posterior band thickening (**Figure 11A**, **B**), anterior band thinning, shortening of the anteroposterior dimension (**Figure 11A**, **B**), and

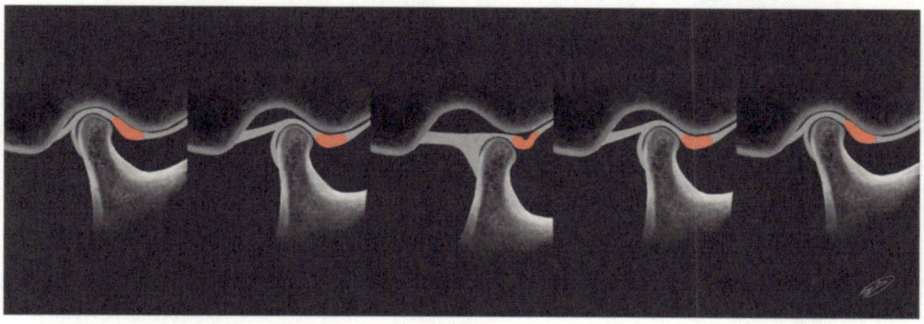

Figure 9.
Diagrammatic representation of disc displacement without reduction.

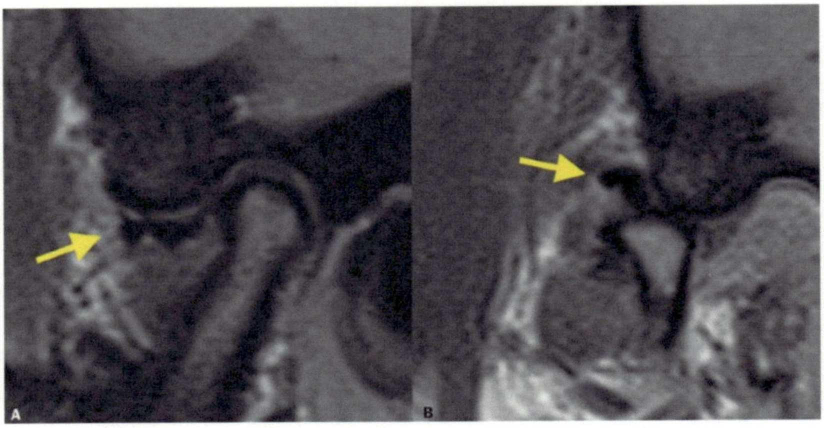

Figure 10.
Anterior disc displacement without reduction. Sagittal PD-weighted image in the closed-mouth position (A), showing the disc anterior to the 11 o'clock position. In the open-mouth position (B), there is no disc recapture. The disc position is indicated by the arrows. Source: Ref. [7] https://pmc.ncbi.nlm.nih.gov/articles/PMC10165975/. License: https://creativecommons.org/licenses/.

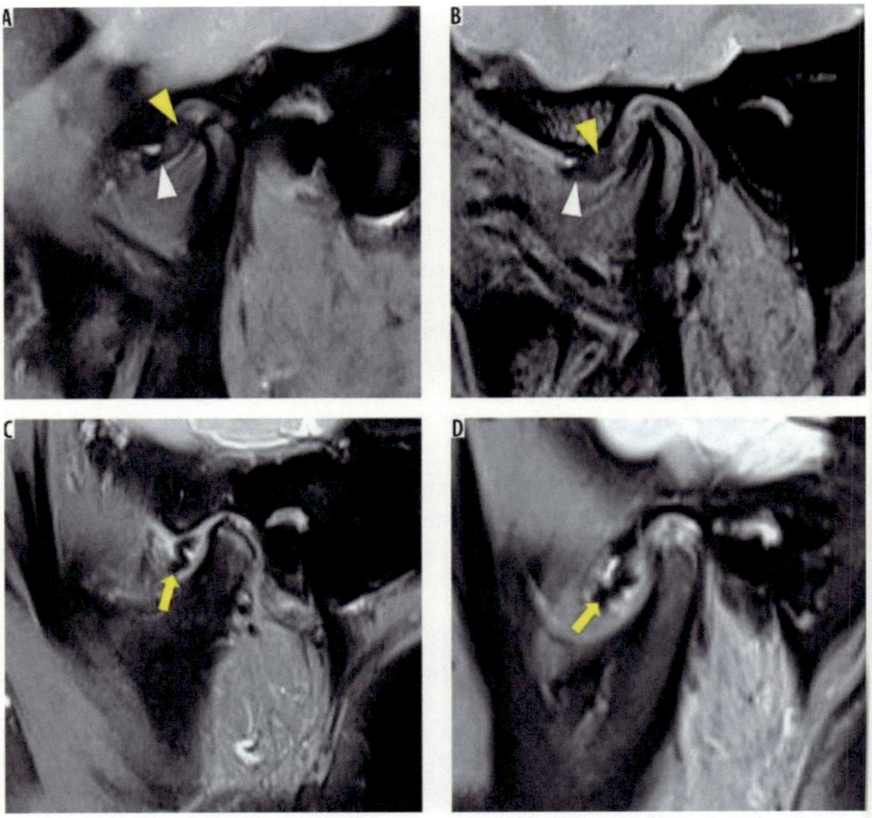

Figure 11.
(A-D) Patterns of altered disc morphology. In 4 different patients with internal derangement, sagittal oblique proton density fat saturation magnetic resonance images show thickening of posterior band (yellow arrowheads) (A, B); shortening of antero-posterior dimension of disc with small intermediate zone (IZ) (A, B); and crumpled disc (yellow arrows) (C, D). Also note the abnormal intermediate signal of disc (A, B). Source: Ref. [26] https://pmc.ncbi.nlm.nih.gov/articles/PMC7016362/. License: http://creativecommons.org/licenses/by-nc-nd/4.0/.

transformation into any of the following configurations: tear-drop, biplanar, flattened, sunglass, amorphous, rounded, or crumpled (**Figures 11C, D** and **12**). In ADDwR, the disc often appears biplanar in the closed-mouth position and becomes biconcave on opening. In contrast, ADDwoR is commonly associated with convex or folded (crumpled) discs that do not change shape during opening. Disc length also fails to increase during opening and remains shorter than in normally positioned discs [40, 41]. Signal characteristics evolve with disease severity. The posterior band typically exhibits higher signal intensity than the anterior band, with progressive increases correlating with advancing derangement. Posterior band thickening is frequently observed, supporting the concept that degeneration begins posteriorly and progresses anteriorly. Histopathologic studies corroborate these findings, demonstrating fibroblast proliferation, neovascularity, and fibrous replacement of normal connective tissue within the posterior attachment [42].

4.2.4 Pesudodisc

In some patients with anterior disc displacement, a pseudodisc may develop within the posterior attachment as an adaptive response. This results from hyalinization and fibrous replacement of the normally vascularized and innervated retrodiscal tissue, producing a band-like structure with hypointense signal on MRI. In certain cases, the pseudodisc can function similarly to the native disc (**Figure 13D**) [9, 20].

4.2.5 Stuck disc

The "stuck disc" or anchored disc phenomenon refers to an immobile disc in both open- and closed-mouth positions, typically resulting from intra-articular adhesions

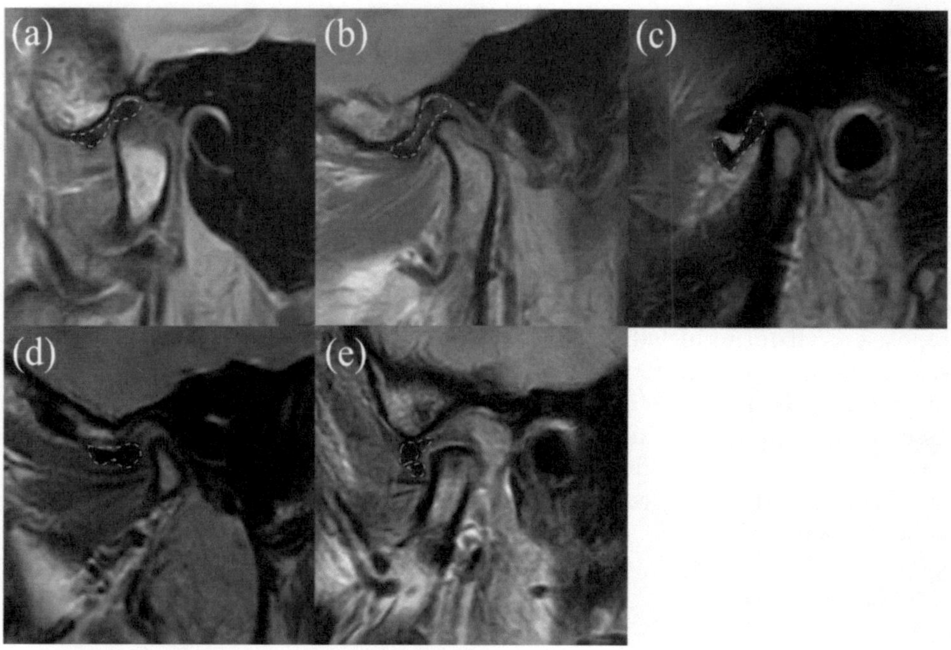

Figure 12.
Disc shapes depicted on sagittal oblique proton density images (dotted lines) (a) Biconcave; (b) Flattened; (c) Folded; (d) Sunglass; (e) Amorphous. Source: Ref. [40] https://www.nature.com/articles/s41598-025-06045-2. License: http://creativecommons.org/licenses/by-nc-nd/4.0/.

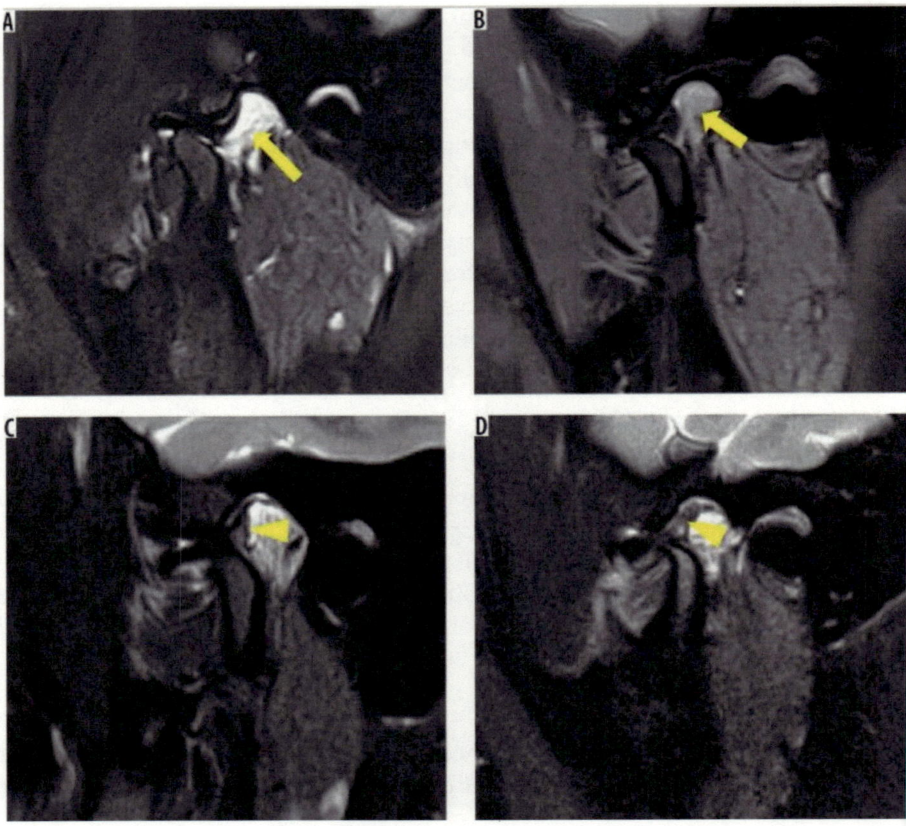

Figure 13.
Posterior attachment remodeling. Sagittal oblique T2W-FS (A) and proton density fat saturation (B) images demonstrate normal posterior attachment (yellow arrow). In two different patients with long-standing internal derangement (C, D), sagittal oblique T2-FS images show a hypointense signal in anterior part of posterior attachment (PA) suggesting fibrosis (remodeling). In the second patient (D), this gives a pseudo-disc appearance. Source: Ref. [26] https://pmc.ncbi.nlm.nih.gov/articles/PMC7016362/. License: http://creativecommons.org/licenses/by-nc-nd/4.0/.

(**Figure 14**). Adhesions occur in up to 20% of advanced internal derangement cases, most commonly in the anterior recess of the superior joint compartment. They may be pseudowall-like (vascularized fibrosynovial) or band-like (collagen-based). Proposed mechanisms include fibrin deposition associated with synovitis, mechanical overloading, or scar tissue formation after hematoma healing. Clinically, this condition presents with restricted condylar translation, pain, and dysfunction, and may be missed without both open- and closed-mouth MRI evaluation. Sagittal oblique cine sequences can demonstrate disc immobility, but MRI is limited in directly identifying adhesions; arthroscopy remains the most definitive diagnostic and therapeutic method [9, 43].

4.2.6 Double disc sign

The superior belly of the lateral pterygoid contributes to mouth closure and retrusion, whereas the inferior belly facilitates mouth opening and protrusion [9]. In internal derangement, the inferior belly may become hyperactive to stabilize and guide the condyle–disc complex, leading to thickening of its attachment. When this

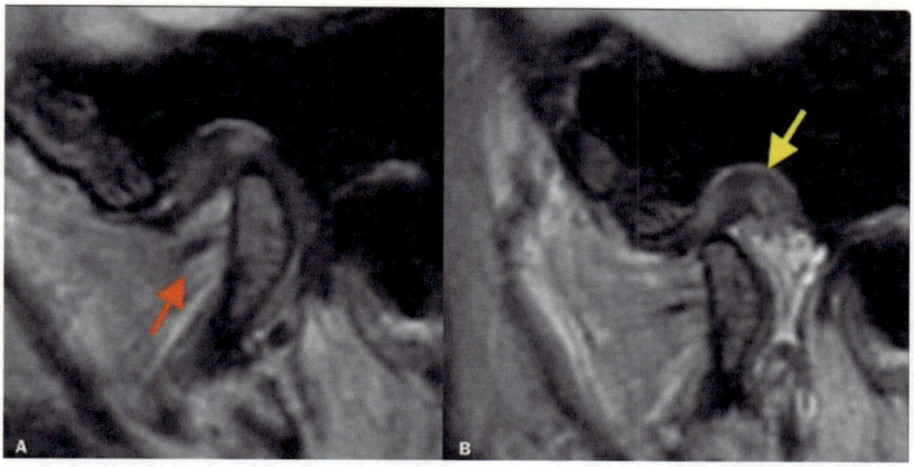

Figure 14.
Disc adhesion. PD-weighted sagittal images in the closed-mouth and open-mouth positions (A and B, respectively), showing alteration of the signal in the posterior band and intermediate zone of the articular disc, together with thickening of the retrodiscal tissue (yellow arrow). Note that the disc remains in the same location in the closed-mouth and open-mouth positions, which is characteristic of disc adhesion (stuck disc). Note also the thickening at the insertion of the lateral pterygoid muscle belly (red arrow), forming the double-disc sign. Source: Ref. [7] https://pmc.ncbi.nlm.nih.gov/articles/PMC10165975/. License: https://creativecommons.org/licenses/.

thickened tendon runs parallel to an anteriorly displaced disc, it creates the characteristic "double disc" sign (**Figure 14**). Electromyographic studies have demonstrated increased activity in the inferior lateral pterygoid attachment in such cases [2, 4, 5, 9]. Recognition of this sign on MRI is important to avoid misinterpreting a thickened LPM attachment as the articular disc.

4.2.7 Hypermobility

TMJ hypermobility, or subluxation, is characterized by excessive forward translation of the condyle–disc complex during mouth opening, such that the condyle moves beyond the articular eminence (**Figure 15**). Unlike dislocation, the condyle returns to the glenoid fossa spontaneously or with minimal assistance. Clinically, it may present as abrupt anterior condylar displacement during the later phase of opening, producing an excessively wide mouth opening. Anatomical variation, particularly a steep articular eminence with a short posterior and elongated anterior slope, is thought to predispose individuals by permitting early disc rotation relative to condylar translation. Systemic and local factors also contribute, including generalized connective tissue disorders (e.g., Ehlers–Danlos and Marfan syndromes), generalized joint hypermobility, iatrogenic trauma (such as after extractions, intubation, or endoscopic procedures), and intrinsic triggers such as excessive yawning, wide mouth opening, or seizure episodes [44].

4.2.8 Perforated disc

The articular disc lacks mesenchymal cell–mediated regenerative or adaptive capacity, and progressive abrasive loss may predispose its thinner regions to perforation (**Figure 16**). Disc perforations occur most frequently in the bilaminar zone and the lateral aspect of the disc [44]. Perforation disrupts the normal lubricating

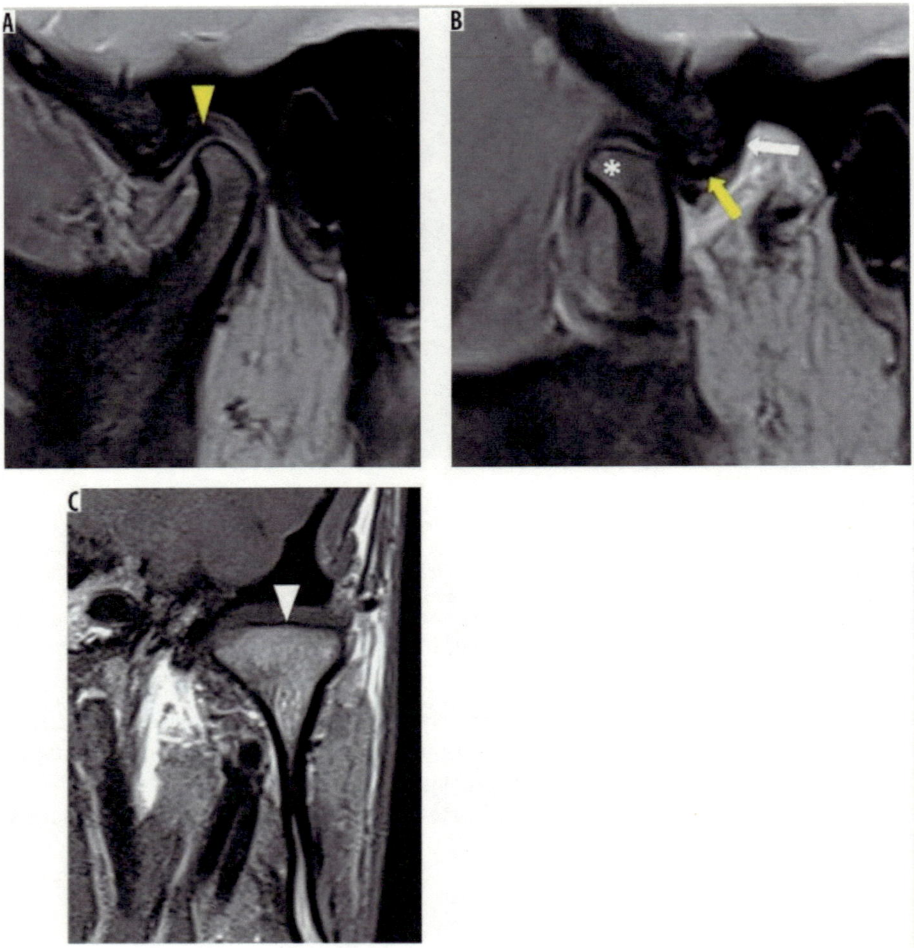

Figure 15.
Hypermobile temporomandibular joint. (A) In a 25-year-old patient who presented with multiple episodes of open lock on left side, closed mouth sagittal oblique proton density fat saturation image reveals a normal disc (yellow arrowhead). (B) Open mouth sagittal oblique proton density image shows increased range of motion where the condyle (asterisk) is seen reaching antero-superiorly to the crest of articular eminence (yellow arrow). Steep (vertical) posterior slope of AE (white arrow) is also noted. (C) Coronal oblique T1W image shows flattening of condyle (white arrowhead). Source: Ref. [26] https://pmc.ncbi.nlm.nih.gov/articles/PMC7016362/. License: http://creativecommons.org/licenses/by-nc-nd/4.0/.

function of synovial fluid, increasing friction and direct loading of the articular surfaces, which may contribute to cartilage hypertrophy [45]. Normally, the disc distributes synovial fluid uniformly across articular interfaces; perforation alters this mechanism and increases frictional and shear stresses between the temporal and condylar components [46]. Histopathologic studies describe osteophyte formation during proliferative phases, followed by reduced activity associated with condylar flattening [47].

Diagnosis is challenging because clinical signs are nonspecific and MRI sensitivity is limited. Fat-suppressed T2-weighted sagittal and coronal images may occasionally demonstrate perforations, particularly when effusion is present [9]. Arthroscopy remains the most reliable diagnostic and therapeutic method. Conventional and MR arthrography may assist by demonstrating contrast passage into both joint

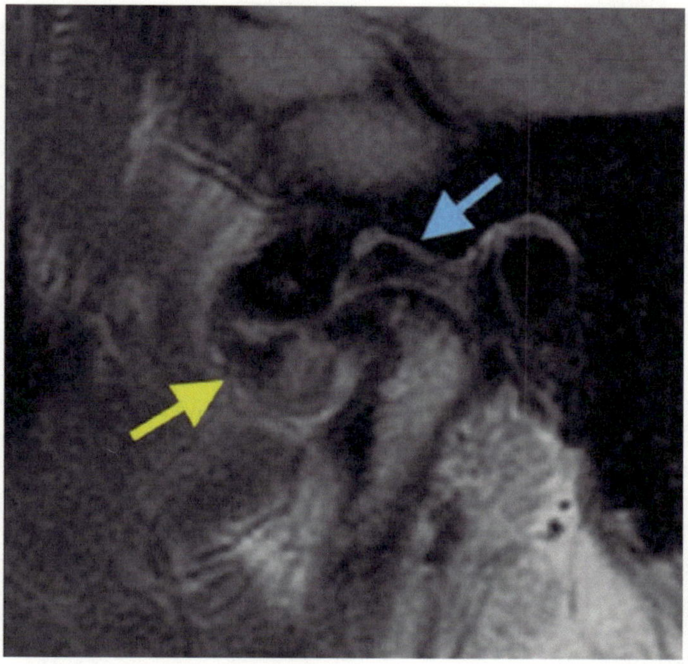

Figure 16.
Disc perforation. Sagittal PD-weighted image showing discontinuity of the articular disc, with separation of the anterior band (yellow arrow) and posterior band (blue arrow). Note also the subcortical sclerosis with an anterior marginal osteophyte in the mandibular condyle. Source: Ref. [7] https://pmc.ncbi.nlm.nih.gov/articles/PMC10165975/. License: https://creativecommons.org/licenses/.

compartments after injection into the lower compartment. A lack of posterior temporal disc attachment stretching during mouth opening is another supportive indicator [39].

4.2.9 Lateral pterygoid muscle changes

The role of the lateral pterygoid muscle in TMJ function remains debated. MRI studies have demonstrated morphological and signal alterations in both the superior and inferior bellies in patients with anterior disc displacement, with or without reduction. These changes include hypertrophy, atrophy, and contracture, and may be associated with symptoms such as pain and restricted mandibular opening. Anterior disc displacement appears more closely related to attachment of the superior LPM to the disc rather than to the condyle. Early changes, such as increased fluid content in the superior head, manifest as T2 hyperintensity, whereas chronic or fatty atrophic changes demonstrate T1 hyperintensity with relative T2 hypointensity. Muscle spasm or edema can result in increased thickness, while atrophy leads to thinning. These imaging features reflect structural and compositional changes within the LPM, although their clinical significance remains uncertain [48, 49].

4.3 Bone marrow changes

MRI characterizes bone marrow changes in the mandibular condyle into two primary patterns: edema and osteonecrosis, based on corresponding histological findings.

- *Bone marrow edema* appears as low signal on T1-weighted or proton-density sequences and high signal on T2-weighted images (**Figure 17**). It has been associated with pain and may represent an early stage in the evolution toward osteonecrosis, particularly in younger patients [50, 51]. Bone marrow abnormalities are generally absent in asymptomatic individuals. Fat-suppressed T2-weighted and fluid-attenuated inversion recovery (FLAIR) sequences improve detection and may show higher signal intensity in painful joints. Although marrow edema correlates with joint effusion and pain [50–52], longitudinal studies indicate that marrow signal does not necessarily parallel symptom severity, and its precise role in TMJ pain remains uncertain [53].

- *Osteonecrosis*, encompassing osteochondritis dissecans (OCD) and avascular necrosis (AVN), shows decreased signal on T1-weighted images with variable T2 appearance depending on stage and associated reparative changes. Early AVN may be hyperintense on T2-weighted imaging, whereas acute OCD typically demonstrates a hypointense central fragment with a hyperintense rim. MRI yields moderate sensitivity (78%) and specificity (84%) for AVN, although advanced condylar sclerosis may mimic necrosis and limit positive predictive value (54%) [54].

4.4 Joint effusion

Joint effusion refers to excess intra-articular fluid and occurs more frequently in symptomatic joints. T2-weighted sequences provide the greatest sensitivity (**Figure 18**). Early effusions often localize anteriorly, while larger collections may occupy both joint compartments. Prominent effusions can aid diagnosis by outlining

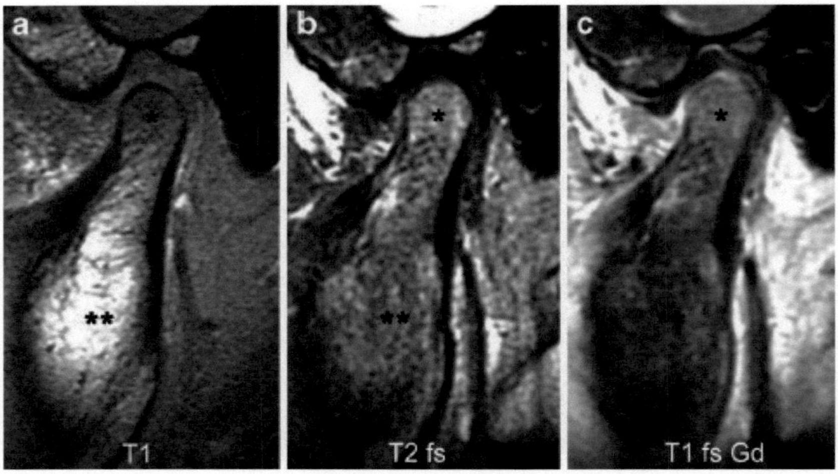

Figure 17.
Bone marrow oedema and enhancement (grade 1) of the mandibular condyle in a 9-year-old boy. (a–c) When compared to the mandibular ramus (**) there is lower signal from the mandibular condyle (*) on the T1-weighted gradient echo sagittal image without fat saturation (TR/TE 300/4.2 ms, flip angle 80°, (a), and slightly increased signal on fat-saturated T2-weighted image (TR/TE 5400/77 ms, (b) and on postcontrast fat-saturated T1-weighted sagittal image (TR/TE 670/10 ms, (c) images, Note mild joint enhancement with high signal intensity (hyperintense to muscle) in the posterior superior joint recess and lower joint compartment on postcontrast fat-saturated T1-weighted image (c). Source: Ref. [52] https://pmc.ncbi.nlm.nih.gov/articles/PMC5823950/. License: http://creativecommons.org/licenses/by/4.0/.

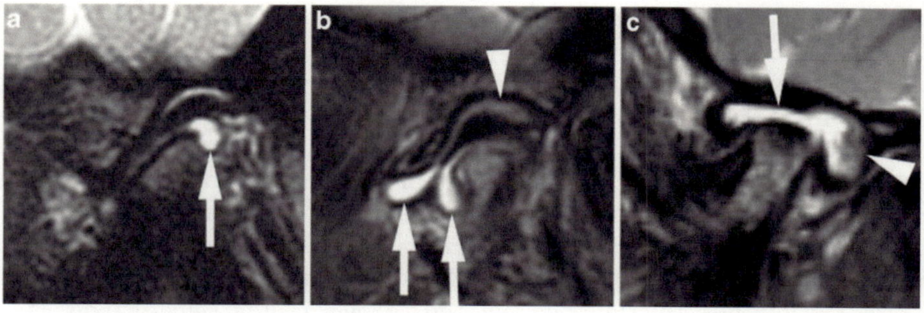

Figure 18.
Large joint effusion (grade 2) on sagittal oblique images. a-c Effusion exceeding 2-mm width (arrows) on fat-saturated T2-weighted fast spin echo images (TR/TE 5400/77 ms) in the posterior recess in a 15-year-old girl (a), in the anterior recesses in a 13-year-old boy (b) and with bulging of the upper joint compartment in a 7-year-old girl (c). Note thickened synovium with intermediate signal intensity (arrowheads) on these posteriorly in (b) and (c). Source: Ref. [52] https://pmc.ncbi.nlm.nih.gov/articles/PMC5823950/. License: http://creativecommons.org/licenses/by/4.0/.

the disc, highlighting perforations, and delineating retrodiscal tissue, producing an "arthrographic effect." On contrast-enhanced T1-weighted imaging, synovitis enhances whereas joint fluid remains non-enhancing, aiding differentiation in inflammatory arthropathies (**Figure 19**) [9, 20].

4.5 MRI features of arthropathies

TMJ can be affected by various inflammatory conditions, such as juvenile idiopathic arthritis, rheumatoid arthritis, septic arthritis, psoriatic arthritis, arthritis secondary to calcium pyrophosphate crystal deposition, and pigmented villonodular synovitis [25].

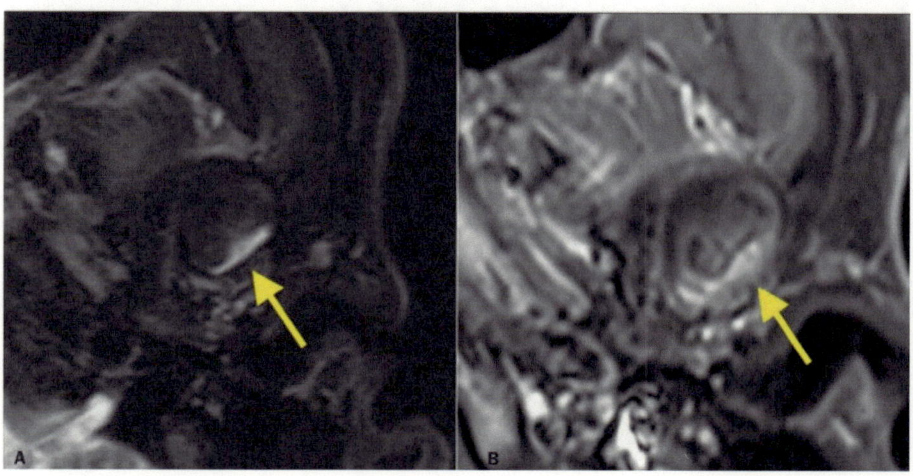

Figure 19.
Synovitis. Axial T2-weighted image with fat saturation (A) and contrast-enhanced T1-weighted image (B), showing synovial thickening with enhancement consistent with synovitis, which should not be confused with joint effusion. Source: Ref. [7] https://pmc.ncbi.nlm.nih.gov/articles/PMC10165975/. License: https://creativecommons.org/licenses/.

4.5.1 Juvenile idiopathic arthritis

Juvenile idiopathic arthritis (JIA) is a chronic inflammatory disorder presenting before age 16 [55, 56]. Genetic susceptibility, environmental triggers, and distinct autoinflammatory pathways contribute to disease onset and subtype variability [56–58]. TMJ involvement occurs in up to half of patients, either unilaterally or bilaterally. Clinical features include joint pain, swelling, tenderness, morning stiffness, and limited mandibular mobility. Severe bilateral TMJ disease can impair mandibular growth, resulting in retrognathia, posteroinferior mandibular rotation, decreased posterior facial height, anterior open bite, and a convex profile. Unilateral disease often produces facial asymmetry and mandibular deviation toward the affected side [55]. Histopathologic changes originate in the synovium, which becomes hyperplastic and vascularized with lymphoplasmacytic infiltration, leading to pannus formation and subsequent osteochondral destruction [59, 60].

4.5.1.1 Imaging features

MRI is the preferred modality and is sensitive for early synovitis and bone marrow edema. Gadolinium-enhanced imaging should be obtained within the first 4 minutes to distinguish synovitis from effusion (**Figure 20**) [55]. Acute findings include effusion, marrow edema, and synovial enhancement (**Figure 21**). Chronic changes include condylar flattening, erosions, hypertrophic bone formation, ramus shortening, disc abnormalities, and pannus [55]. The JAMRIS-TMJ scoring system standardizes evaluation of acute and chronic features (**Table 2**) [52]. While the JAMRIS-TMJ scoring system standardizes the evaluation of acute and chronic inflammatory changes, additional features such as pannus formation and retrodiscal tissue alterations, though not formally included in the scoring system, are increasingly recognized as relevant imaging findings in JIA [61].

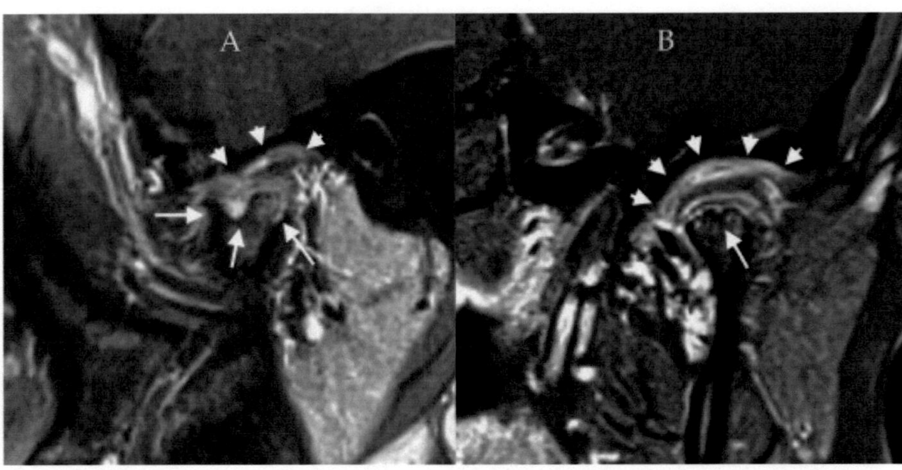

Figure 20.
Juvenile idiopathic arthritis. Post-contrast T1W fat-saturated sagittal (A) and coronal (B) images of the TMJ demonstrate flattening and irregularity of the condyle with erosions (longtail arrows), resulting in an irregular foreshortened appearance from chronic inflammation. Jointeffusion is noted with surrounding synovial enhancement (short tail arrows), consistent with anacute JIA flair. Source: Ref. [3] https://pmc.ncbi.nlm.nih.gov/articles/PMC9031630/. License: http://creativecommons.org/licenses/by/4.0/.

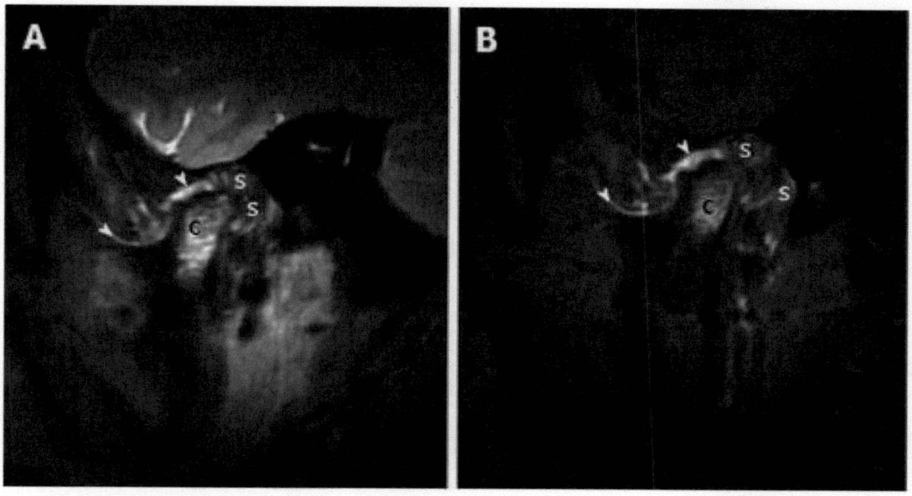

Figure 21.
Juvenile idiopathic arthritis. A: Sagittal proton density weighted magnetic resonance imaging (MRI) in the closed mouth position demonstrates increased signal at the mandibular condyle (the letter, c), extensive thickening of the synovium (the letter, s) in the retrodiscal regions. It can be noted that the thickening and increased signal of the synovium at other places (arrowheads); B: Sagittal fat suppressed post contrast T1 weighted MRI in the closed mouth position demonstrates enhancement of signal at the mandibular condyle (the letter, c), enhancement and extensive thickening of the synovium (the letter, s) in the retrodiscal regions. There is thickening and enhancement of the synovium at other places (arrowheads). Source: Ref. [31] https://www.wjgnet.com/1949-8470/full/v6/i8/567.htm?appgw_azwaf_jsc=Edpoad8rB8m1jwKpLl3k9cTe6n9LK33hO7vnig6xHwc. License: http://creativecommons.org/licenses/by/4.0/.

Item	Definition	Grade 0	Grade 1	Grade 2
(A) Inflammatory domain				
Bone marrow edema	Hyperintense marrow signal in the condyle compared with mandibular ramus on fluid-sensitive sequences, and/or hypointense signal on non–fat-suppressed T1-weighted images	Absent	Present	—
Bone marrow enhancement	Post-contrast hyperintense marrow signal in the condyle relative to mandibular ramus on fat-suppressed T1-weighted images	Absent	Present	—
Joint effusion	Excess intra-articular fluid with signal similar to cerebrospinal fluid on fluid-sensitive sequences	≤1 mm (absent)	Small: >1–≤2 mm in recess or full compartment	Large: >2 mm in recess or full compartment
Synovial thickening	Thickened synovial lining with intermediate signal intensity on fluid-sensitive images	None (≤1 mm)	Mild: >1–≤2 mm at thickest point	Moderate/severe: >2 mm at thickest point

Item	Definition	Grade 0	Grade 1	Grade 2
Joint enhancement	Post-contrast synovial/capsular signal greater than muscle on fat-suppressed T1-weighted images	Normal: confined to physiologic fluid perimeter	Mild: focal signal beyond physiologic perimeter	Diffuse: extensive involvement of one/both compartments
(B) Damage domain				
Condylar flattening	Alteration of the normal rounded or slightly angular condylar contour (sagittal oblique view)	Absent	Mild: partial surface flattening	Moderate/severe: entire surface flattened or condylar height reduced
Erosions	Cortical irregularities or breaks of the articular surface	Absent	Mild: irregularities affecting part of the articular surface	Moderate/severe: deep subchondral defects in two planes or entire surface irregular
Disc abnormalities	Any alteration of the articular disc (flattening, displacement, or destruction)	Absent	Present	—

Table 2.
Juvenile idiopathic arthritis magnetic resonance imaging scoring system for the temporomandibular joint (JAMRIS-TMJ) [52].

Pannus formation: Pannus represents abnormal soft tissue within the joint compartment, typically showing iso- to hypointense signal on T1- and fat-suppressed T2-weighted sequences. Unlike acute synovitis, pannus seldom enhances following contrast administration. In the context of JAMRIS-TMJ, pannus may be reflected indirectly by the coexistence of minimal or absent joint enhancement and moderate to severe synovial thickening [55, 62].

Retrodiscal tissue changes: Retrodiscal tissue signal alterations may reflect hypervascularity, edema, or fibrosis. Studies have shown that patients with TMJ-related pain often demonstrate higher signal intensity in the retrodiscal tissue on dynamic contrast-enhanced, T2-weighted, and FLAIR sequences. Hyperintensity generally corresponds to hypervascularity and edema, while low signal may indicate fibrotic changes. Standardized evaluation of retrodiscal signal alterations in JIA could provide an additional marker of inflammatory activity once validated [55, 62].

New bone formation and secondary osteoarthritis may occur in long-standing disease, although the incidence has declined with biologic therapy. Heterotopic ossification has been reported after intra-articular corticosteroids [55, 62].

4.5.2 Rheumatoid arthritis

Rheumatoid arthritis (RA) is a systemic inflammatory disease that commonly affects periarticular tissues, with TMJ involvement in approximately 50–75% of patients, typically after systemic diagnosis [31]. TMJ involvement is often characterized by deep preauricular pain, exacerbated by mastication, together with the limited range of motion and morning stiffness. Progressive disease may cause trismus, facial deformity, and chronic loss of function [3].

4.5.2.1 Imaging features

Common MRI findings include synovial thickening and enhancement, joint space narrowing, articular erosions, reduced condylar height, restricted condylar motion, disc deformation, and, in advanced cases, disc displacement. Unlike osteoarthritis, disc displacement in RA tends to occur later and is usually secondary to bony resorption rather than intrinsic disc pathology. Although a standardized radiologic grading system for RA in the TMJ has not been established, studies have shown that condylar dimensions decrease with increasing disease activity [3, 51].

4.5.3 Septic arthritis

Septic arthritis of the TMJ is rare and most commonly caused by *Staphylococcus aureus*, through hematogenous spread or local extension (e.g., otitis media) [3].

4.5.3.1 Imaging features

MRI demonstrates synovial enhancement, effusion, adjacent soft tissue swelling, bone marrow edema, and osteomyelitis (**Figure 22**). Clinical differentiation from other arthritis relies on the abrupt onset of severe pain and systemic symptoms such as fever and malaise [63].

4.5.3.2 Psoriatic arthritis

Psoriatic arthritis occurs in 5–8% of patients with psoriasis [2]. TMJ involvement is uncommon but resembles RA, showing condylar flattening, erosions, restricted motion, effusion, and disc abnormalities. CT may show condylar resorption with new bone formation. Other seronegative arthropathies (e.g., ankylosing spondylitis, systemic lupus erythematosus) may produce similar imaging features [25].

4.5.4 Calcium pyrophosphate crystal deposition

Calcium pyrophosphate deposition disease (CPPD), also referred to as *tophaceous pseudogout*, is a noninfectious inflammatory arthropathy caused by the accumulation of calcium pyrophosphate crystals within articular and periarticular tissues. Two clinical forms have been identified, the common type and the tumoral or tophaceous type, with the latter more frequently affecting the TMJ.

4.5.4.1 Imaging features

On radiographs and computed tomography (CT), CPPD may present with chondrocalcinosis of the articular disc, narrowing of the joint space, osteophytosis, subchondral cysts, and in some cases, erosive changes of the condyle and temporal bone that may resemble tumor-like lesions. On MRI, CPPD is usually identified as periarticular low signal intensity on T2-weighted sequences with heterogeneous enhancement and post-contrast T1 hyperintensity, features that can mimic aggressive conditions such as chondrosarcoma (**Figure 23**). The definitive diagnosis of CPPD is established through joint aspiration and fluid analysis demonstrating calcium pyrophosphate crystals [64].

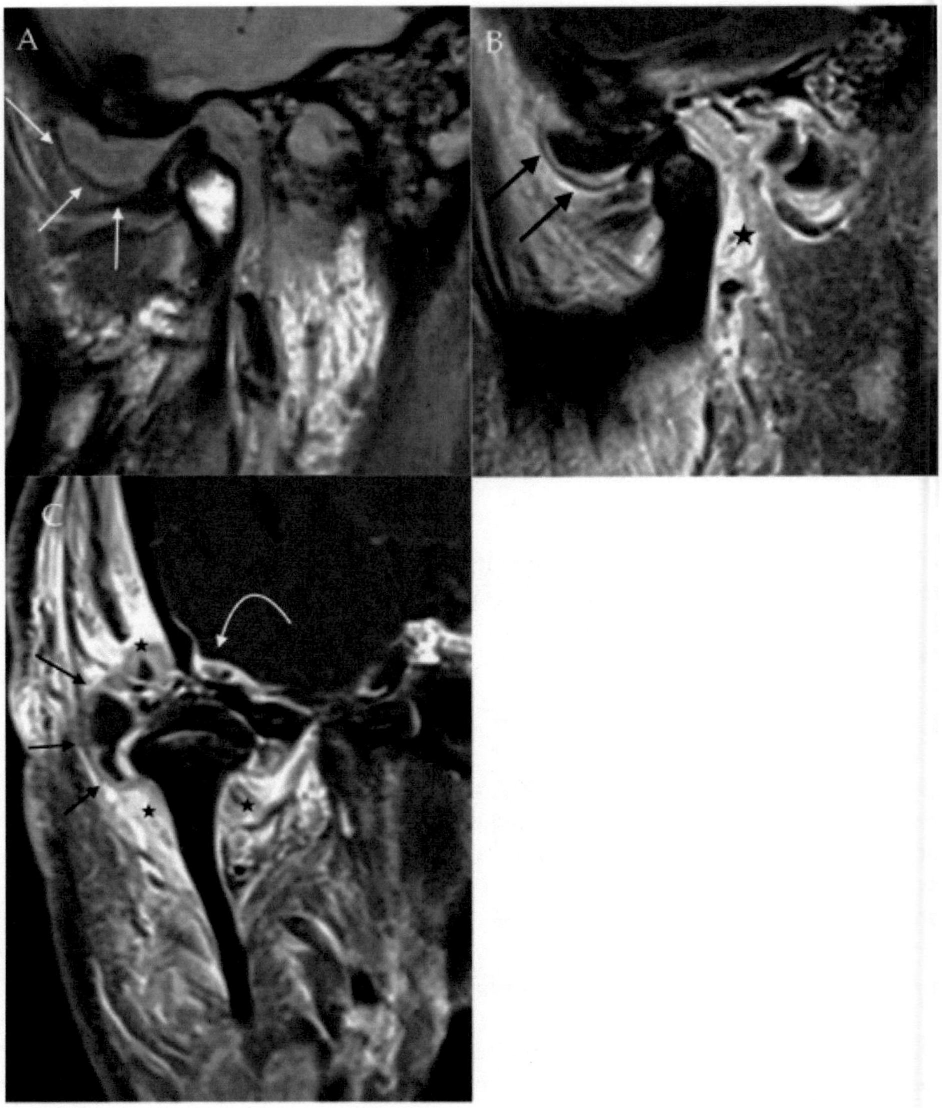

Figure 22.
Septic arthritis. Proton density sagittal image of the TMJ (A) demonstrates a large joint effusion expanding the space between the articular disc and articular tubercle (straight white arrow). Post-contrast T1Wfat-saturated sagittal (B) and coronal (C) images demonstrate extensive surrounding synovial enhancement (black arrows) and soft tissue enhancement (star). Also noted is enhancement along the dura of the right temporal lobe (curved arrow), indicating the intracranial extension of infection. Source: Ref. [3] https://pmc.ncbi.nlm.nih.gov/articles/PMC9031630/. License: http://creativecommons.org/licenses/by/4.0/.

4.5.5 Pigmented villonodular synovitis

Pigmented villonodular synovitis (PVNS) is the preferred term for a spectrum of benign proliferative and inflammatory disorders originating from the synovium of joints, bursae, and tendon sheaths. PVNS has locally aggressive potential, characterized by abnormal synovial proliferation and recurrent intra-articular hemorrhage. Primary involvement of the TMJ is uncommon. Based on its extent, PVNS is classified into nodular and diffuse forms [30].

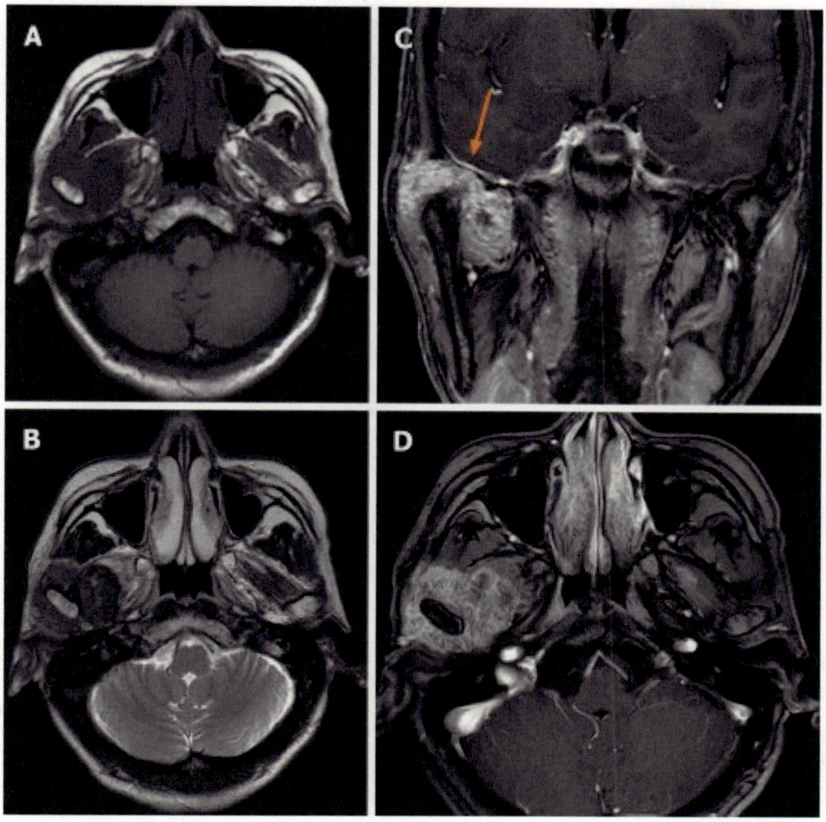

Figure 23.
Calcium pyrophosphate deposition disease - Magnetic resonance imaging images 1. Axial T1-weighted image (A) and T2-weighted image (B) showed a hypointense mass. The lesion was markedly enhanced after enhancement (C and D) and in contact with the dura mater on the inferior surface (C, arrow). Source: Ref. [64] https://pmc.ncbi.nlm.nih.gov/articles/PMC8040178/. License: http://creativecommons.org/licenses/by/4.0/.

4.5.5.1 Imaging features

CT typically reveals a hyperattenuating intra-articular mass that may produce erosive changes on both articular surfaces of the TMJ. In advanced cases, the expanding lesion can breach the skull base and extend intracranially. MRI demonstrates characteristic findings related to hemosiderin (low-intensity) (**Figure 24**) deposition within the lesion. Signal intensity is generally intermediate to low on T1-weighted, T2-weighted, and proton-density sequences. This effect is particularly pronounced on gradient-echo (GRE) or T2* sequences, which are highly sensitive to magnetic field inhomogeneities. These sequences exaggerate the susceptibility artifact, producing a characteristic blooming effect that is considered highly suggestive of PVNS and serves as a valuable diagnostic hallmark [65].

4.6 MRI features of cyst-like and tumor-like lesions

4.6.1 Ganglion and synovial cyst

Ganglion and synovial cysts are rare fluid-filled lesions of the TMJ that present similarly, most often with preauricular swelling and pain, but they differ

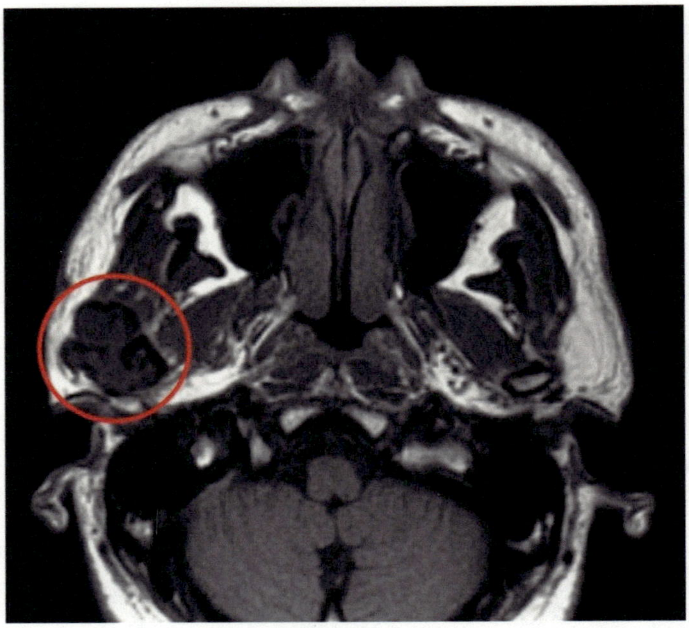

Figure 24.
Pigmented villonodular synovitis (PVNS) - The axial T1-weighted image of magnetic resonance imaging shows the intermediate signal intensity with peripheral low signal intensity rim (hemosiderin depsoits) Source: Ref. [65] https://pmc.ncbi.nlm.nih.gov/articles/PMC4095812/. License: http://creativecommons.org/licenses/by-nc/3.0/.

histopathologically. Ganglion cysts arise from capsular degeneration and contain a connective tissue lining without communication to the joint cavity, whereas synovial cysts have a synovial cell lining that may or may not connect with the joint space. Synovial cysts are more commonly associated with elevated intra-articular pressure from trauma or inflammatory disease [66, 67].

4.6.1.1 Imaging features

Imaging assists in characterization but is not definitive. Panoramic radiographs are usually unremarkable, and ultrasound may help evaluate the parotid gland in cases of preauricular swelling. On multidetector computed tomography (MDCT), these cysts appear as well-circumscribed, hypodense, spherical lesions along the lateral joint surface and typically measure between 1.5 and 2.5 cm. Less frequently, they may occur anteriorly or posteriorly and may cause mild cortical effacement. MRI demonstrates well-defined, thin-walled lesions with T1 hypointensity and T2 hyperintensity (**Figures 25** and **26**). Synovial cysts may show a thin stalk-like connection to the joint on T2-weighted imaging (**Figure 26**). Histopathologic evaluation remains essential for definitive diagnosis, and D2-40 immunostaining is useful in distinguishing synovial from ganglion cysts [66, 67].

4.6.2 Subchondral pseudocyst

Subchondral pseudocysts, also called geodes, are degenerative lesions most commonly associated with osteoarthritis. In the TMJ, they are usually

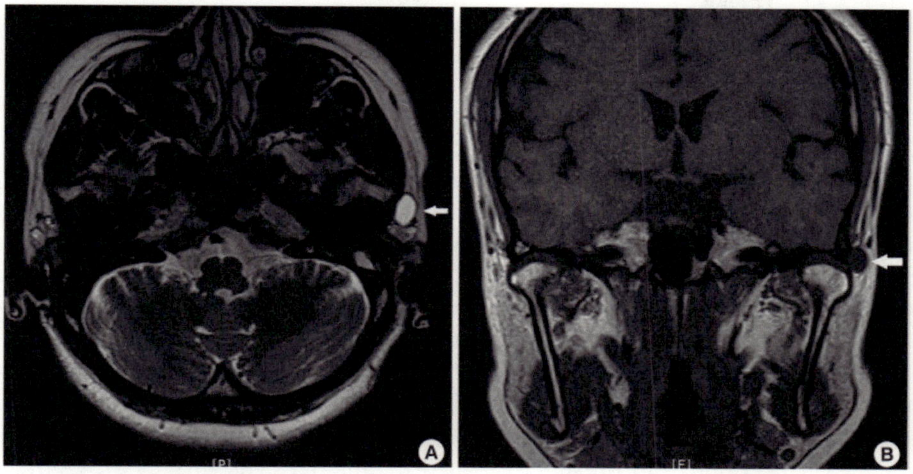

Figure 25.
(A) Axial T2-weighted magnetic resonance image. (B) Coronal T1-weighted magnetic resonance image shows a ganglion cyst (white arrows) lateral to the left condyle. Source: Ref. [66] https://pmc.ncbi.nlm.nih.gov/articles/PMC4228227/. License: http://creativecommons.org/licenses/by-nc/3.0/.

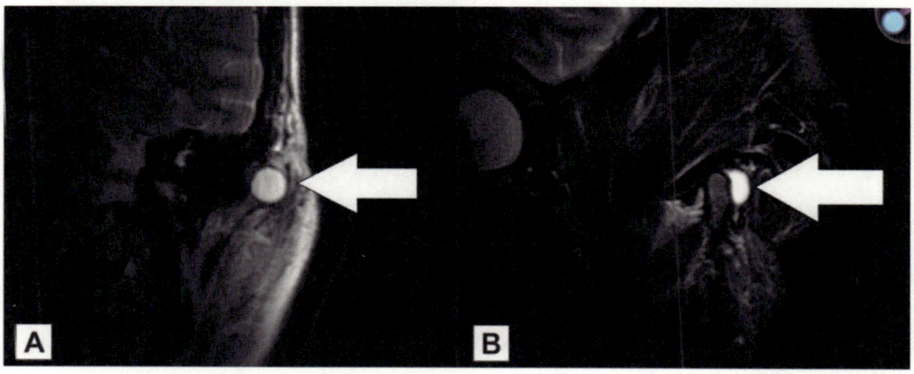

Figure 26.
(A) Coronal section T2-weighted MRI (B) Sagittal section T2-weighted MRI depicting synovial cyst marked by white arrow. The cyst lumen is fluid-filled, making the cyst lumen bright on T2- weighted MRI. Source: Ref. [67] https://pmc.ncbi.nlm.nih.gov/articles/PMC6498815/. License: http://creativecommons.org/licenses/by-nc/3.0/.

asymptomatic and do not cause visible swelling or pain, but their presence reflects late-stage degenerative joint disease. Clinically, they may contribute indirectly to joint dysfunction when accompanied by other degenerative changes such as erosion, osteophyte formation, or generalized sclerosis. Their development has been explained by two main mechanisms. (1) Synovial fluid intrusion theory: It involves intrusion of synovial fluid into the subchondral bone through defects in the articular cartilage, leading to the development of a cystic cavity. However, histological correlation studies in the knee joint have shown that only a minority of cysts occur beneath full-thickness cartilage defects. This suggests that cartilage breach, while contributory, is not always essential for cyst formation. (2) Bone contusion theory: The second mechanism attributes cyst formation to repetitive mechanical loading that produces microfractures, localized bone necrosis, and subsequent cystic degeneration [68].

4.6.2.1 Imaging features

On CT and CBCT, pseudocysts appear as well-defined subcortical radiolucent cavities bordered by a thin sclerotic rim. They usually measure 2 to 3 mm, though some may exceed 1 cm. The cortical outline is generally preserved, but small cortical discontinuities or narrow tracts connecting the pseudocyst to the articular surface may be seen and are sometimes described as a tail-like extension. Their presence is considered a hallmark of TMJ osteoarthritis, particularly when accompanied by osteophyte formation or cortical erosions. On MRI, subchondral cysts are usually seen as well-circumscribed areas of hyperintense or intermediate signal on T2-weighted and short-TI inversion recovery (STIR) sequences (**Figure 27**). In contrast, they demonstrate low to intermediate signal intensity on proton density and T1-weighted images. Bone marrow edema–like changes, when present, are most effectively detected on fat-suppressed T2-weighted or STIR sequences. The concurrent presence of these edema patterns with cystic changes further supports the role of mechanical stress in the development of subchondral cysts [68, 69].

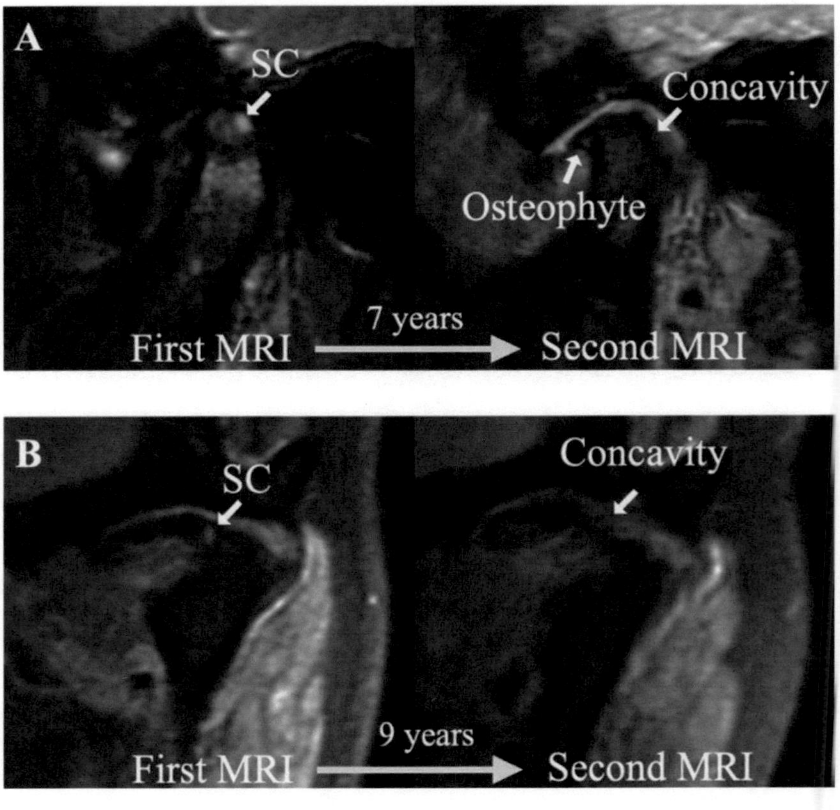

Figure 27.
Two examples of temporal changes of the joints with subchondral cysts (SCs). A: On the sagittal plane, the second MRI showed concavity on the surface of the condyle, where the SC was present on the first MRI as a hyper intensity on T2 - weighted image. Osteophytes were observed in the anterior part of the condyle in the second MRI scan. B: On the coronal plane, the second MRI showed concavity on the surface of the condyle, where the SC was present on the first MRI as a intermediate intensity on T2 - weighted image. Source: Ref. [69] https://pubmed.ncbi.nlm.nih.gov/36288977/. License: http://creativecommons.org/licenses/by/4.0/.

4.6.3 Simple bone cyst

Simple bone cysts (SBCs), also known as traumatic bone cysts, are traditionally described as empty intraosseous cavities, and more than half of reported cases in systematic reviews contain no detectable material. However, this interpretation has been questioned. In one clinical series of nineteen patients, fluid was present in every case on both imaging and intraoperative evaluation. The composition of this fluid remains uncertain. Some reports have described blood or serous fluid, although no study has demonstrated complete equivalence between cyst fluid and blood. Intraoperative introduction of blood during surgical access has been suggested as a possible explanation for hemorrhagic aspirates. Typically, fluid aspirated from SBCs appears clear initially, with blood more often encountered toward the end of aspiration, likely originating from the cyst wall. Cytological examinations have shown variable concentrations of blood-derived elements, with eosinophils and basophils consistently detected. Previous studies of SBCs have also reported eosinophils, leading to speculation that eosinophilic recruitment may be mediated by mast cell–derived factors and may contribute to bone resorption. Despite occasional inflammatory cells, SBCs are generally considered non-inflammatory lesions.

The etiology of SBCs remains uncertain. Proposed mechanisms include trauma-induced intramedullary hemorrhage, vascular obstruction, and impaired bone repair. Biochemical analyses of cyst fluid demonstrate electrolyte and protein similarities to serum, although total protein concentrations are consistently lower, supporting the interpretation of the fluid as a transudate. Passive fluid accumulation through plasma diffusion across the cyst wall has been proposed, and studies of other jaw cysts suggest that electrolyte gradients may contribute to this process [70].

4.6.3.1 Imaging features

Imaging features of SBCs differ from those of subcortical pseudocysts. SBCs are typically larger, lack a sclerotic margin, and show smooth, uninterrupted borders without cortical micro-communication. On panoramic radiographs and CT, they appear as radiolucent defects. On MRI they usually demonstrate intermediate signal intensity on T1-weighted sequences and high signal intensity on T2-weighted images (**Figure 28**) [70].

4.6.4 Aneurysmal bone cyst

Aneurysmal bone cysts (ABCs) are benign, expansile lesions that are neither true cysts nor aneurysms and do not behave as neoplasms despite their potential for rapid growth. They occur predominantly in long bones, and jaw involvement is rare, accounting for approximately 2% of cases. When present in the jaws, the mandible is affected more often than the maxilla, and TMJ involvement is particularly uncommon. ABCs of the jaw typically present as painless swelling, facial asymmetry, or, when affecting the TMJ, dental malocclusion or mandibular deviation. They occur most frequently in children and young adults with no consistent sex predilection, although reported cases range from early childhood through the fourth decade of life.

The etiology of ABCs is not fully understood. Proposed mechanisms include trauma-related changes, reactive vascular phenomena, and secondary development within preexisting lesions such as fibrous dysplasia, ossifying fibroma, or

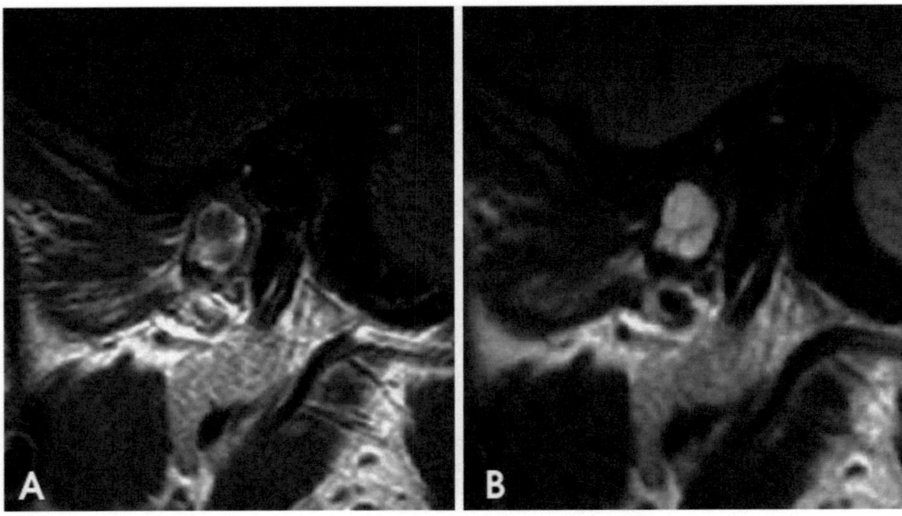

Figure 28.
Simple Bone Cyst - MRI shows homogeneous intermediate SI on the T1-weighted sagittal image (A) and homogeneous high SI on the T2-weighted sagittal image (B). Source: Ref. [70] https://pmc.ncbi.nlm.nih.gov/articles/PMC3604371/. License: http://creativecommons.org/licenses/by-nc/3.0/.

osteosarcoma. Histologically, ABCs exhibit sinusoidal blood-filled spaces without endothelial lining, intermixed solid areas with osteoid formation, and multinucleated giant cells. The absence of an epithelial lining distinguishes them from true cystic lesions [71, 72].

4.6.4.1 Imaging features

Imaging features are variable. Radiographically, ABCs range from unilocular to multilocular in appearance. Cross-sectional imaging typically shows a well-defined expansile lesion with cortical thinning and outward ballooning. MRI demonstrates heterogeneous T1 signal and fluid–fluid levels on T2-weighted imaging (**Figure 29**). Because imaging findings may overlap with those of hemangioma, angiography can help identify feeding vessels. Recurrence is possible and most often occurs within the first postoperative year, warranting follow-up imaging [71, 72].

4.6.5 Synovial chondromatosis

Synovial chondromatosis (SC) is a benign proliferative disorder characterized by synovial metaplasia with formation of multiple cartilaginous nodules that may undergo calcification or ossification. Although the etiology is uncertain, SC is believed to arise from metaplastic transformation of synovial stromal cells. The condition primarily affects large joints, and TMJ involvement is rare. Bilateral involvement is uncommon. SC most often affects the superior joint compartment, with inferior compartment involvement occurring mainly after disc perforation. Rarely, SC may cause condylar erosion, temporal bone involvement, or intracranial extension. Patients typically present with preauricular discomfort, swelling, crepitus, or limited mandibular motion, and symptoms frequently resemble myofascial pain dysfunction. SC most commonly occurs after the third decade of life and shows a modest female predominance [31].

DOI: http://dx.doi.org/10.5772/intechopen.1013684

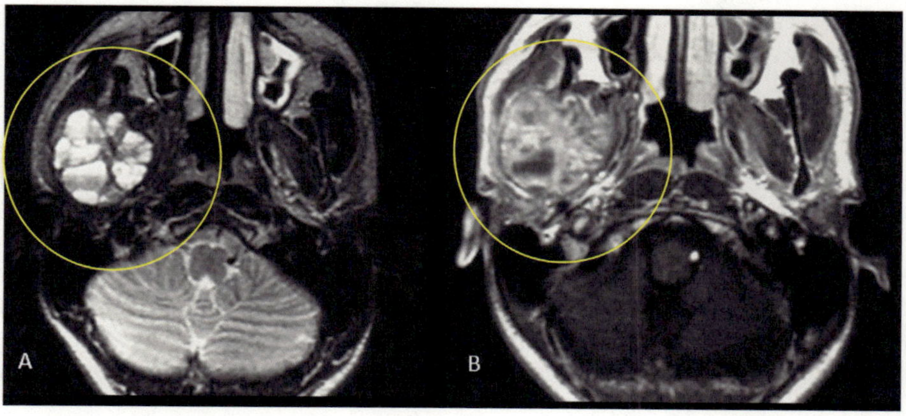

Figure 29.
Aneurysmal bone cyst - (A) T2- weighted MRI axial section depicting fluid-fluid level (B) T1- weighted MRI axial section depicting heterogeneous signal. Source: Ref. [71] https://dtjournal.org/articles/252. License: http://creativecommons.org/licenses/by/4.0/.

4.6.5.1 Imaging features

Imaging features include calcified loose bodies, joint space widening, condylar and glenoid fossa irregularity, subchondral sclerosis, and soft tissue swelling. CT typically shows multiple calcified nodules surrounding the condyle. MRI provides superior assessment of both calcified and non-calcified nodules and allows visualization of the disc without ionizing radiation. Calcified nodules appear hypointense on T1- and T2-weighted images, whereas associated joint effusion is hyperintense on T2-weighted sequences, and proliferative synovium enhances after contrast administration (**Figure 30**). MRI is therefore preferred for characterization and treatment planning [31]. Detached osseous fragments from degenerative osteophytes may mimic SC and represent secondary synovial chondromatosis. These fragments occur in late-stage osteoarthritis and are accompanied by other degenerative changes such as sclerosis, articular flattening, and joint space narrowing. Secondary SC differs in

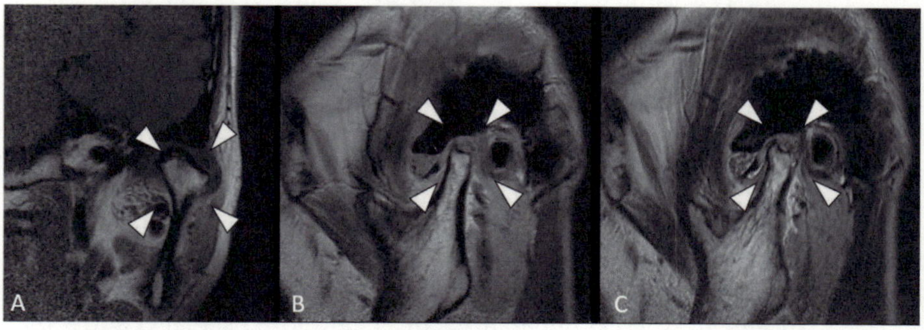

Figure 30.
Synovial chondromatosis- MR images (a (coronal), b (sagittal)) T1-weighted image; (c) T2-weighted sagittal image. T1-weighted images show deformity of the left mandibular condyle and anterior disc displacement without reduction, and T2-weighted images show areas of small, nodular hypo intensity around the left mandibular condyle. Source: Ref. [73] https://onlinelibrary.wiley.com/doi/10.1155/2021/5927215. License: https://creativecommons.org/licenses/by/4.0/.

pathogenesis from primary SC and reflects advanced degenerative joint disease rather than primary synovial metaplasia [73].

4.7 Malignancy

4.7.1 Osteosarcoma

Multiple sarcoma subtypes may involve the TMJ, but all are exceedingly rare, with osteosarcoma being the most frequent primary malignant tumor in this region. Compared with long-bone osteosarcoma, maxillofacial involvement tends to occur later in life and generally demonstrates slower progression and more favorable prognosis. The chondroblastic subtype is reported as the most common in the maxillofacial region [74].

4.7.1.1 Imaging features

On imaging, TMJ osteosarcoma typically appears as a mixed lytic–sclerotic lesion with an expansile soft-tissue component that may distort or erode adjacent joint structures. Mineralization varies from fine punctate calcifications to dense sclerotic foci. Periosteal reaction is characteristic and may appear as radiating spicules producing a sunburst or hair-on-end pattern. More compact or lamellated periosteal new bone formation can also be present. These features are best depicted with CT, which provides detailed characterization of osseous architecture. MRI is more sensitive for evaluating marrow infiltration and spread into adjacent soft tissues. Typical findings include heterogeneous signal intensity: areas of low signal on both T1- and T2-weighted images corresponding to mineralized tumor matrix, and intermediate T1 and high T2 signal within the soft tissue component. Following gadolinium administration, the non-calcified portions of the tumor demonstrate variable enhancement (**Figure 31**) [75].

4.7.2 Chondrosarcoma

Chondrosarcoma is the second most common primary malignant bone tumor, though TMJ involvement is extremely uncommon. It is a malignant neoplasm of cartilage-producing cells, typically low-grade and more frequently reported in females. Tumors may arise de novo or, rarely, evolve from preexisting conditions such as synovial chondromatosis or osteochondroma [76].

4.7.2.1 Imaging features

On imaging, chondrosarcoma demonstrates heterogeneous appearance due to the combination of bone destruction, chondroid matrix, and variable mineralization. Reported TMJ cases consistently show expansile masses arising from the condyle with cortical and marrow destruction. On MRI, non-calcified cartilage appears markedly hyperintense on T2-weighted images and corresponds to regions with minimal enhancement, whereas mineralized areas show lower signal (**Figure 32**). Calcifications may display punctate or confluent patterns, with ring-and-arc morphology considered characteristic for cartilaginous matrix mineralization. Periosteal reaction, when present, may be solid, spiculated, or linear. Low-grade lesions can mimic benign cartilage tumors, but focal solid enhancement or enhancing septa should raise suspicion for malignancy [77, 78].

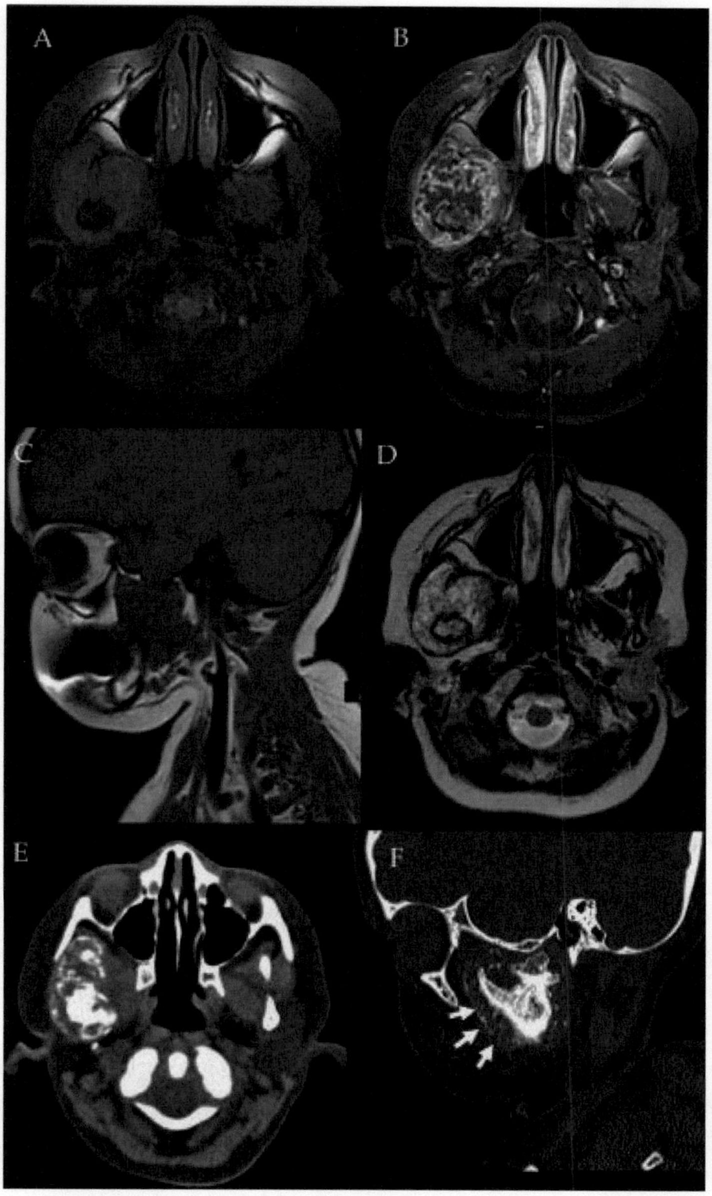

Figure 31.
Condylar chondroblastic osteosarcoma. Axial pre-contrast (A) and post-contrast T1W (B), sagittal pre-contrast T1W (C), and axial T2W (D) images demonstrate a heterogeneously enhancing and T2-hyperintense right condylar mass in a nine-year-old patient. Axial (E) and sagittal (F) CT images show a soft tissue mass with mineralized matrix and aggressive periosteal reaction (small arrows) at the TMJ. Source: Ref. [3] https://pmc.ncbi.nlm.nih.gov/articles/PMC9031630/. License: http://creativecommons.org/licenses/by/4.0/.

4.7.3 Metastasis

Metastatic involvement of the jaws is uncommon and typically favors the posterior mandible, particularly the molar region. Extension to the TMJ is very rare. Adenocarcinoma is the most common histologic type, with primary tumors most often arising from the breast, lung, kidney, or prostate (**Figure 33**) [79, 80].

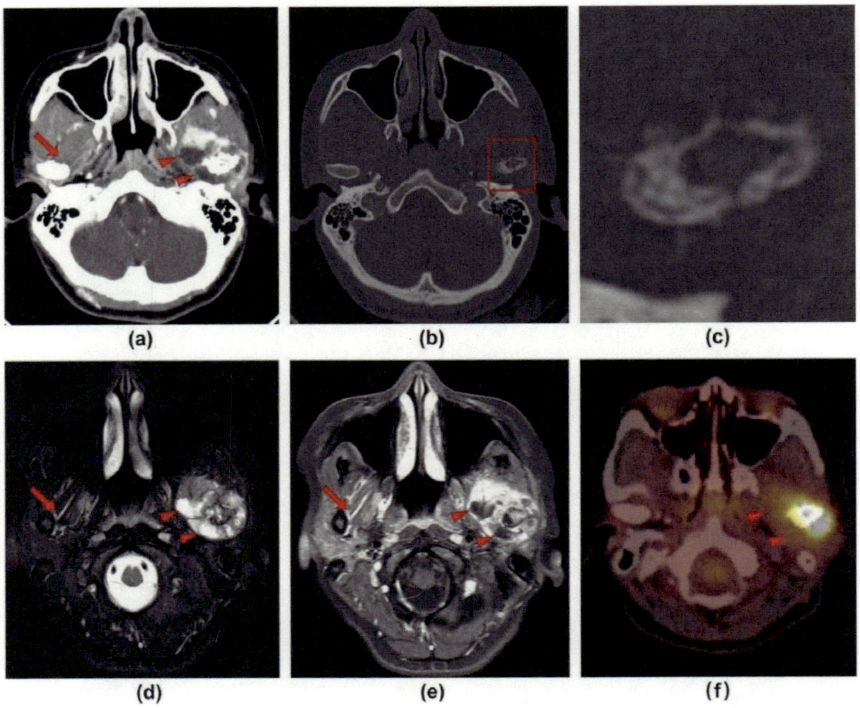

Figure 32.
A 16-year-old female patient with grade III chondrosarcoma. (a, b, c [magnified image of the red box in b]) CT images show a large mass surrounding the left mandibular condyle. Note the severely destroyed mandibular condyle with prominent periosteal reaction, indicating that the direction of lesion growth is outward from the mandibular condyle. At the anterior aspect of the left mandibular condyle, complete infiltration into the tendon of the lateral pterygoid muscle in the pterygoid fovea by the mass is observed, whereas intact tendon of the lateral pterygoid muscle (red arrow) on the right side. (d, e) Axial fat-suppressed T2-weighted and contrast-enhanced T1-weighted MRI images show markedly hyperintense T2 signal portion without enhancement (red arrowheads). (f) PET/CT image shows markedly increased FDG uptake; however, FDG uptake less than that of mediastinal blood pool is observed in the medial and posterior aspect to the mandibular condyle (red arrowheads), which corresponds to the portion of markedly hyperintense T2 signal portion without enhancement in (d) and (e). Source: Ref. [77] https://pubmed.ncbi.nlm.nih.gov/32843140/. License: http://creativecommons.org/licenses/by/4.0/.

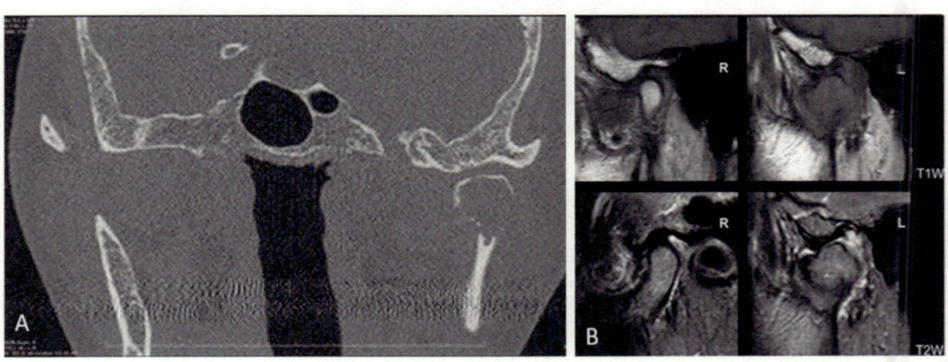

Figure 33.
Metastatic Breast Cancer - (A) Computed tomography Image (coronal plane). A low-density destructive lesion of the left condyle. The cortical bones thin and perforated. (B) The upper images are T1-weighted MRI and the lower images are T2-weighted MRI. The shape of the right condyle is normal. An isointense soft-tissue mass is observed in the left condylar region. Despite the presence of this mass on left side, the articular disc maintains its normal shape. Source: Ref. [79] https://pmc.ncbi.nlm.nih.gov/articles/PMC5688695/. License: http://creativecommons.org/licenses/by/4.0/.

4.7.3.1 Imaging features

Panoramic radiographs may show larger or multifocal lesions, but smaller or purely articular metastases are often missed on two-dimensional imaging. Most TMJ metastases are osteolytic and cause destruction of cortical and cancellous bone, although osteoblastic metastases can produce sclerosis or periosteal reaction. CT and MRI typically reveal bone destruction with associated soft-tissue masses and extension into adjacent structures such as masticatory muscles, parotid gland, ear canal, or skull base. Although these findings are nonspecific, correlation with known malignancy is crucial. PET/CT is particularly valuable for detecting occult primary tumors and evaluating systemic metastatic burden [81].

4.8 Trauma

MRI is a central modality for evaluating TMJ trauma and must be interpreted alongside a detailed clinical history and thorough examination. Several characteristic findings help establish the diagnosis:

Joint effusion is best visualized on T2-weighted sequences, where fluid demonstrates high signal intensity relative to surrounding fat. Effusion reflects a combination of acute hemarthrosis followed by sustained synovial inflammation marked by hypertrophy, hyperemia, and increased vascular permeability. Persistence of effusion for up to 2 weeks after injury highlights the role of ongoing inflammatory activity rather than isolated acute bleeding. Effusion is encountered more frequently in high condylar fractures and in fractures associated with dislocation, whereas subcondylar fractures without dislocation show a lower incidence. Notably, effusion is seldom observed in contralateral, unfractured joints, suggesting that transmitted mechanical forces are insufficient to induce detectable intra-articular fluid accumulation. The presence and extent of effusion therefore provide meaningful insight into the severity of condylar injury [82, 83].

Traumatic disc displacement is most commonly anteromedial and often reflects the pull of the lateral pterygoid muscle. Differentiation between acute and chronic displacement relies on associated findings. Bone marrow edema, ligamentous edema, and absence of degenerative features support a recent traumatic event. When preexisting degenerative alterations are present, pronounced retrodiscal signal changes may indicate an additional acute component. Long-standing displacement may demonstrate disc degeneration and loss of normal disc height.

Disc rupture, when observed without evidence of chronic degeneration, strongly supports an acute traumatic mechanism. Injury to the bilaminar zone appears as marked hyperintensity on fat-suppressed sequences due to the vascular nature of this region. Loss of definition of the superior retrodiscal lamina, which anchors the disc to the temporal bone, is an important indicator of injury. Loss of continuity within this structure can be biomechanically equivalent to disc rupture. Capsular tears frequently accompany retrodiscal injury because the disc, bilaminar zone, capsule, and associated ligaments function as an interconnected complex. These injuries may present with altered appearance of capsule–ligament attachments at the condyle. On coronal views, collateral ligaments may appear indistinct, while sagittal images may reveal altered attachment patterns anterior to the articular tubercle.

Bone marrow edema of the condyle is not consistently observed in TMJ trauma and occurs less frequently in isolated capsule–ligament injuries. However, its presence warrants careful evaluation, as associated fibrocartilage deterioration and periosteal reaction, in the context of hemarthrosis, may predispose to heterotopic ossification and subsequent ankylosis. On MRI, bone edema manifests as a hyperintense signal on fat-suppressed sequences [82, 83].

5. Recent advancements of MRI techniques

5.1 Dynamic or real-time MRI

Dynamic or real-time MRI provides rapid, continuous acquisition with immediate reconstruction, allowing direct visualization of disc–condyle motion during voluntary mandibular opening and closing [84]. This approach overcomes the limitations of pseudo-dynamic imaging by capturing physiologic muscle activity. Gradient-echo (GRE) sequences are commonly used because short repetition times (TR) and low flip angles support high temporal resolution. Coherent steady-state free precession (SSFP) sequences (e.g., fast imaging with steady-state precession [FISP], true FISP) generate strong contrast between the disc and surrounding joint fluid, whereas spoiled GRE techniques (e.g., fast low-angle shot [FLASH]) provide reliable anatomic detail and functional assessment [85]. SSFP-based methods can demonstrate disc displacement, reduction events, and morphologic changes before and after reduction. Radial k-space sampling and tiny–golden-angle reconstruction improves temporal resolution and minimize motion artifacts, although geometric distortion may occur when these methods are combined with balanced SSFP [86, 87]. Multislice FLASH with advanced reconstruction (e.g., nonlinear inverse algorithms) has enabled bilateral imaging with frame rates as fast as 25.5 ms, preserving disc contrast while allowing functional evaluation of both joints [88, 89]. Challenges include incomplete depiction of rapid movements, susceptibility to motion-related artifacts, and a dependence on computationally intensive reconstruction that frequently requires multi-GPU systems. These factors currently restrict broader clinical implementation [84].

5.2 Ultrashort echo time and zero echo time MRI

The TMJ disc, fibrocartilage, and subchondral bone exhibit short or ultrashort T2 values, making them poorly visualized on conventional MRI sequences [90, 91]. UTE techniques address this limitation by using extremely short RF pulses followed immediately by data acquisition along radial k-space trajectories, preserving signal before rapid transverse decay. ZTE sequences apply gradients prior to RF excitation, effectively minimizing the echo time (TE) to near zero and improving both SNR and acquisition efficiency relative to UTE [15, 92, 93].

UTE and ZTE improve visualization of fibrocartilage, cortical bone, subchondral structures, and the disc–condyle interface. Quantitative parameter mapping (T2, T2*, T1ρ) derived from these techniques correlates with biochemical alterations associated with early TMD, and elevated UTE-based T2* values have been reported in symptomatic patients. ZTE demonstrates strong agreement with CT and micro-CT for assessing condylar morphology, including flattening, osteophytes, and subcortical sclerosis [93]. When integrated with routine MRI, these ultrashort-TE approaches may allow comprehensive hard- and soft-tissue characterization while avoiding ionizing radiation [94–96]. Despite promising early results, broader clinical adoption remains limited due to requirements for specialized hardware, longer acquisition times, and insufficient data defining normal versus pathologic appearances in TMJ imaging [97].

5.3 Diffusion-weighted imaging

Diffusion weighted imaging (DWI) measures the random motion of water molecules and allows calculation of the apparent diffusion coefficient (ADC) to characterize tissue microstructure [95]. Intravoxel incoherent motion (IVIM), which uses a biexponential model to separate true molecular diffusion from perfusion related pseudo-diffusion, extends this capability [96]. In organized tissues such as the temporomandibular joint (TMJ) disc and the masticatory muscles, collagen alignment produces anisotropic diffusion. This makes diffusion tensor imaging (DTI) valuable for assessing directional diffusivity and fiber orientation [97]. Elevated ADC values have been demonstrated in painful masticatory muscles, supporting an association with edema [98]. IVIM parameters have distinguished perfusion related changes in disc displacement and effusion from diffusion related alterations seen in TMJ osteoarthritis [99]. DTI provides fiber orientation maps and quantitative measures such as eigenvalues and fractional anisotropy, with abnormalities correlating with disease state [100]. Functional DTI studies have shown changes in lateral pterygoid muscle (LPM) eigenvalues during clenching and opening [101]. Treatment related diffusion changes, including postoperative increases in fractional anisotropy and alterations following splint therapy, highlight potential use in therapy monitoring [102]. Routine clinical use remains limited by susceptibility related artifacts, geometric distortion, long acquisition times, and lack of standardized b value protocols. Overlapping pathological processes can further complicate interpretation [95].

5.4 T2 mapping

Conventional T2-weighted imaging (T2WI) may reveal signal intensity changes in the TMJ disc, condyle, or masticatory muscles in patients with TMDs. These alterations are thought to reflect disruption of the collagen framework, altered hydration, or other biochemical changes. However, visual assessment of such findings is subjective and may not reliably capture subtle or early abnormalities. T2 mapping was introduced as a quantitative method to overcome these limitations. The technique relies on multi-echo spin-echo sequences, in which images are acquired at multiple echo times within a single repetition time (TR). The signal intensities are fitted to an exponential decay model, allowing T2 relaxation times to be calculated on a pixel-by-pixel basis. The resulting parametric maps display spatial variation in relaxation constants, providing objective information about tissue microstructure. Initially developed for large joints such as the knee, T2 mapping has been adapted for TMJ research and shows promise in evaluating early and subtle disease-related changes [103–106].

6. Conclusion

MRI remains the primary modality for evaluating TMJ disorders, offering high-resolution, multiplanar assessment of osseous and soft-tissue structures without radiation. Conventional protocols continue to underpin diagnosis of internal derangements, inflammatory arthropathies, neoplastic processes, trauma, and differentiation between degenerative and inflammatory disease. Recent advances have broadened diagnostic capability: dynamic cine MRI visualizes disc–condyle kinematics in real time; UTE and ZTE improve delineation of fibrocartilage and cortical bone; and quantitative methods such as T2 mapping, DWI, and DTI enable assessment of microstructural and biochemical alterations. These techniques support earlier detection of pathology, more objective characterization of disease, and reproducible monitoring of treatment response. Persistent challenges include motion artifacts, technical constraints, and lack of standardized acquisition and interpretation protocols across institutions. Continued progress in hardware, sequence design, quantitative analysis, and multicenter protocol harmonization will strengthen MRI's role as a comprehensive platform for structural, functional, and biochemical evaluation of TMJ disorders.

Acknowledgements

We extend our gratitude to Qingyu Meng (NYU Dentistry Class of 2027) for his illustration. For inquiries, he can be reached at qm316@nyu.edu.

Author contributions

Conceptualization: S.K.; Writing—Original Draft Preparation: S.K., P.P., D.T.; Writing—Review & Editing: S.K., P.P., D.T.; Introduction, Anatomy and Protocol Sections: P.P., S.K.; Imaging Features of TMJ Variants and Pathology, Arthropathies, Cyst-like and Tumor-like Lesions, Malignancy, and Trauma: S.K., P.P., D.T.; Recent MRI Advancements: S.K. All authors have read and agreed to the published version of the manuscript.

Conflict of interest

The authors declare no conflict of interest.

Data availability statement

Source data not available for this article.

Author details

Sonam Khurana[1*], Pranav Parasher[2] and Denise Trochesset[1]

1 Department of Oral and Maxillofacial Pathology, Radiology and Medicine, NYU College of Dentistry, New York, USA

2 Resident, Oral and Maxillofacial Radiology, University of Connecticut School of Dental Medicine, Farmington, Connecticut, USA

*Address all correspondence to: sk10542@nyu.edu

References

[1] Salamon NM, Casselman JW. Temporomandibular joint disorders: A pictorial review. Seminars in Musculoskeletal Radiology. 2020;**24**(5):591-607

[2] Petscavage-Thomas JM, Walker EA. Unlocking the jaw: Advanced imaging of the temporomandibular joint. AJR. American Journal of Roentgenology. 2014;**203**(5):1047-1058

[3] Gharavi SM, Qiao Y, Faghihimehr A, Vossen J. Imaging of the temporomandibular joint. Diagnostics (Basel). 2022;**12**(4):1006

[4] Whyte A, Boeddinghaus R, Bartley A, Vijeyaendra R. Imaging of the temporomandibular joint. Clinical Radiology. 2021;**76**(1):e21-e35

[5] Hasan NMA, Abdelrahman TEF. MRI evaluation of TMJ internal derangement: Degree of anterior disc displacement correlated with other TMJ soft tissue and osseous abnormalities. Egyptian Journal of Radiology and Nuclear Medicine. 2014;**45**(3):735-744

[6] Tomas X, Pomes J, Berenguer J, Mercader JM, Pons F, Donoso L. Temporomandibular joint soft-tissue pathology, II: Nondisc abnormalities. Seminars in Ultrasound, CT, and MR. 2007;**28**(3):205-212

[7] de Oliveira LRLB, Alves IDS, Vieira APF, Passos UL, Leite CDC, Gebrim ES. Temporomandibular joint: From anatomy to internal derangement. Radiologia Brasileira. 2023;**56**(2):102-109. DOI: 10.1590/0100-3984.2022.0072-en

[8] Yilmaz D, Kamburoglu K. Comparison of the effectiveness of high-resolution ultrasound with MRI in patients with temporomandibular joint disorders. Dento Maxillo Facial Radiology. 2019;**48**:20180349

[9] Tomas X, Pomes J, Berenguer J, Quinto L, Nicolau C, Mercader JM, et al. MR imaging of temporomandibular joint dysfunction: A pictorial review. Radiographics. 2006;**26**(3):765-781. DOI: 10.1148/rg.263055091

[10] Yoshida M, Honda E, Ozawa E, Inoue-Arai SM, Ohmori H, Moriyama K, et al. Principles of the magnetic resonance imaging movie method for articulatory movement. Oral Radiology. 2019;**35**(2):91-100. DOI: 10.1007/s11282-018-0347-7

[11] Karlo CA, Patcas R, Kau T, Watzal H, Signorelli L, Müller L, et al. MRI of the temporo-mandibular joint: Which sequence is best suited to assess the cortical bone of the mandibular condyle? A cadaveric study using micro-CT as the standard of reference. European Radiology. 2012;**22**(7):1579-1585. DOI: 10.1007/s00330-012-2391-8

[12] Nikkuni Y, Nishiyama H, Hayashi T. Clinical significance of T2 mapping MRI for the evaluation of masseter muscle pain in patients with temporomandibular joint disorders. Oral Radiology. 2013;**29**:50-55

[13] Bae WC, Biswas R, Statum S, Sah RL, Chung CB. Sensitivity of quantitative UTE MRI to the biomechanical property of the temporomandibular joint disc. Skeletal Radiology. 2014;**43**:1217-1223

[14] Shiraishi T, Chikui T, Inadomi D, Kagawa T, Yoshiura K, Yuasa K. Evaluation of diffusion parameters and T2 values of the masseter muscle during jaw opening,

clenching, and rest. Acta Radiologica. 2012;**53**:81-86

[15] Vaddi A, Parasher P, Khurana S. Beyond X-rays: Unveiling the future of dental diagnosis with dental magnetic resonance imaging. Diagnostics (Basel). 2025;**15**(9):1153. DOI: 10.3390/diagnostics15091153

[16] Mezitis M, Rallis G, Zachariades N. The normal range of mouth opening. Journal of Oral and Maxillofacial Surgery. 1989;**47**(10):1028-1029

[17] Nitzan DW, Marmary Y. The "anchored disc phenomenon": A proposed etiology for sudden-onset, severe, and persistent closed lock of the temporomandibular joint. Journal of Oral and Maxillofacial Surgery. 1997;**55**(8):797-802; discussion 802-3

[18] Abou-Atme YS, Chedid N, Melis M, Zawawi KH. Clinical measurement of normal maximum mouth opening in children. Cranio. 2008;**26**(3):191-196

[19] Young AL. Internal derangements of the temporomandibular joint: A review of the anatomy, diagnosis, and management. Journal of Indian Prosthodontic Society. 2015;**15**(1):2-7

[20] Ahmad M, Schiffman EL. Temporomandibular joint disorders and orofacial pain. Dental Clinics of North America. 2016;**60**(1):105-124. DOI: 10.1016/j.cden.2015.08.004

[21] González-García R, Gil-Díez Usandizaga JL, Rodríguez-Campo FJ. Arthroscopic anatomy and lysis and lavage of the temporomandibular joint. Atlas of the Oral and Maxillofacial Surgery Clinics of North America. 2011;**19**(2):131-144

[22] Ramdhan RC, Iwanaga J. Anatomy and variations of the temporomandibular joint. In: Iwanaga J, Tubbs RS, editors. Anatomical Variations in Clinical Dentistry. Cham: Springer; 2019. pp. 87-202. DOI: 10.1007/978-3-319-97961-8_18 [Accessed: December 19, 2023]

[23] Warburton G. Internal derangements of the temporomandibular joint. In: Bonanthaya K, Panneerselvam E, Manuel S, Kumar VV, Rai A, editors. Oral and Maxillofacial Surgery for the Clinician. Singapore: Springer; 2021. pp. 1361-1380. DOI: 10.1007/978-981-15-1346-6_63

[24] Harms SE, Wilk RM. Magnetic resonance imaging of the temporomandibular joint. Radiographics. 1987;**7**(3):521-542. DOI: 10.1148/radiographics.7.3.3448646

[25] Aiken A, Bouloux G, Hudgins P. MR imaging of the temporomandibular joint. Magnetic Resonance Imaging Clinics of North America. 2012;**20**(3):397-412. DOI: 10.1016/j.mric.2012.05.002

[26] Mehndiratta A, Kumar J, Manchanda A, Singh I, Mohanty S, Seth N, et al. Painful clicking jaw: A pictorial review of internal derangement of the temporomandibular joint. Polish Journal of Radiology. 2019;**84**:e598-e615. DOI: 10.5114/pjr.2019.92287

[27] Drace JE, Young SW, Enzmann DR. TMJ meniscus and bilaminar zone: MR imaging of the substructure—Diagnostic landmarks and pitfalls of interpretation. Radiology. 1990;**177**(1):73-76. DOI: 10.1148/radiology.177.1.2399341

[28] Scapino RP, Obrez A, Greising D. Organization and function of the collagen fiber system in the human temporomandibular joint disk and its attachments. Cells, Tissues, Organs. 2006;**182**(3-4):201-225

[29] Katzberg RW, Hatcher D, Ethier J. Overview of Disc Displacements. In:

Tamimi D, Hatcher D, editors. Specialty Imaging: Temporomandibular Joint. 1st ed. Philadelphia: Elsevier; 2016. pp. 490-496

[30] Alomar X, Medrano J, Cabratosa J, et al. Anatomy of the temporomandibular joint. Seminars in Ultrasound, CT, and MR. 2007;**28**(3):170-183

[31] Bag AK, Gaddikeri S, Singhal A, Hardin S, Tran BD, Medina JA, et al. Imaging of the temporomandibular joint: An update. World Journal of Radiology. 2014;**6**(8):567-582. DOI: 10.4329/wjr.v6.i8.567

[32] Rao VM, Bacelar MT. MR imaging of the temporomandibular joint. Magnetic Resonance Imaging Clinics of North America. 2002;**10**(4):615-630. DOI: 10.1016/S1064-9689(02)00011-9

[33] Chen CA, Kijowski R, Shapiro LM, Tuite MJ, Davis KW, Klaers JL, et al. Cartilage morphology at 3.0T: Assessment of three-dimensional magnetic resonance imaging techniques. Journal of Magnetic Resonance Imaging. 2010;**32**(1):173-183. DOI: 10.1002/jmri.22213

[34] Chen M, Herregods N, Jaremko JL, Carron P, Elewaut D, Van den Bosch F, et al. Diagnostic performance for erosion detection in sacroiliac joints on MR T1-weighted images: Comparison between different slice thicknesses. European Journal of Radiology. 2020;**133**:109352. DOI: 10.1016/j.ejrad.2020.109352

[35] Burlak K, So TY, Maclaurin WA, Dixon AF. Foramen tympanicum with symptomatic temporomandibular joint herniation. Radiology Case Reports. 2018;**13**(4):822-824. DOI: 10.1016/j.radcr.2018.05.009

[36] Salé H, Bryndahl F, Isberg A. Temporomandibular joints in asymptomatic and symptomatic nonpatient volunteers: A prospective 15-year follow-up clinical and MR imaging study. Radiology. 2013;**267**(1):183-194

[37] Roth C, Ward RJ, Tsai S, Zolotor W, Tello R. MR imaging of the TMJ: A pictorial essay. Applied Radiology. 2005;**34**:9-16

[38] Helms CA, Kaban LB, McNeill C, Dodson T. Temporomandibular joint: Morphology and signal intensity characteristics of the disk at MR imaging. Radiology. 1989;**172**(3):817-820

[39] Larheim TA, Westesson P, Sano T. Temporomandibular joint disk displacement: Comparison in asymptomatic volunteers and patients. Radiology. 2001;**218**(2):428-432. DOI: 10.1148/radiology.218.2. r01fe11428

[40] Kim JY, Lee C, Lee JH, et al. Comparison of the maximum standardized uptake value and magnetic resonance imaging characteristics between temporomandibular joint osteoarthrosis and osteoarthritis. Scientific Reports. 2025;**15**:23542. DOI: 10.1038/s41598-025-06045-2

[41] Arayasantiparb R, Tsuchimochi M, Mitrirattanakul S. Transformation of temporomandibular joint disc configuration in internal derangement patients using magnetic resonance imaging. Oral Science International. 2012;**9**(2):43-48. DOI: 10.1016/S1348-8643(12)00025-0

[42] Orhan K, Nishiyama H, Tadashi S, Murakami S, Furukawa S. Comparison of altered signal intensity, position, and morphology of the TMJ disc in MR images corrected for variations in surface coil sensitivity. Oral Surgery, Oral Medicine, Oral Pathology, Oral Radiology, and Endodontics.

2006;**101**(4):515-522. DOI: 10.1016/j.tripleo.2005.04.004

[43] Schellhas KP, Wilkes CH. Temporomandibular joint inflammation: Comparison of MR fast scanning with T1- and T2-weighted imaging techniques. AJR. American Journal of Roentgenology. 1989;**153**(1):93-98. DOI: 10.2214/ajr.153.1.93

[44] Liu XM, Zhang SY, Yang C, Chen MJ, Cai XY, Haddad MS, et al. Correlation between disc displacements and locations of disc perforation in the temporomandibular joint. Dento Maxillo Facial Radiology. 2010;**39**(3):149-156. DOI: 10.1259/dmfr/72395946

[45] Lang TC, Zimny ML, Vijayagopal P. Experimental temporomandibular joint disc perforation in the rabbit: A gross morphologic, biochemical, and ultrastructural analysis. Journal of Oral and Maxillofacial Surgery. 1993;**51**(10):1115-1128. DOI: 10.1016/s0278-2391(10)80451-3

[46] Helmy E, Bays R, Sharawy M. Osteoarthrosis of the temporomandibular joint following experimental disc perforation in *Macaca fascicularis*. Journal of Oral and Maxillofacial Surgery. 1988;**46**(11):979-990. DOI: 10.1016/0278-2391(88)90335-7

[47] Muñoz-Guerra MF, Rodríguez-Campo FJ, Escorial V, Naval L. Temporomandibular joint disc perforation: Long-term results after operative arthroscopy. Journal of Oral and Maxillofacial Surgery. 2013;**71**(4):667-676. DOI: 10.1016/j.joms.2012.08.026

[48] Yura S, Nobata K, Shima T. Diagnostic accuracy of fat-saturated T2-weighted magnetic resonance imaging in the diagnosis of perforation of the articular disc of the temporomandibular joint. The British Journal of Oral & Maxillofacial Surgery. 2012;**50**(4):365-368. DOI: 10.1016/j.bjoms.2011.05.017

[49] Finden SG, Enochs WS, Rao VM. Pathologic changes of the lateral pterygoid muscle in patients with derangement of the temporomandibular joint disk: Objective measures at MR imaging. AJNR. American Journal of Neuroradiology. 2007;**28**(8):1537-1539. DOI: 10.3174/ajnr.A0590

[50] Larheim TA, Westesson PL, Hicks DG, Eriksson L, Brown DA. Osteonecrosis of the temporomandibular joint: Correlation of magnetic resonance imaging and histology. Journal of Oral and Maxillofacial Surgery. 1999;**57**(7):888-898. DOI: 10.1016/s0278-2391(99)90001-0

[51] Sano T, Westesson PL, Yamamoto M, Okano T. Differences in temporomandibular joint pain and age distribution between marrow edema and osteonecrosis in the mandibular condyle. Cranio. 2004;**22**:283-288. DOI: 10.1179/crn.2004.035

[52] Kellenberger CJ, Junhasavasdikul T, Tolend M, Doria AS. Temporomandibular joint atlas for detection and grading of juvenile idiopathic arthritis involvement by magnetic resonance imaging. Pediatric Radiology. 2018;**48**:411-426

[53] Chiba M, Kumagai M, Fukui N, Echigo S. The relationship of bone marrow edema pattern in the mandibular condyle with joint pain in patients with temporomandibular joint disorders: Longitudinal study with MR imaging. International Journal of Oral and Maxillofacial Surgery. 2006;**35**:55-59. DOI: 10.1016/j.ijom.2005.04.020

[54] Schellhas KP, Wilkes CH, Fritts HM, Omlie MR, Lagrotteria LB. MR of

osteochondritis dissecans and avascular necrosis of the mandibular condyle. AJR. American Journal of Roentgenology. 1989;**152**:551-560. DOI: 10.2214/ajr.152.3.551

[55] Navallas M, Inarejos EJ, Iglesias E, et al. MR imaging of the temporomandibular joint in juvenile idiopathic arthritis: Technique and findings. Radiographics. 2017;**37**:595-612

[56] Ravelli A, Martini A. Juvenile idiopathic arthritis. Lancet. 2007;**369**:767-778

[57] Glass DN, Giannini EH. Juvenile rheumatoid arthritis as a complex genetic trait. Arthritis and Rheumatism. 1999;**42**:2261-2268

[58] Prakken B, Albani S, Martini A. Juvenile idiopathic arthritis. Lancet. 2011;**377**:2138-2149

[59] Gregorio A, Gambini C, Gerloni V, et al. Lymphoid neogenesis in juvenile idiopathic arthritis correlates with ANA positivity and plasma cells infiltration. Rheumatology (Oxford, England). 2007;**46**:308-313

[60] Gattorno M, Gerloni V, Morando A, et al. Synovial membrane expression of matrix metalloproteinases and tissue inhibitor 1 in juvenile idiopathic arthritides. The Journal of Rheumatology. 2002;**29**:1774-1779

[61] Kodama S, Otonari-Yamamoto M, Sano T, Sakamoto J, Imoto K, Wakoh M. Signal intensity on fluid-attenuated inversion recovery images of condylar marrow changes correspond with slight pain in patients with temporomandibular joint disorders. Oral Radiology. 2014;**30**:212-218. DOI: 10.1007/s11282-014-0165-5

[62] Inarejos Clemente EJ, Tolend M, Navallas M, Doria AS, Meyers AB. MRI of the temporomandibular joint in children with juvenile idiopathic arthritis: Protocol and findings. Pediatric Radiology. 2023;**53**:1498-1512. DOI: 10.1007/s00247-023-05616-7. Epub 2023 Mar 22

[63] Leighty SM, Spach DH, Myall RW, Burns JL. Septic arthritis of the temporomandibular joint: Review of the literature and report of two cases in children. International Journal of Oral and Maxillofacial Surgery. 1993;**22**:292-297. DOI: 10.1016/S0901-5027(05)80519-3

[64] Tang T, Han FG. Calcium pyrophosphate deposition disease of the temporomandibular joint invading the middle cranial fossa: Two case reports. World Journal of Clinical Cases. 2021;**9**:2662-2670. DOI: 10.12998/wjcc.v9.i11.2662

[65] Kim IK, Cho HY, Cho HW, Seo JH, Lee DH, Peng W. Pigmented villonodular synovitis of the temporomandibular joint—Computed tomography and magnetic resonance findings: A case report. Journal of the Korean Association of Oral and Maxillofacial Surgeons. 2014;**40**:140-146. DOI: 10.5125/jkaoms.2014.40.3.140. Epub 2014 Jun 27

[66] Lee YT, Kwon SB, Cho SH, Eo S, Rhee SC. A ganglion cyst of the temporomandibular joint. Archives of Plastic Surgery. 2014;**41**:777-780. DOI: 10.5999/aps.2014.41.6.777. Epub 2014 Nov 3

[67] Maribo Y, Stokbro K, Aagaard E Larsen SR, Thygesen T. Synovial cysts in the temporomandibular joint: A case report and critical review of the literature. Journal of Oral & Maxillofacial Research. 2019;**10**:e4. DOI: 10.5037/jomr.2019.10104

[68] Nozawa M, Ogi N, Ariji Y, Kise Y, Nakayama M, Nishiyama M,

et al. Reliability of diagnostic imaging for degenerative diseases with osseous changes in the temporomandibular joint with special emphasis on subchondral cyst. Oral Radiology. 2020;**36**:156-162

[69] Takaoka R, Koishi Y, Kuyama K, Ueda Y, Ishigaki S, Uchiyama Y, et al. Cross-sectional and longitudinal assessment of subchondral cysts in temporomandibular joints: Clinical and MRI study with a mean follow-up of 66 months. Journal of Prosthodontic Research. 2023;**67**:392-399. DOI: 10.2186/jpr.JPR_D_22_00089. Epub 2022 Oct 26

[70] Kim KA, Koh KJ. Recurrent simple bone cyst of the mandibular condyle: A case report. Imaging Science in Dentistry. 2013;**43**:49-53. DOI: 10.5624/isd.2013.43.1.49

[71] Dhaif G, Dhaif M, Sethi A. Giant aneurysmal bone cyst of the mandibular condyle mimicking parotid tumor: A case report and 22-year follow-up. Journal of Diagnostics and Treatment of Oral and Maxillofacial Pathology. 2023;**7**(6):51-62. DOI: 10.23999/j.dtomp.2023.6.1

[72] Omami G, Mathew R, Gianoli D, et al. Enormous aneurysmal bone cyst of the mandible: Case report and radiologic-pathologic correlation. Oral Surgery, Oral Medicine, Oral Pathology, Oral Radiology. 2012;**114**(1):e75-e79

[73] Matsusue Y, Yamamoto K, Yamakawa N, Yamamoto I, Matsuda S, Yoshimura H, et al. A case of synovial chondromatosis of temporomandibular joint with numerous loose bodies. Case Reports in Dentistry. 2021;**2021**:5927215. DOI: 10.1155/2021/5927215

[74] Lee RJ, Arshi A, Schwartz HC, et al. Characteristics and prognostic factors of osteosarcoma of the jaws: A retrospective cohort study. JAMA Otolaryngology. Head & Neck Surgery. 2015;**141**(5):470-477

[75] Uchiyama Y, Matsumoto K, Murakami S, et al. MRI in a case of osteosarcoma in the temporomandibular joint. Dento Maxillo Facial Radiology. 2014;**43**(5):20130280

[76] Faro TF, Martins-de-Barros AV, Lima GTWF, et al. Chondrosarcoma of the temporomandibular joint: Systematic review and survival analysis of cases reported to date. Head and Neck Pathology. 2021;**15**(3):923-934

[77] Jang BG, Huh KH, Kang JH, Kim JE, Yi WJ, Heo MS, et al. Imaging features of chondrosarcoma of the temporomandibular joint: Report of nine cases and literature review. Clinical Radiology. 2020;**75**(11):878.e1-878.e12. DOI: 10.1016/j.crad.2020.07.016. Epub 2020 Aug 22

[78] Gómez-León N, Galán-González I, Moreno-Casado MJ, et al. Chondroid tumors: Review of salient imaging features and update on the WHO classification. Current Problems in Diagnostic Radiology. 2023;**52**(2):197-211. DOI: 10.1067/j.cpradiol.2022.06.00

[79] Dodo M, Kumagai M, Kato Y, Hirakawa H, Koseki T. Metastasis in the mandibular condyle: A case report. Journal of Medical Case Reports. 2017;**11**:323. DOI: 10.1186/s13256-017-1450-9

[80] Kruse AL, Luebbers HT, Obwegeser JA, et al. Temporomandibular disorders associated with metastases to the temporomandibular joint: A review of the literature and 3 additional cases. Oral Surgery, Oral Medicine, Oral Pathology, Oral Radiology, and Endodontics. 2010;**110**(6):e21-e28. DOI: 10.1016/j.tripleo.2010.06.193

[81] Oliver C, Mouallem G, Dutot-Philipeau N, et al. A case report of condyle metastasis and a review of

the literature. Journal of Stomatology, Oral and Maxillofacial Surgery. 2022;**123**(4):360-363. DOI: 10.1016/j.jormas.2021.09.010

[82] Wang P, Yang J, Yu Q. MR imaging assessment of temporomandibular joint soft tissue injuries in dislocated and nondislocated mandibular condylar fractures. AJNR. American Journal of Neuroradiology. 2009;**30**(1):59-63. DOI: 10.3174/ajnr.A1313. Epub 2008 Oct 8

[83] Takahashi T, Ohtani M, Sano T, et al. Magnetic resonance evidence of joint effusion of the temporomandibular joint after fractures of the mandibular condyle: A preliminary report. Cranio. 2004;**22**:124-131

[84] Uecker M, Zhang S, Voit D, Merboldt KD, Frahm J. Real-time MRI: Recent advances using radial FLASH. Imaging in Medicine. 2012;**4**:461-476

[85] Zhang S, Block KT, Frahm J. Magnetic resonance imaging in real time: Advances using radial FLASH. Journal of Magnetic Resonance Imaging. 2010;**31**:101-109

[86] Sun Q, Du M-J, Tang X-F, Yu Q, Li K-C, Yang C. Dynamic MR imaging of temporomandibular joint: An initial assessment with fast imaging employing steady-state acquisition sequence. Magnetic Resonance Imaging. 2015;**33**:270-275

[87] Uecker M, Zhang S, Voit D, Karaus A, Merboldt KD, Frahm J. Real-time MRI at a resolution of 20 ms. NMR in Biomedicine. 2010;**23**:986-994

[88] Frahm J, Voit D, Uecker M. Real-time magnetic resonance imaging: Radial gradient-echo sequences with nonlinear inverse reconstruction. Investigative Radiology. 2019;**54**:757-766

[89] Krohn S, Joseph AA, Voit D, Michaelis T, Merboldt KD, Buergers R, et al. Multi-slice real-time MRI of temporomandibular joint dynamics. Dento Maxillo Facial Radiology. 2019;**48**(1):20180162. DOI: 10.1259/dmfr.20180162. Epub 2018 Jul 20

[90] Reichert IL, Robson MD, Gatehouse PD, et al. Magnetic resonance imaging of cortical bone with ultrashort TE pulse sequences. Magnetic Resonance Imaging. 2005;**23**:611-618

[91] Carl M, Sanal HT, Diaz E, et al. Optimizing MR signal contrast of the temporomandibular joint disk. Journal of Magnetic Resonance Imaging. 2011;**34**:1458-1464

[92] Weiger M, Pruessmann K. MRI with zero echo time. eMagRes. 2012;**1**:311-322

[93] Sanal HT, Bae WC, Pauli C, Du J, Statum S, Znamirowski R, et al. Magnetic resonance imaging of the temporomandibular joint disc: Feasibility of novel quantitative magnetic resonance evaluation using histologic and biomechanical reference standards. Journal of Orofacial Pain. 2011 Fall;**25**(4):345-353

[94] Chang EY, Du J, Chung CB. UTE imaging in the musculoskeletal system. Journal of Magnetic Resonance Imaging. 2015;**41**:870-883

[95] Khoo MM, Tyler PA, Saifuddin A, Padhani AR. Diffusion-weighted imaging (DWI) in musculoskeletal MRI: A critical review. Skeletal Radiology. 2011;**40**(6):665-681. DOI: 10.1007/s00256-010-1030-

[96] Le Bihan D. What can we see with IVIM MRI? NeuroImage. 2019;**187**:56-67. DOI: 10.1016/j.neuroimage.2017.12.062

[97] Oudeman J, Nederveen AJ, Strijkers GJ, Maas M, Luijten PR,

Froeling M. Techniques and applications of skeletal muscle diffusion tensor imaging: A review. Journal of Magnetic Resonance Imaging. 2016;**43**(4):773-788

[98] Chikui T, Shiraishi T, Ichihara T, et al. Effect of clenching on T2 and diffusion parameters of the masseter muscle. Acta Radiologica. 2010;**51**(1):58-63

[99] Ngamsom S, Nakamura S, Sakamoto J, Kotaki S, Tetsumura A, Kurabayashi T. The intravoxel incoherent motion MRI of masticatory muscle: A quantitative analysis in patients with temporomandibular joint disorders. Dento Maxillo Facial Radiology. 2017;**46**(1):20160424

[100] Benavides E, Bilgen M, Al-Hafez B, Alrefae T, Wang Y, Spencer P. High-resolution magnetic resonance imaging and diffusion tensor imaging of the porcine temporomandibular joint disc. Dento Maxillo Facial Radiology. 2009;**38**(3):148-155

[101] Liu S, Wang M, Ai T, et al. In vivo morphological and functional evaluation of the lateral pterygoid muscle: A diffusion tensor imaging study. The British Journal of Radiology. 2016;**89**(1060):20160041

[102] Nastro E, Bonanno L, Catalfamo L, et al. Diffusion tensor imaging reveals morphological alterations of the lateral pterygoid muscle in patients with mandibular asymmetry. Dento Maxillo Facial Radiology. 2018;**47**(2):20170129

[103] Gold GE, Chen CA, Koo S, Hargreaves BA, Bangerter NK. Recent advances in MRI of articular cartilage. AJR. American Journal of Roentgenology. 2009;**193**(3):628-638

[104] Nikkuni Y, Nishiyama H, Hayashi T. The relationship between masseter muscle pain and T2 values in temporomandibular joint disorders. Oral Surgery, Oral Medicine, Oral Pathology, Oral Radiology. 2018;**126**(4):349-354

[105] Shigeno K, Sasaki Y, Otonari-Yamamoto M, Ohata H, Shibahara T. Evaluating the mandibular condyles of patients with osteoarthritis for bone marrow abnormalities using magnetic resonance T2 mapping. Oral Radiology. 2019;**35**(3):272-279

[106] Cao Y, Xia C, Wang S, He S, Wamalwa P, Chen S. Application of magnetic resonance T2 mapping in the temporomandibular joints. Oral Surgery, Oral Medicine, Oral Pathology, Oral Radiology. 2012;**114**(5):644-649

Chapter 3

Bruxism: Innovative Perspectives in Assessment and Therapy

Elvin Gunel and Huseyin Kurtulmus

Abstract

Bruxism is a prevalent parafunctional behavior marked by involuntary clenching, grinding, bracing, or thrusting of the mandible during wakefulness or sleep, whose cumulative mechanical load can surpass the adaptive capacity of dental and musculoskeletal tissues and precipitate tooth wear, orofacial pain, and temporomandibular disorders. Reported prevalence estimates range 3.5–96%, reflecting heterogeneity in diagnostic definitions, assessment methods, and study populations, with adult rates averaging approximately 7% and pediatric estimates spanning 3.5–40.6%. Etiologically, bruxism emerges from the interplay of peripheral factors—such as facial morphology and occlusal discrepancies—central neuromuscular dysregulation, psychosocial stressors, pharmacological influences, and genetic predisposition. An integrated diagnostic schema—categorizing cases as possible, probable, or definite based on self-report, clinical examination, electromyography, and polysomnography—enhances consistency across settings. Management prioritizes reversible measures, such as patient education, behavioral modification, physical therapy, pharmacotherapy, and occlusal splint therapy, to reduce parafunctional load, with occlusal adjustment, botulinum toxin injections, or surgical intervention reserved for refractory presentations.

Keywords: bruxism, sleep bruxism, temporomandibular disorders, occlusal splint therapy, pathophysiology of bruxism

1. Introduction

Bruxism is a general term referring to involuntary clenching or grinding movements of the teeth that result from non-functional activation of the masticatory muscles, either during sleep or wakefulness [1]. "Clenching" describes tonic contractions resulting in sustained contact between the upper and lower teeth, whereas "grinding" refers to rhythmic chewing-like movements occurring in the absence of food. First described in the early twentieth century under the term *la bruxomania*, the condition was later renamed "bruxism" and has since undergone evolving definitions, highlighting its complexity and clinical relevance [2].

The concept of parafunction encompasses all movements of the masticatory system that do not serve a physiological purpose, among which bruxism is the most common and clinically significant example [3–6]. Even brief episodes of excessive force can result in damage to the periodontal ligament and alveolar bone, while some patients may remain asymptomatic, underscoring the importance of careful evaluation of dental surface wear, masticatory muscle tone, and temporomandibular joint (TMJ) function during oral examinations [7–11].

The prevalence of bruxism varies widely due to differences in definitions, diagnostic criteria, and populations studied. Overall, the prevalence tends to increase from adolescence to young adulthood, with considerable interindividual variability [12, 13].

The historical variability in the clinical definitions of bruxism also contributes to its heterogeneity. While Zarb and Carlsson define bruxism strictly as tooth clenching or grinding that occurs during sleep [14], Walsh reported that such behavior can also be observed during wakefulness [15]. Attanasio distinguished between static and dynamic relationships: clenching, representing a static relationship that involves sustained contact between the maxilla and mandible in centric or eccentric positions; in contrast, grinding reflects a dynamic relationship, characterized by forceful contact during lateral or protrusive movements of the mandible [16].

The historical variability in bruxism definitions illustrates its heterogeneity. Modern definitions emphasize its involuntary nature and the need for clinical management. For example, the American Academy of Prosthodontics defines bruxism as an "involuntary habit of clenching or grinding the teeth" [17], while the American Academy of Orofacial Pain stresses that these parafunctional activities can occur both nocturnally and diurnally [18]. The most recent definition by Kato et al. describes bruxism as "a condition characterized by excessive forceful and prolonged involuntary contact or friction between the upper and lower teeth, which must be monitored and managed" [19]. This perspective not only clarifies the mechanism of bruxism but also highlights the necessity for precise diagnostics and innovative management approaches in contemporary clinical practice.

Understanding the neuroanatomical mechanisms underlying bruxism, including central cortico-cerebellar arousals and dopaminergic dysfunction, along with peripheral, genetic, and psychosocial factors, is essential for developing effective management strategies. Although no definitive treatment currently exists to eliminate bruxism permanently, clinical management aims to reduce the parafunctional load, protect dental and jaw structures, prevent pain and TMJ dysfunction, and improve patient quality of life [20].

2. Epidemiology and prevalence

Most adults, including children, exhibit nocturnal bruxism of varying intensity at some point in their lives. Although the tissues of the masticatory system generally adapt to this parafunctional activity, in some individuals, the cumulative forces may exceed physiological limits, leading to pain and functional impairment [20].

To date, the use of subjective assessment criteria has hindered the establishment of a globally standardized diagnostic protocol for bruxism. This issue also applies to determine its prevalence.

Consistent findings regarding the prevalence and characteristics of bruxism episodes remain elusive due to methodological variability among studies, including differences in diagnostic criteria, age groups, and sample types. As a result, reported prevalence rates in both adult and pediatric populations range widely from 7% to 88% [20].

In adults, bruxism is estimated to affect approximately 7.4% of the general population [21]. In studies focusing on sleep bruxism, particularly in children, prevalence rates have been reported to range from 3.5% to 40.6%, with a general trend of decline observed with advancing age [4]. In older populations, prevalence rates may drop as low as 3% [22].

There is also no clear consensus regarding sex-related differences. Some studies report that bruxism is three to nine times more prevalent in females compared to males [19, 23], whereas others have found no statistically significant difference between sexes [2, 4].

Polysomnographic studies reveal that the frequency and duration of bruxism episodes throughout the night vary significantly among individuals. On average, approximately five episodes occur during an 8-hour sleep period, with each episode lasting around 8 seconds. Consequently, a duration of 8–9 seconds has become the generally accepted range for a bruxism episode in the literature [20, 24]. However, some studies have reported that longer episodes may also occur. Furthermore, in individuals with temporomandibular disorders (TMDs), the cumulative duration of tooth contact during an 8-hour sleep period may reach up to 38.7 minutes, whereas in health controls, this average remains limited to 5.4 minutes [25]. These findings demonstrate that the duration and intensity of bruxism activity can vary widely depending on both physiological and pathological conditions, and that the resulting load may exceed the adaptive capacity of the musculoskeletal system.

3. Etiology

The origin of bruxism remains not fully understood, and current evidence suggests that it has a multifactorial etiology [3, 7, 26]. These factors are generally categorized into two groups: morphological (peripheral) and central [27]. Peripheral factors include facial morphology, condylar asymmetry, variations in dental arch form, malocclusion, discrepancies between centric relation and maximum intercuspation, and general occlusal irregularities. Central factors encompass psychological, pathophysiological, neurological, genetic, and systemic elements, as well as side effects of medications. Recent review studies indicate that pathophysiological components account for nearly 70% of bruxism cases, psychosocial factors account for approximately 20%, and morphological factors account for about 10%.

3.1 Morphological factors

Although skeletal deviations and occlusal discrepancies were initially considered the primary causes of bruxism, they are now believed to play only a limited role. No reliable association has been established between occlusal interferences and bruxism, and the elimination of these interferences has not been shown to affect parafunctional activity [28, 29] significantly. Nonetheless, achieving harmony between centric relation and maximum intercuspation is considered clinically beneficial [30].

3.2 Psychosocial factors

Although psychological factors have long been proposed as potential triggers for bruxism, no consistent personality profile unique to "bruxists" has yet been defined [31]. Questionnaire-based and self-reported studies suggest that individuals with a history of clenching or grinding may be more prone to anxiety, hyperactivity, or aggression, although these findings lack consistency [32, 33]. The current theoretical framework posits that daily life stressors may increase both the frequency and severity of bruxism episodes. This model suggests that the limbic system and hypothalamus may trigger parafunctional activity by sending unnecessary stimuli to the masticatory muscles via the gamma-efferent pathway [34]. Indeed, isolated EMG recordings have shown a notable increase in masseter muscle activity during stressful periods, such as exams, arguments, or high workloads; however, these observations are mostly case-based, and their interpretation remains at a hypothetical level [35].

The lack of large-scale polysomnography-supported studies limits our understanding of the actual impact of psychological stress on nocturnal bruxism. Therefore, while stress, anxiety, and personality traits are accepted as potential contributors, their precise role in the development of bruxism has yet to be quantified. Further objective, longitudinal, and multi-center studies are needed to clarify these associations.

3.3 Pathophysiological factors

Sleep is divided into two primary phases: non-rapid eye movement (NREM) and REM, which alternate cyclically throughout the night [32, 36–38]. Polysomnographic data demonstrate that bruxism-related masticatory muscle activity can occur in all stages of the sleep cycle. However, approximately 60–80% of bruxism episodes in adults are concentrated in the first two stages of NREM sleep (N1–N2) [32, 36–38]. Although episodes occurring during the REM phase are less frequent, they are considered the most destructive form due to the intensity of muscle contractions and their prolonged duration [39].

It has been suggested that autonomic arousal and cortical reactivation during micro-arousals may trigger nocturnal bruxism by stimulating the masticatory muscles. Moreover, shortening of slow-wave sleep (N3) has been reported to facilitate this triggering [40, 41]. In individuals with snoring or obstructive sleep apnea syndrome (OSAS), both of which cause sleep fragmentation, bruxism risk has been shown to increase significantly [42, 43].

Recent studies highlight that centrally mediated autonomic nervous system mechanisms, modulated by psychological stress, play a more substantial role in the pathophysiology of bruxism than previously assumed [29, 30].

3.4 Drug-related side effects

Various studies have suggested that the side effects of substances, such as alcohol, caffeine, tobacco, and prescription medications for systemic diseases may contribute to the development of bruxism [44–46]. Lobbezoo et al. reported a reduction in bruxism activity in patients receiving low doses of levodopa. In contrast, long-term use of levodopa, particularly in conditions such as Parkinson's disease, was associated with increased clenching and grinding [47]. The same research group also proposed that selective serotonin reuptake inhibitors (SSRIs) may trigger bruxism when used long term [48]. Although there is a widespread belief regarding the adverse effect of SSRIs on bruxism, controlled clinical data confirming this association remain insufficient.

3.5 Genetic factors

Evidence concerning the genetic predisposition to bruxism appears to be conflicting. An extensive survey involving over 4,000 twin pairs reported that 39–64% of the

DOI: http://dx.doi.org/10.5772/intechopen.1012570

variance in bruxism could be attributed to genetic factors [49]. In contrast, another study with 250 twin pairs found no evidence of heritability [50]. On a molecular level, a specific polymorphism in the HTR2A gene has been associated with an increased susceptibility to sleep bruxism [51]. Additionally, between 20% and 50% of individuals with nocturnal bruxism report a family history of teeth grinding [31]. A meta-analysis reviewing 10 genetic studies supports the hypothesis that bruxism is partially heritable [52].

4. Diagnosis

Bruxism can be challenging to diagnose due to the lack of awareness by the patient or their surroundings, as well as the clinician's limited attention to subtle signs and symptoms.

The American Academy of Sleep Medicine (AASM) updated its diagnostic criteria in 2014, summarized as follows (**Table 1**) [53]:

Due to the lack of a universally accepted diagnostic standard, an international consensus meeting was held in 2013 to address this uncertainty. The expert panel defined bruxism as "a repetitive jaw-muscle activity characterized by clenching or grinding of the teeth and/or by bracing or thrusting of the mandible." The consensus also emphasized the circadian classification of bruxism into two distinct types: sleep bruxism and awake bruxism. To facilitate use in both clinical and research settings, a three-level diagnostic grading system was proposed (**Table 2**) [54].

Since no single test is considered sufficient to confirm the diagnosis of bruxism, multiple approaches are often used in combination. According to Koyano et al. [55, 56], five main diagnostic strategies are commonly employed in clinical practice.

4.1 Questionnaires

Questionnaires are widely used in both clinical practice and field studies to screen for bruxism. Their primary advantage is their ability to assess large populations in a short time. The most frequently used formats include yes/no responses to questions such as:

- Do you feel pain or fatigue in your jaw muscles upon waking?
- Do you experience tooth pain in the morning?
- Has anyone ever noticed that you grind your teeth during sleep?

Criterion	Description / Clinical sign
A—sleep sound	Repetitive or regular grinding/clenching sounds during sleep, reported by a bed partner or observer.
B—clinical findings *(at least one must accompany A)*	1. Pathological teeth consistent with sleep bruxism
	2. Morning jaw muscle pain or fatigue, or temporal headache
	3. Sensation of jaw locking or tightness upon awakening

Table 1.
Diagnostic criteria for sleep bruxism (American Academy of Sleep Medicine, 2014).

Level	Basis of diagnosis
Possible	Self-report only (questionnaire or interview)
Probable	Self-report + clinical examination showing bruxism-specific findings
Definite	Self-report + clinical signs + polysomnography (preferably with audio-video recording)

Table 2.
International consensus-based grading of bruxism.

- Have you ever noticed yourself grinding your teeth during the day?
- Do you catch yourself clenching your teeth during the day?
- Do you experience temporal headaches upon awakening?

According to Pintado et al., individuals clinically identified as bruxists answered "yes" to at least two of the six questions above. However, it is important to note that these diagnoses were not always confirmed using additional objective methods [57].

4.2 Clinical examination

The clinical diagnosis of bruxism is typically based on a combination of patient-reported symptoms and morphological and functional findings observed during examination. Key indicators that may support suspicion of parafunctional activity include:

- Reported grinding or clenching sounds during sleep by others
- Masseter muscle hypertrophy
- Morning masticatory muscle pain, fatigue, or temporal headache
- Temporomandibular joint clicking or locking
- Thermal sensitivity and pathological tooth wear
- Mucosal indentations on the cheek or tongue (**Figure 1**)
- Wear patterns consistent with normal or eccentric mandibular movements.

Sleep bruxism is most often brought to clinical attention by the patient's partner or family member. During a clinical examination, the presence of pathological wear on the incisal-labial and palatal surfaces of the anterior teeth, or the occlusal surfaces of the posterior teeth, typically supports the diagnosis. The severity of tooth wear can range from small, polished spots on the enamel to deep surface loss exposing secondary dentin (**Figure 2**). Experimental data have shown that intra-tissue fluid pressure increases during bruxism episodes, leading to muscle edema, which is expected to contribute to pain perception [58].

Another common objective sign is masseter muscle hypertrophy (**Figure 3**) [55]. While hypertrophy typically appears as a bilateral and symmetrical enlargement, unilateral cases have also been reported. Therefore, to determine whether the observed hypertrophy is indeed related to bruxism, a comprehensive clinical examination is necessary, and ambiguous cases should be referred to the appropriate medical specialty.

DOI: http://dx.doi.org/10.5772/intechopen.1012570

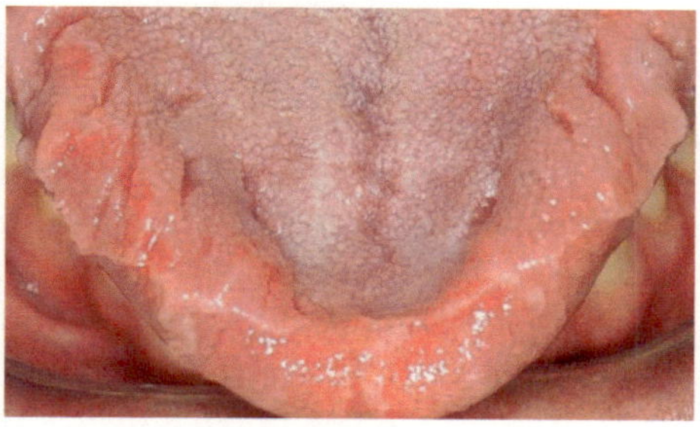

Figure 1.
Scalloped tongue (indentation marks on the lateral side).

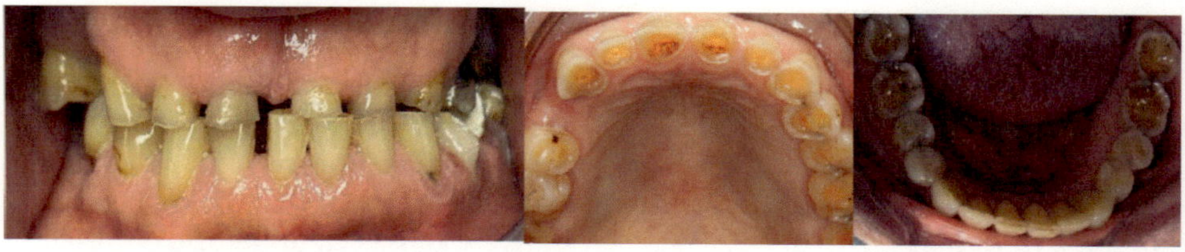

Figure 2.
Pathological wear patterns on incisal-labial and palatal surfaces of anterior teeth and occlusal surfaces of posterior teeth.

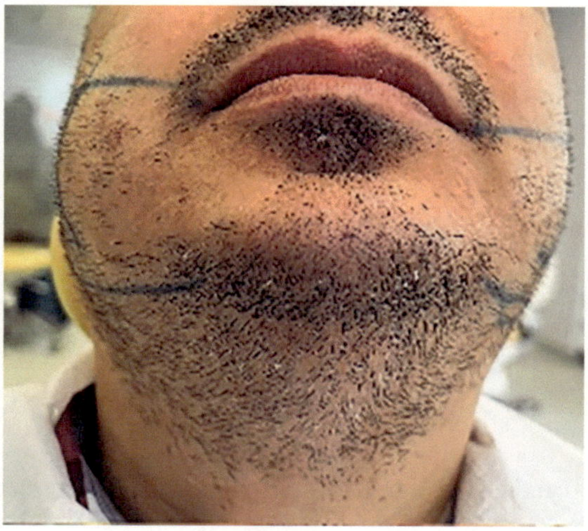

Figure 3.
Masseter muscle hypertrophy.

4.3 Objective measurement with intraoral appliances

To strengthen the diagnosis of bruxism in research settings, objective data beyond clinical observation are required. One such method involves analyzing wear marks on occlusal splints, which can provide quantitative insights into the presence and severity of bruxism [59, 60]. In more advanced setups, pressure sensors embedded in the splints dynamically record biting force, offering a detailed profile of parafunctional activity [61, 62]. These approaches improve diagnostic accuracy by enabling both wear pattern analysis and real-time force measurement.

4.4 Polysomnographic assessment

Polysomnography (PSG) is regarded as the gold standard for diagnosing bruxism. However, its use is limited by high equipment costs and the requirement for a sleep laboratory setting, which may alter the patient's natural parafunctional behavior due to the unfamiliar environment [55, 63]. The primary diagnostic marker for nocturnal bruxism in PSG is the electromyographic (EMG) activity of the jaw muscles. Additionally, PSG enables differentiation between bruxism and other orofacial activities, such as snoring, swallowing, or coughing, and can detect co-existing sleep disorders, such as obstructive sleep apnea (OSA) or insomnia. Furthermore, PSG allows for the simultaneous monitoring of cardiovascular and respiratory changes associated with sleep bruxism [38, 64, 65].

5. Treatment

The management of bruxism primarily targets three anatomical and functional domains: the masticatory muscles, the TMJ, and the dentition. Disorders originating from the TMJ or masticatory muscles are collectively classified under the umbrella term temporomandibular disorder. The origins of this concept trace back to James Costen's description of otological symptoms associated with TMJ dysfunction. Later, Ramfjord and Ash proposed categorizing these conditions as functional joint disorders [66]. Both the American Academy of Orofacial Pain (AAOP) and the American Dental Association (ADA) have adopted the term TMD to encompass all dysfunctions of the masticatory system.

According to the classification framework developed by J.P. Okeson, which is widely used for diagnostic and therapeutic guidance, TMDs are grouped into four major categories:

a. Masticatory muscle disorders

b. Temporomandibular joint disorders

c. Chronic mandibular hypomobility

d. Developmental anomalies.

The treatment of bruxism is tailored based on which of these groups is predominantly involved. For instance, in cases of muscle hyperactivity, physical therapy, biofeedback, or botulinum toxin injections may be utilized. When joint dysfunction is evident, occlusal splints, manual therapy, or intra-articular injections may be indicated. In the presence of tooth wear or malocclusion, occlusal adjustment or restorative approaches may be necessary. Treatment protocols should be individualized based on symptom severity, distribution of etiological factors, and the patient's general health status.

Given the multifactorial nature of TMD, no single therapy is sufficient for all cases, and interdisciplinary collaboration is often essential. A comprehensive treatment plan combining non-invasive and invasive strategies is typically required.

5.1 Reversible therapies

- Patient education and habit modification

DOI: http://dx.doi.org/10.5772/intechopen.1012570

- Physical therapy interventions
- Pharmacotherapy
- Psychological support
- Occlusal splint therapy.

5.2 Irreversible (invasive) interventions

- Occlusal adjustment
- Surgical procedures.

5.3 Alternative techniques

- Botulinum toxin
- Biofeedback therapy
- Hypnotherapy
- Anti-snoring devices.

This stepwise protocol advocates initiating treatment with low-risk conservative methods, progressing to more extensive interventions only when necessary.

5.4 Reversible treatment approaches

5.4.1 Patient education and behavioral modification

Patients are educated to recognize their bruxism habits and taught self-monitoring and behavioral control techniques. Exercises involving the tongue and palate, as well as stress reduction strategies, such as yoga or psychotherapy, may be recommended [67, 68].

5.4.2 Physical therapy

Modalities such as transcutaneous electrical nerve stimulation (TENS), ultrasound, and massage may improve muscle relaxation and circulation [69].

5.4.3 Psychiatric support

Counseling or psychotherapy focused on anxiety and stress management can enhance the patient's awareness of parafunctional habits, thereby helping reduce the frequency of clenching and grinding [68].

5.4.4 Pharmacotherapy

Medications such as muscle relaxants, benzodiazepines, and tricyclic antidepressants are commonly used for orofacial pain and sleep bruxism. In some cases, dopamine agonists, propranolol, or botulinum toxin A may be added. However, the number of well-controlled studies supporting their efficacy remains limited [70].

5.4.5 Occlusal splint therapy

Among conservative treatments for the masticatory system, the use of interocclusal appliances (occlusal splints or night guards) is the most common approach [9]. Initially developed by Karolyi in 1901, splint design has evolved, with rigid acrylic appliances now preferred over soft materials due to superior stability, wear resistance, and adjustability [71, 72]. Soft splints are prone to deformation, discoloration, and lack of retention, leading to reduced clinical longevity [73–78].

The primary therapeutic goals of splints include [71–79]:

- Eliminating premature contacts
- Protecting teeth from wear
- Promoting muscle relaxation
- Reducing TMJ stress
- Supporting proper condylar positioning
- Monitoring adaptation to occlusal or vertical changes.

Their effect stems from occlusal redistribution, reduced proprioceptive drive, joint stabilization, and increased behavioral awareness. A minor vertical increase promotes muscle relaxation by restoring optimal fiber length. The perception of the splint as a "treatment device" may also elicit a placebo effect (Hawthorne effect) [80].

According to Laskin's classification, four main types are used clinically: stabilization splints, anterior/posterior bite plates, anterior repositioning splints, and soft splints [81].

5.4.5.1 Stabilization splints

Made of hard acrylic and covering the entire arch, these splints—referred to in the literature as Michigan, Fox, Tanner, flat-plane, or Ramfjord appliances—promote stable centric occlusion and provide anterior guidance during dynamic movements. While typically applied to the arch with more missing teeth, selection depends on skeletal and arch morphology [82]. It is one of the first options in temporomandibular disorders accompanied by pain and functional limitations [83].

5.4.5.2 Anterior bite plates

These thin acrylic appliances cover the upper anterior teeth and contact only the mandibular anterior teeth. By eliminating posterior contacts, they effectively reduce muscle hyperactivity in a short period. They are typically used for 3–6 days during initial therapy. Extended use may cause supraeruption of posterior teeth, leading to anterior open bite [11].

5.4.5.3 Anterior repositioning splints

These full-arch appliances guide the mandible slightly forward and downward from the intercuspal position, stabilizing the condyle-disc complex and allowing time for retrodiscal tissue adaptation. Some authors recommend continuous wear (including during meals) for 6–7 weeks, while others suggest nighttime-only use for 2–6 months [82].

5.4.5.4 Soft splints

Soft splints are appliances made of thermoplastic material. They have a specific thickness and do not require balancing or adjustment with opposing teeth. They maintain continuous contact with the opposing teeth. This splint is used for urgent intervention in patients with pain and dysfunction. Wright reported that occlusal changes occur in users of soft splints, and symptoms increase in patients using non-adjusted appliances. Additionally, it is noted that soft splints may trigger parafunctional activity [84, 85].

5.5 Alternative techniques

5.5.1 Botulinum toxin

Botulinum toxin (Botox) is an exotoxin produced by *Clostridium botulinum*. This toxin causes temporary inactivation of muscles and glands by blocking the release of acetylcholine at the neuromuscular junction, also known as the cholinergic motor nerve terminals. In the treatment of bruxism, Botox injections are typically applied to the masseter muscle. However, in studies considering the synergistic effect of the masseter and temporal muscles, injections have been administered to both muscles.

Treatment option	Indications	Evidence level	Notes
Behavioral counseling	Mild bruxism, awake episodes	Moderate	First-line approach; includes patient education, stress management, and habit reversal techniques
Physical therapy	Muscle pain, hyperactivity	Moderate	Jaw exercises, relaxation techniques, and posture correction, often combined with behavioral therapy
Occlusal splints (stabilization splints)	Sleep bruxism, tooth wear, TMJ overload	High	Reversible, protective; reduces dental wear and may alleviate muscle hyperactivity
Botulinum toxin injections	Resistant muscular hyperactivity, severe jaw pain	Low to moderate	Adjunctive therapy; effects are temporary and require repeat administration
Pharmacological therapy	Severe cases with pain or comorbidities	Low	Analgesics, muscle relaxants, or anxiolytics; use with caution due to side effects
Surgical intervention	Rare, severe TMJ dysfunction	Very low	Last resort; irreversible and high-risk; limited supporting evidence

Table 3.
Summary of bruxism treatment options, indications, and evidence levels.

There is a lack of sufficient studies comparing these two approaches. In recent years, the use of Botox in the treatment of both daytime and sleep bruxism has been a topic of discussion. It has been proven that botulinum toxin reduces bruxism symptoms [86]. The toxin inhibits the release of acetylcholine, a neurotransmitter responsible for glandular secretion and muscle contraction. This results in a reduction in muscle tone in the injected area. The substance effectively weakens the muscle for 3–4 months [87].

Table 3 summarizes the primary treatment modalities, their clinical indications, and levels of supporting evidence to aid clinical decision-making.

6. Conclusion

Bruxism is a multifactorial, dynamic condition influenced by anatomical, neurological, psychological, and genetic components [3, 7, 26]. Recent diagnostic advances, including classification systems and technological tools, have improved diagnostic accuracy and therapeutic targeting [53–55].

Conservative approaches—such as behavioral therapy, physical rehabilitation, and stabilization splints—remain the foundation of treatment [9, 66, 71]. In cases resistant to conventional methods, botulinum toxin serves as a viable adjunct [86]. Pharmacologic and surgical interventions are reserved for specific, severe presentations.

A multidisciplinary, personalized treatment plan based on the patient's clinical and psychological profile is essential for long-term success.

Future research on bruxism should aim to clarify the neurophysiological pathways involved in both sleep and awake forms, using longitudinal study designs that capture variation over time. The integration of wearable diagnostic technologies, including EMG sensors and bite force detectors, may offer real-time, ecologically valid data. Additionally, advances in genetic analysis and neuroimaging can enhance precision diagnostics and help define personalized treatment pathways. Standardization of outcome measures and longer follow-up periods is essential to assess the durability and safety of both conventional and emerging therapies.

Conflict of interest

The authors declare no conflict of interest.

DOI: http://dx.doi.org/10.5772/intechopen.1012570

Author details

Elvin Gunel[1*] and Huseyin Kurtulmus[2]

1 Institute of Prosthodontics, Eskisehir, Turkey

2 Institute of Prosthodontics, University of Tinaztepe, Izmir, Turkey

*Address all correspondence to: elvingn3@gmail.com

References

[1] Manfredini D, Lobbezoo F. Role of psychosocial factors in the etiology of bruxism. Journal of Orofacial Pain. 2009;**23**(2):153-166

[2] Bader G, Lavigne G. Sleep bruxism; an overview of an oromandibular sleep movement disorder. Sleep Medicine Reviews. 2000;**4**(1):27-43

[3] Shetty S, Pitti V, Satish Babu CL, Surendra Kumar GP, Deepthi BC. Bruxism: A literature review. Journal of Indian Prosthodontic Society. 2010;**10**(3):141-148

[4] Manfredini D, Restrepo C, Diaz-Serrano K, Winocur E, Lobbezoo F. Prevalence of sleep bruxism in children: A systematic review of the literature. Journal of Oral Rehabilitation. 2013;**40**(8):631-642

[5] Carlsson GE, Egermark I, Magnusson T. Predictors of bruxism, other oral parafunctions, and tooth wear over a 20-year follow-up period. Journal of Orofacial Pain. 2003;**17**(1):50-57

[6] Guo H, Wang T, Niu X, Wang H, Yang W, Qiu J, et al. The risk factors related to bruxism in children: A systematic review and meta-analysis. Archives of Oral Biology. 2018;**86**:18-34

[7] Lobbezoo F, Jacobs R, De Laat A, Aarab G, Wetselaar P, Manfredini D. Chewing on bruxism. Diagnosis, imaging, epidemiology and aetiology. Nederlands Tijdschrift voor Tandheelkunde. 2017;**124**(6):309-316

[8] Jokubauskas L, Baltrušaitytė A, Pileičikienė G. Oral appliances for managing sleep bruxism in adults: A systematic review from 2007 to 2017. Journal of Oral Rehabilitation. 2018;**45**(1):81-95

[9] Reddy SV, Kumar MP, Sravanthi D, Mohsin AH, Anuhya V. Bruxism: a literature review. 2014;**6**(6):105-109

[10] Grobet P, Gilon Y, Bruwier A, Nizet JL. Sleep bruxism: State of the art and management. Revue Médicale de Liège. 2017;**72**(9):410-415

[11] McNeill C. Management of temporomandibular disorders: Concepts and controversies. The Journal of Prosthetic Dentistry. 1997;**77**(5):510-522

[12] Lobbezoo F, Ahlberg J, Manfredini D, Winocur E. Are bruxism and the bite causally related? Journal of Oral Rehabilitation. 2012;**39**(7):489-501

[13] Strausz T, Ahlberg J, Lobbezoo F, Restrepo CC, Hublin C, Ahlberg K, et al. Awareness of tooth grinding and clenching from adolescence to young adulthood: A nine-year follow-up. Journal of Oral Rehabilitation. 2010;**37**(7):497-500

[14] Zarb GA, Carlsson GE. Temporomandibular disorders: Osteoarthritis. Journal of Orofacial Pain. 1999;**13**(4):295-306

[15] Walsh JP. The psychogenesis of bruxism. Journal of Periodontology. 1965;**36**(5):417-420

[16] Attanasio R. An overview of bruxism and its management. Dental Clinics of North America. 1997;**41**(2):229-241

[17] AAoO P. Guidelines for Assessment, Diagnosis, and Management. American Academy of Orofacial Pain. Chicago: Quintessence Publishing; 1996

[18] de la Hoz-Aizpurua JL, Díaz-Alonso E, LaTouche-Arbizu R,

Mesa-Jiménez J. Sleep bruxism. Conceptual review and update. Medicina Oral, Patología Oral y Cirugía Bucal. 2011;**16**(2):e231-e238

[19] Bruksizm KO. Tanı ve tedavi. İstanbul: Quintessence Yayıncılık; 2012

[20] Attanasio R. Nocturnal bruxism and its clinical management. Dental Clinics of North America. 1991;**35**(1):245-252

[21] Maluly M, Andersen ML, Dal-Fabbro C, Garbuio S, Bittencourt L, de Siqueira JT, et al. Polysomnographic study of the prevalence of sleep bruxism in a population sample. Journal of Dental Research. 2013;**92**(Suppl. 7):97s-103s

[22] Lavigne GJ, Montplaisir JY. Restless legs syndrome and sleep bruxism: Prevalence and association among Canadians. Sleep. 1994;**17**(8):739-743

[23] Johansson A, Unell L, Carlsson GE, Söderfeldt B, Halling A. Gender difference in symptoms related to temporomandibular disorders in a population of 50-year-old subjects. Journal of Orofacial Pain. 2003;**17**(1):29-35

[24] Christensen LV. Jaw muscle fatigue and pains induced by experimental tooth clenching: A review. Journal of Oral Rehabilitation. 1981;**8**(1):27-36

[25] Trenouth MJ. The relationship between bruxism and temporomandibular joint dysfunction as shown by computer analysis of nocturnal tooth contact patterns. Journal of Oral Rehabilitation. 1979;**6**(1):81-87

[26] Klasser GD, Rei N, Lavigne GJ. Sleep bruxism etiology: The evolution of a changing paradigm. Journal of the Canadian Dental Association. 2015;**81**:f2

[27] B AC. Bruksizm Tanı ve Tedavisinde Güncel Yaklaşımlar. Kırıkkale Üniversitesi Tıp Fakültesi Dergisi. 2012;**14**:20-25

[28] Clark GT, Adler RC. A critical evaluation of occlusal therapy: Occlusal adjustment procedures. Journal of the American Dental Association (1939). 1985;**110**(5):743-750

[29] Lobbezoo F, Naeije M. Bruxism is mainly regulated centrally, not peripherally. Journal of Oral Rehabilitation. 2001;**28**(12):1085-1091

[30] Lobbezoo F, Brouwers JE, Cune MS, Naeije M. Dental implants in patients with bruxing habits. Journal of Oral Rehabilitation. 2006;**33**(2):152-159

[31] Reding GR, Rubright WC, Zimmerman SO. Incidence of bruxism. Journal of Dental Research. 1966;**45**(4):1198-1204

[32] Reding GR, Zepelin H, Robinson JE Jr, Zimmerman SO, Smith VH. Nocturnal teeth-grinding: All-night psychophysiologic studies. Journal of Dental Research. 1968;**47**(5):786-797

[33] Satoh T, Harada Y. Electrophysiological study on tooth-grinding during sleep. Electroencephalography and Clinical Neurophysiology. 1973;**35**(3):267-275

[34] Nicholson RA, Lakatos CA, Gramling SE. EMG reactivity and oral habits among facial pain patients in a scheduled-waiting competitive task. Applied Psychophysiology and Biofeedback. 1999;**24**(4):235-247

[35] Intrieri RC, Jones GE, Alcorn JD. Masseter muscle hyperactivity and myofascial pain dysfunction syndrome: A relationship under stress. Journal of Behavioral Medicine. 1994;**17**(5):479-500

[36] Sjöholm T, Lehtinen II, Helenius H. Masseter muscle activity in diagnosed

sleep bruxists compared with non-symptomatic controls. Journal of Sleep Research. 1995;**4**(1):48-55

[37] Macaluso GM, Guerra P, Di Giovanni G, Boselli M, Parrino L, Terzano MG. Sleep bruxism is a disorder related to periodic arousals during sleep. Journal of Dental Research. 1998;**77**(4):565-573

[38] Bader GG, Kampe T, Tagdae T, Karlsson S, Blomqvist M. Descriptive physiological data on a sleep bruxism population. Sleep. 1997;**20**(11):982-990

[39] Ö N. Temporomandibuler Bozuklukların Psikiyatrik Yönü ve Bruksizm. Klinik Psikiyatri Dergisi. 2007;**10**:148-156

[40] Kato T, Rompré P, Montplaisir JY, Sessle BJ, Lavigne GJ. Sleep bruxism: An oromotor activity secondary to micro-arousal. Journal of Dental Research. 2001;**80**(10):1940-1944

[41] Nagels G, Okkerse W, Braem M, Van Bogaert PP, De Deyn B, Poirrier R, et al. Decreased amount of slow wave sleep in nocturnal bruxism is not improved by dental splint therapy. Acta Neurologica Belgica. 2001;**101**(3):152-159

[42] Ohayon MM, Li KK, Guilleminault C. Risk factors for sleep bruxism in the general population. Chest. 2001;**119**(1):53-61

[43] Sjöholm TT, Lowe AA, Miyamoto K, Fleetham JA, Ryan CF. Sleep bruxism in patients with sleep-disordered breathing. Archives of Oral Biology. 2000;**45**(10):889-896

[44] Winocur E, Gavish A, Voikovitch M, Emodi-Perlman A, Eli I. Drugs and bruxism: A critical review. Journal of Orofacial Pain. 2003;**17**(2):99-111

[45] Ahlberg J, Savolainen A, Rantala M, Lindholm H, Könönen M. Reported bruxism and biopsychosocial symptoms: A longitudinal study. Community Dentistry and Oral Epidemiology. 2004;**32**(4):307-311

[46] Lobbezoo F, Van Der Zaag J, Naeije M. Bruxism: Its multiple causes and its effects on dental implants—An updated review. Journal of Oral Rehabilitation. 2006;**33**(4):293-300

[47] Lobbezoo F, Soucy JP, Montplaisir JY, Lavigne GJ. Striatal D2 receptor binding in sleep bruxism: A controlled study with iodine-123-iodobenzamide and single-photon-emission computed tomography. Journal of Dental Research. 1996;**75**(10):1804-1810

[48] Lobbezoo F, van Denderen RJ, Verheij JG, Naeije M. Reports of SSRI-associated bruxism in the family physician's office. Journal of Orofacial Pain. 2001;**15**(4):340-346

[49] Hublin C, Kaprio J, Partinen M, Koskenvuo M. Sleep bruxism based on self-report in a nationwide twin cohort. Journal of Sleep Research. 1998;**7**(1):61-67

[50] Michalowicz BS, Pihlstrom BL, Hodges JS, Bouchard TJ Jr. No heritability of temporomandibular joint signs and symptoms. Journal of Dental Research. 2000;**79**(8):1573-1578

[51] Abe Y, Suganuma T, Ishii M, Yamamoto G, Gunji T, Clark GT, et al. Association of genetic, psychological and behavioral factors with sleep bruxism in a Japanese population. Journal of Sleep Research. 2012;**21**(3):289-296

[52] Lobbezoo F, Visscher CM, Ahlberg J, Manfredini D. Bruxism and genetics: A review of the literature. Journal of Oral Rehabilitation. 2014;**41**(9):709-714

[53] Sateia MJ. International classification of sleep disorders-third edition: Highlights and modifications. Chest. 2014;**146**(5):1387-1394

[54] Lobbezoo F, Ahlberg J, Glaros A, Kato T, Koyano K, Lavigne G, et al. Bruxism defined and graded: An international consensus. Journal of Oral Rehabilitation. 2013;**40**(1):2-4

[55] Koyano K, Tsukiyama Y, Ichiki R, Kuwata T. Assessment of bruxism in the clinic. Journal of Oral Rehabilitation. 2008;**35**(7):495-508

[56] Santamato A, Panza F, Di Venere D, Solfrizzi V, Frisardi V, Ranieri M, et al. Effectiveness of botulinum toxin type a treatment of neck pain related to nocturnal bruxism: A case report. Journal of Chiropractic Medicine. 2010;**9**(3):132-137

[57] Pintado MR, Anderson GC, DeLong R, Douglas WH. Variation in tooth wear in young adults over a two-year period. The Journal of Prosthetic Dentistry. 1997;**77**(3):313-320

[58] Zeldow LL. Treating clenching and bruxing by habit change. Journal of the American Dental Association (1939). 1976;**93**(1):31-33

[59] Pierce CJ, Gale EN. Methodological considerations concerning the use of Bruxcore plates to evaluate nocturnal bruxism. Journal of Dental Research. 1989;**68**(6):1110-1114

[60] Korioth TW, Bohlig KG, Anderson GC. Digital assessment of occlusal wear patterns on occlusal stabilization splints: A pilot study. The Journal of Prosthetic Dentistry. 1998;**80**(2):209-213

[61] Onodera K, Kawagoe T, Sasaguri K, Protacio-Quismundo C, Sato S. The use of a bruxchecker in the evaluation of different grinding patterns during sleep bruxism. Cranio. 2006;**24**(4):292-299

[62] Baba K, Clark GT, Watanabe T, Ohyama T. Bruxism force detection by a piezoelectric film-based recording device in sleeping humans. Journal of Orofacial Pain. 2003;**17**(1):58-64

[63] Lobbezoo F, van der Zaag J, van Selms MK, Hamburger HL, Naeije M. Principles for the management of bruxism. Journal of Oral Rehabilitation. 2008;**35**(7):509-523

[64] Manfredini D, Lobbezoo F. Relationship between bruxism and temporomandibular disorders: A systematic review of literature from 1998 to 2008. Oral Surgery, Oral Medicine, Oral Pathology, Oral Radiology, and Endodontics. 2010;**109**(6):e26-e50

[65] Lavigne GJ, Guitard F, Rompré PH, Montplaisir JY. Variability in sleep bruxism activity over time. Journal of Sleep Research. 2001;**10**(3):237-244

[66] Costen JB. A syndrome of ear and sinus symptoms dependent upon disturbed function of the temporomandibular joint. 1934. The Annals of Otology, Rhinology, and Laryngology. 1997;**106**(10 Pt 1):805-819

[67] Johansson A, Omar R, Carlsson GE. Bruxism and prosthetic treatment: A critical review. Journal of Prosthodontic Research. 2011;**55**(3):127-136

[68] Cadden S. Orofacial pain. Guidelines for assessment, diagnosis, and management, 4th edition (2008). European Journal of Orthodontics. 2009;**31**:216-217

[69] JP. O. Management of Temporomandibular Disorders and

Occlusion. 3rd ed. Florida, USA: Mosby; 1992

[70] Wahlund K, List T, Larsson B. Treatmentoftemporomandibulardisorders among adolescents: A comparison between occlusal appliance, relaxation training, and brief information. Acta Odontologica Scandinavica. 2003;**61**(4):203-211

[71] Okeson JP. Orofacial Pain: Guidelines for Assessment, Diagnosis, and Management. Chicago, IL: Quintessence Publishing Co; 1996

[72] Allen DL. Accurate occlusal bite guards. Periodontics. 1967;**5**(2):93-95

[73] Greenwald AS. The bruxism appliance and its varied application: Outline of procedure. The New York Journal of Dentistry. 1968;**38**(10):443

[74] Askinas SW. Fabrication of an occlusal splint. The Journal of Prosthetic Dentistry. 1972;**28**(5):549-551

[75] Gabriele P. A double night guard retainer. The New York State Dental Journal. 1986;**52**(1):30-31

[76] Ordene NM. A modified bruxism appliance. The New York State Dental Journal. 1989;**55**(1):40-41

[77] Perel ML. Parafunctional habits, nightguards, and root form implants. Implant Dentistry. 1994;**3**(4):261-263

[78] Cowie RR. The clinical use of night guards: Occlusal objectives. Dentistry Today. 2004;**23**(9):4-5

[79] Waltimo A, Könönen M. A novel bite force recorder and maximal isometric bite force values for healthy young adults. Scandinavian Journal of Dental Research. 1993;**101**(3):171-175

[80] De Boever JA, McCall WD Jr, Holden S, Ash MM Jr. Functional occlusal forces: An investigation by telemetry. The Journal of Prosthetic Dentistry. 1978;**40**(3):326-333

[81] Roy W. Temporomandibular disorders: An evidence-based approach to diagnosis and treatment. Physical Therapy. 2006;**86**:1451a-14512a

[82] Kreiner M, Betancor E, Clark GT. Occlusal stabilization appliances. Evidence of their efficacy. Journal of the American Dental Association (1939). 2001;**132**(6):770-777

[83] Yap AU. Effects of stabilization appliances on nocturnal parafunctional activities in patients with and without signs of temporomandibular disorders. Journal of Oral Rehabilitation. 1998;**25**(1):64-68

[84] Laskin DMGC, Hylander WL. Clinical Management. An Evidence-Based Approach to Diagnosis and Treatment. Texasz: Quintessence Publishing Co.; 2006

[85] Egermark I, Carlsson GE, Magnusson T. A 20-year longitudinal study of subjective symptoms of temporomandibular disorders from childhood to adulthood. Acta Odontologica Scandinavica. 2001;**59**(1):40-48

[86] Gu W, Yang J, Zhang F, Yin X, Wei X, Wang C. Efficacy of biofeedback therapy via a mini wireless device on sleep bruxism contrasted with occlusal splint: A pilot study. Journal of Biomedical Research. 2015;**29**(2):160-168

[87] Nayyar P, Kumar P, Nayyar PV, Singh A. BOTOX: Broadening the horizon of dentistry. Journal of Clinical and Diagnostic Research. 2014;**8**(12):Ze25-Ze29

Chapter 4

Otological Presentation and Temporomandibular Joint Disorders

Toye Gabriel Olajide, Oyebanji Anthony Olajuyin, Atilade Waheed Adegbiji and Segun Mathew Agboola

Abstract

Temporomandibular joint (TMJ) is a hinge joint that occur between the jaw and temporal bone with an articular disc separating the two structures. The disorders associated with TMJ are due to problems involving the muscles of mastication, the temporomandibular joint itself, and associated structures such as the ear. The most frequent otological manifestations in relation to temporomandibular disorder (TMD) are, hearing loss, otalgia, tinnitus, ear fullness, and vertigo. The objective of this review is to highlight the various otological manifestations of temporomandibular joint disorders (TMD). Although the mechanisms that are responsible for these manifestations are not fully known, the various theories reported by researchers are as follows: the inflammatory process near the TMJ, the shared innervation pathways, muscle spasms on the tympanic membrane, auditory perception as modulated by central neural process, pressure changes and compression of nerves. Most of these disrupt Eustachian tube function causes its blockage and results in various hearing-related symptoms. Management of the condition is usually involved thorough evaluation with contribution from pure tone audiometry, tympanometry, and occasionally computerized tomography scan or magnetic resonance image examinations. A multidisciplinary approach (ENT, Dentists, Physiotherapy and Oral and Maxillofacial) is therefore recommended in the management. Usually, most of the affected individuals normally respond to conservative treatment, physical therapy and analgesics. Otological presentations of TMD are common and need a high index of suspicion to arrive at a diagnosis and treatment. There is a need for more studies to further reveal the association between temporomandibular disorders and neuro-otologic manifestations.

Keywords: disorders, otological, temporomandibular, hearing loss, joint

1. Introduction

Temporomandibular joint (TMJ) is a hinge joint that occurs between the jaw and the temporal bone with an articular disc separating the two structures [1]. The TMJ is very important in performing the function of jaw movement, which may include propulsion, laterality, yawning, chewing, biting, and opening and closing of the mouth [2–4]. The muscles of mastication are primarily responsible for the movement of this joint. Temporomandibular joint disorders (TMJD) are a major cause of non-dental pain in the orofacial region. TMJ also aids the Eustachian tube opening during its various movements. The disorders associated with TMJ are due to problems involving the muscles of mastication, the temporomandibular joint itself, and associated structures such as the ear [5]. The causes of TMJD are multifactorial and include excessive masticatory muscle activity, harmful habits, TMJ trauma, degenerative disorders, and psychosocial factors [6, 7]. Others are a combination of genetics, clenching or grinding of the teeth (bruxism), arthritis, autoimmune diseases, dental surgery, and infections [8]. These disorders are said to be common among women and Caucasians than in African Americans [9].

Barreto et al. and Pita et al., in their literature reviews on TMDs and the relationship with auditory symptoms, concluded that there is a link between the stomatognathic system and the auditory system [10, 11]. Studies have also postulated that the pathophysiology of otological symptoms in TMD patients may be due to the anatomical proximity of the TMJ, muscles innervated by the trigeminal nerve, and the ear structures [12].

Epidemiological findings generally have reported that the prevalence of ear symptoms in the general population may be in the range of 10–31%; however, this may increase to 85% in patients with TMD. It was also noted that 50% of those patients referred due to otological complaints may not present with problems in the ear [13, 14]. However, there are some problems that are associated with this disorder, namely difficulty in chewing, dizziness, facial pain, headaches, jaw pain, stiffness in the neck or shoulders and trismus. The most cited otological symptoms in the literature that are related to TMJD in various studies were tinnitus, otalgia, ear fullness, hearing loss and vertigo [15, 16]. Population-based studies show that TMD affects 10–15% of adults, but only 5% usually seek treatment [17, 18].

The incidence of TMD peaks from 20 to 40 years of age; it is twice as common in women as in men and carries a significant financial burden from loss of work [19]. Symptoms can range from mild discomfort to debilitating pain, including limitations of jaw movement. Multifactorial diversity that can lead to the onset of TMJDs makes it difficult to identify a single cause for the presence of ear complaints in such a population [20].

In a study of the relationship between otological symptoms and TMD conducted by Pamela et at, it was shown that the number of female patients was higher than male, with a ratio of 78.54% to 21.45%, respectively. Regarding the age groups, the highest prevalence of otological symptoms occurred in the 41–50 years-old group (37%) followed by the 51–60 years-old group (32%) [2]. The findings also indicated that the prevalence of otological symptoms such as tinnitus, deafness, dizziness, ear fullness, and imbalance was 87% regardless of sex and age, but when they studied the presence of symptoms alone, it was observed that tinnitus had the highest prevalence of 42%, followed by ear fullness 39% [2]. When relating the symptoms they presented with the participant's gender, there were significant relationships ($p < 0.05$) in symptoms of tinnitus and dizziness [2].

The association of TMD and the origin of otologic symptoms is not yet fully understood, but there were some studies that show the relation between otological symptoms and TMD [21, 22].

Manfredini et al. noted that the frequency of TMD signs and symptoms in general population ranged between 5% and 50%, however many epidemiological studies evaluated the prevalence of TMD in different population, among them are Caucasian (17–20%), Hongkong Chinese (21%), Native American (23–26%) [23]. The prevalence of TMD in the study conducted by Mohammed was 20.5%, as reported by him [24].

As noted above, patients with various type of temporomandibular disorder (TMD) present with several symptoms in their temporomandibular joints, masticatory muscles and associated structures, and also might have otological symptoms such as tinnitus, ear fullness, ear pain, hearing loss, hyperacusis, and vertigo, which are due to the anatomical proximity between the temporomandibular joint, muscles innervated by the trigeminal nerve, and the ear structures as noted by Caria et al. [7]. We therefore review some of these symptoms as they occur in temporomandibular disorders with emphasis on the pathophysiology and mechanism, evaluation and treatment.

2. Hearing loss and temporomandibular joint disorder

Temporomandibular joint disorder is a relatively common condition and affects people of all ages, with about one-third of adults experiencing the symptoms. Hearing loss is one of the complaints associated with this disorder, and it is said to be noticed in 1 out of 10 people with TMD [25]. There are some symptoms that are related to hearing loss in this disorder. Some of the symptoms are muffled hearing, ringing in the ears, otalgia, sensation of fullness in the ear, and popping or clicking sounds during movement of the jaw [25]. The level of hearing loss may depend on the severity of the TMJ disorder. A study conducted by Kitsoulis et al. reported that those who had the most symptoms, including jaw stiffness, were more likely to experience hearing problems [26].

2.1 Pathophysiology and mechanisms of hearing loss in TMD

Since the TMJ is situated very close to the middle ear, disorders of TMJ can affect hearing, although the exact reason is not clear, but thought to be due to inflammation and pressure from the joint, which can affect the nerves and muscles at the site and subsequently lead to blockage of the Eustachian tubes [26].

Other researchers thought that it was due to altered middle-ear/inner-ear pressure equilibrium [27]. Tinnitus and hearing loss may also be due to improper drainage of fluid from the middle ear by the Eustachian tube [28]. Identifying TMJ-related hearing loss can be challenging, as the symptoms may overlap with other conditions. Individuals experiencing TMJ-related hearing loss may report a combination of the following symptoms: ear fullness or pressure, tinnitus (ringing or buzzing in the ears), reduced hearing sensitivity, ear pain or discomfort, muffled or distorted hearing, dizziness or imbalance. Another theory proposes that common innervation of the tensor veli palatini, tensor tympani, masseter, temporalis and pterygoid muscles by the motor nucleus of the trigeminal nerve is the underlying cause of the aural symptomatology in TMD patients [29].

It is important to note that sensorineural hearing loss is uncommon; however, there were transient or subjective hearing changes which was reported in a significant number of TMD patients. The following mechanisms or theories were said to have been involved in hearing loss and TMD. However, further investigations are necessary to fully comprehend the underlying mechanisms and establish a definitive causal relationship.

2.1.1 Eustachian tube dysfunction

The two muscles, namely, the tensor veli palatini and tensor tympani, which are innervated by the mandibular branch of the trigeminal nerve, also supply the TMJ. The muscles play a major role in Eustachian tube function and middle ear pressure regulation. Abnormal function of those nerves may affect hearing [30]. Eustachian tube is responsible for equalizing pressure in the middle ear. Its inflammation can affect and cause Eustachian tube dysfunction, which can lead to a sensation of fullness, pressure, and potentially conductive hearing loss [31].

It has been reported that TMD patients cannot open their mouths wide (trismus) to yawn which was due to inflammation and subsequently led to poor Eustachian tube function [29]. The end result may be otitis media with effusion and hearing loss. Chronic muscle tension from TMJ disorders can also affect the Eustachian tube, causing it to become blocked, which can lead to middle ear effusion. Also, as a result of muscle hyperactivity or dysfunction, there may be negative middle ear pressure, conductive hearing loss and sensation of "ear fullness" [32].

2.1.2 Proximity, potential mechanisms and ossicular chain vibration disturbance

Another possible theory for the association between TMJ disorders and hearing loss is the close proximity of the temporomandibular joint to the middle ear. The middle ear contains the ossicles, which transmit sound vibrations from the eardrum to the inner ear. The thin bony wall separating the temporomandibular joint and the middle ear, known as the tympanic plate, leaves room for potential influences on middle ear function and hearing [27].

2.1.3 Shared neural pathways, referred neural effects and muscle dysfunction

Another theory proposes that the muscles involved in TMJ disorders, including those responsible for jaw movement and those connected to the middle ear, share neural pathways or have interconnected reflexes. Abnormal functioning in these muscles could impair the normal activity of the auditory system and subsequently lead to hearing-related symptoms. In this mechanism, it was projected that shared innervation pathways (the trigeminal nerve) between the TMJ and auditory structures may affect auditory perception through central neural modulation [33].

2.1.4 Inflammation, swelling and nerve compression

One theory focuses on the inflammation and swelling commonly associated with TMJ disorders. Inflammation in the temporomandibular joint and surrounding tissues can spread to nearby structures, including the middle ear. This inflammation may disrupt the delicate structures of the middle ear, such as the ossicles or the eardrum, and interfere with their ability to transmit sound vibrations effectively, leading to a variety of symptoms such as ear fullness, pressure, and potential hearing loss.

The inflammation-induced disruption can impede the movement of air and fluid in the Eustachian tube—the tube that connects the middle ear to the back of the throat, leading to changes in middle ear pressure and impaired sound transmission to the inner ear [3, 34].

The misalignment or dysfunction of the jaw joint in TMJ disorders can result in nerve compression. The nerves that supply the ear, including the trigeminal nerve and its branches, pass through or near the temporomandibular joint. When the jaw joint is misaligned, excessive pressure or tension can be exerted on these nerves, affecting their normal function [33]. The compression of these nerves can disrupt the transmission of auditory signals from the ear to the brain, resulting in various hearing-related symptoms. This compression can affect the auditory pathway, potentially leading to sensorineural hearing loss, where the nerve itself is affected. Tinnitus, a ringing or buzzing sensation in the ears, reduced hearing sensitivity, and a feeling of blocked or muffled hearing are among the potential auditory symptoms that may arise from nerve compression [35]. It is important to note that the relationship between TMJ-related inflammation, nerve compression, and hearing loss is complex and multifaceted. Further research is needed to gain a more comprehensive understanding of the underlying mechanisms and the extent of their impact on auditory function. Additionally, individual variations in the presentation of TMJ disorders and associated hearing symptoms should be considered, as the severity and specific mechanisms can vary from person to person.

2.1.5 Direct impact on middle ear structures and pressure changes

Direct effect on the ossicular bone in the middle ear can occur as those ossicles are attached to the TMJ *via* ligaments. Inflammation and muscle spasms can affect the tension of the tympanic membrane, potentially disrupting sound transmission [27]. Other contributing factors like tinnitus can also cause hearing loss in patients with TMJ disorders. Muscle tension and pressure changes can cause tinnitus, which can make it difficult to hear or concentrate. The TMJ's movement can create pressure changes that directly affect the cochlea (inner ear structure).

2.2 Prevalence and characteristics

Hearing loss associated with TMJ disorders has been found to occur in 5–30% of TMD patients, depending on the diagnostic criteria [36]. Also, the hearing loss was said to be unilateral or bilateral in nature and may be fluctuating rather than progressive. It was mostly conductive or mixed in nature and more often than not can be associated with ear fullness, tinnitus and ear ache.

2.3 Evaluation of hearing loss associated with TMD

Evaluation of patients with hearing loss associated with TMJ disorders mainly consists of getting detailed and comprehensive history from the patients followed by a thorough general or physical and clinical examination of the Ear, Nose, Throat, Head and Neck. Such examinations are to exclude primary ear pathology. Emphasis should be more on otoscopy, palpation of the TMJ and related muscles and bones. Otoscopy may be normal in TMJ—related hearing loss.

2.4 Investigations

The following investigations should be carried out

i. ENT evaluation

ii. Pure tone audiometry (PTA)—it may show mild conductive hearing loss

iii. Tympanometry—to rule out middle ear pathology

iv. Magnetic resonance imaging (MRI)—useful for identifying internal derangement of TMJ (e.g., disc displacement)

2.5 Treatment of hearing loss from TMD

Treatment is usually directed to the cause or suspected cause of hearing loss.

Although ENT surgeons will not personally initiate surgical treatment once the diagnosis of TMD has been made, they are integral in commencing conservative management and involving a multidisciplinary care team [18].

By ordinarily treating the underlying TMD, most of the hearing symptoms would resolve. However, the following modes of treatment are employed depending on the findings:

i. Occlusal splints to reduce joint pressure.

ii. Physical therapy for muscle relaxation and posture.

iii. NSAIDs or muscle relaxants to reduce inflammation or spasm.

iv. Behavioral therapy for stress-related bruxism or clenching.

v. Myofunctional therapy to improve muscle coordination affecting the Eustachian tube.

3. Tinnitus and temporomandibular disorders

Tinnitus otherwise known as ringing or buzzing in the ears is one of the extra-articular symptoms often associated with TMD. This symptoms can significantly affect quality of life and are frequently misdiagnosed, often leading to referrals to ENT specialists before the TMJ origin is considered.

Epidemiologic studies have demonstrated tinnitus to be a common symptom in the general population, but with a higher prevalence in patients with TMD symptoms [37]. Israel et al. in their study reported the incidence of tinnitus to be 10–31% of the general population and up to 85% in the population of patients with TMD symptoms [38]. Another study done by Morais et al. reported a prospective and cross-sectional study seeking to characterize tinnitus in individuals with normal hearing and its relationship with TMD. They found that 70% of the individuals were women with an average age between 20 and 55 years [39]. Tinnitus related to TMD is thought to be produced by the lateral pterygoid muscles and the discomalleolar ligament [29].

3.1 Mechanism and pathophysiology of tinnitus in TMD

The tinnitus in TMD is described as a subjective type and non-pulsatile, and it has been reported to be due to the following mechanism

i. *Muscle hyperactivity*—when there is spasm or hypertonicity in the muscles of mastication or cervical muscles, it will have an effect on the middle ear muscles, for example, tensor tympani, leading to altered auditory perception.

ii. The neural pathways of the trigeminal nerve and auricuo temporal nerve seem to overlap, which may cause referred auditory sensations.

iii. TMJ-middle ear connection: The close anatomical relationship between the TMJ and the ear canal (especially the anterior wall of the external auditory canal) can transmit abnormal joint motion or inflammation, potentially impacting ear structures.

iv. Somatosensory tinnitus: Stimulation of the somatosensory system (jaw movements, pressure on masticatory muscles) can modulate auditory perception in the brainstem.

v. Tinnitus related to TMD is thought to be produced by the lateral pterygoid muscles and the discomalleolar ligament [29].

Tinnitus is reported in 30–60% of TMD patients. Many of these patients lack any primary ear pathology, and ENT evaluations may be normal.

4. Otalgia and temporomandibular disorder

This type of ear pain is called referred or secondary earache. It has no identifiable otologic cause that comes from TMD. Usually, the pain is from the masticatory muscles, TMJ and associated structures according to Miller and Wyrwa [40].

Salvetti et al. suggest that disposition of the joint disk during jaw movement increases pressure in the Eustachian tube, the ear structures, the auriculotemporal and masseteric nerve and some branches of the deep posterior temporal nerve. The auriculotemporal nerve innervates the TMJ, the tympanic membrane, the anterosuperior part of the external ear and the tragus, and its stimulation gives the sense of otalgia [41].

4.1 Mechanisms

This type of pain has a possible mechanism through one of the following ways [42, 43]:

i. *Shared innervation:* The auriculotemporal branch of the mandibular division of the trigeminal nerve (V3) innervates both the TMJ and the external auditory canal. Irritation or dysfunction in the TMJ can be perceived as ear pain.

ii. *Myofascial pain referral:* Trigger points in masticatory muscles (especially the masseter and lateral pterygoid) may refer pain to the ear region.

iii. *Joint inflammation or internal derangement:* These may exert pressure or inflammatory effects on adjacent tissues, contributing to otalgia.

4.2 Epidemiology

i. Otalgia is reported in 40–70% of TMD cases, especially in those with disc displacement or joint inflammation [32].

ii. Many of these patients lack any primary ear pathology, and ENT evaluations may be normal.

4.3 Clinical evaluation

In evaluating a patient for otalgia, whether primary or secondary the following steps should be follow.

1. Detailed history must be obtained from the patient, as it relates to the location, duration, jaw locking, and trauma.

2. A comprehensive general or physical and clinical examination of ear, nose and throat is done. Emphasis should be laid on palpation of TMJ and surrounding structures, muscles of mastication and bone. Jaw movement and deviations are also noted. The diagnosis of pain-related TMD is made on history and physical examination findings alone [32].

3. Investigation that should be done are audiological testing, which comprises pure tone audiometry and tympanometry. Magnetic resonance imaging (MRI) should be carried out under certain conditions. Usually, the hearing may be normal and the absence of diseases in the middle or inner ear.

4. Treatment of otalgia associated with TMD should be based on:

a. Conservative management (first-line): by applying any of the following, depending on findings

i. Occlusal splints (bite guards). This is to reduce joint loading and bruxism.

ii. Physical therapy, like TMJ exercises, postural correction.

iii. Pharmacologic: Non-steroidal anti-inflammatory drugs (NSAIDs), muscle relaxants, low-dose tricyclic antidepressants.

iv. Cognitive behavioral therapy (CBT): Stress and pain management.

v. Dietary modifications like a Soft diet, avoiding chewing gum.

b. Advanced management:

i. Trigger point injections or botulinum toxin for myofascial pain.

ii. TMJ arthrocentesis or surgery (rarely needed).

c. For tinnitus, the following measures should be applied

i. Somatosensory tinnitus modulation techniques: for example, jaw exercises.

ii. Sound therapy or tinnitus retraining therapy (TRT) if persistent.

5. Vertigo and temporomandibular disorder

Vertigo is a subjective sensation of imbalance where a patient feels like either he/she or the environment is moving when it is not. It is a specific type of dizziness that can significantly impact balance and make everyday tasks difficult.

5.1 The possible mechanisms through which a patient with TMD may have vertigo are as follows

i. *Anatomical proximity:* The TMJ is very close to the inner ear and vestibular apparatus. With inflammation or malfunction in the TMJ, it can affect nearby structures through mechanical or inflammatory means [27].

ii. *Auriculotemporal nerve irritation:* This nerve supplies the TMJ and parts of the external ear and may affect balance perception if irritated.

iii. *Tensor veli palatini and tensor tympani muscle dysfunction:* These muscles, innervated by the mandibular nerve (V3), are involved in auditory tube and middle ear function. Also, muscle hyperactivity or spasm due to TMD can impair Eustachian tube function, causing pressure changes and dizziness [31].

iv. *Cervicogenic components:* TMD is often associated with cervical spine abnormality (especially C1–C3), which may contribute to dizziness *via* proprioceptive disturbances.

5.2 Clinical presentation

i. *Prevalence*: Studies suggest that up to 40.8% of TMD patients report dizziness or vertigo [32].

ii. *Symptoms overlap*: TMD-related vertigo is often associated with ear fullness, tinnitus, headache, and neck pain.

5.3 Diagnosis

This is based on the history, general or physical and clinical examination with emphasis on TMJ palpation for pain, clicking, or crepitus. Also, evaluation of associated muscle tenderness (masseter, temporalis and sternocleidomastoid).

The following test should be carried out:

i. *Otologic assessment*: This will rule out vestibular pathologies (e.g., BPPV and Meniere's disease). In addition, the audiometry and vestibular function tests should be carried out.

ii. *Imaging*: TMJ MRI or cone beam computed tomography (CBCT) to assess joint structure and disc displacement.

5.4 Treatment usually will consist of the following steps

a. *Conservative TMD treatments*:

i. Occlusal splints.

ii. Physical therapy for jaw and neck.

iii. Non-steroidal anti-inflammatory drugs (NSAIDs) and muscle relaxants.

iv. Stress management and cognitive behavioral therapy.

b. *Vestibular therapy*:

i. For persistent vertigo symptoms, vestibular rehabilitation exercises may help.

c. *Multidisciplinary approach*:

i. Collaboration between dentists, ENT specialists, neurologists, and physical therapists is often needed.

6. Ear fullness and temporomandibular disorders

Ear fullness — this is the sensation of pressure, blockage, or "stuffiness" in the ear without actual hearing loss or any fluid collection. — It is a common Otological symptom that may be linked not only to ear-related conditions (like Eustachian tube dysfunction) but also to temporomandibular disorders (TMD).

6.1 Causes of ear fullness

Dalla-Bona et al. show that their data clearly suggest a link between aural fullness and TMD. It is not clear how TMD causes aural fullness, although it has been proposed that TMD patients with a clenching habit might have dysfunctional masticatory muscles and tensor tympani muscles, leading to aural fullness [44]. Cox, in his study, reported that ear fullness was experienced by 13.5% of TMD and 4.7% of non-TMD patients [RR = 2.87] [45]. In the study done by Youngxin et al. [46], Aural fullness was completely resolved or significantly improved in 67 and 34 patients, respectively, following treatments aimed at improving TMD, with a combined effectiveness of 90.2% (101/112)

The temporomandibular joint is located very close to the ear canal and middle ear structures. Dysfunction in this joint or surrounding muscles can lead to symptoms perceived in the ear due to:

i. *Anatomical proximity:* The TMJ lies just anterior to the external auditory canal.

ii. *Shared nerve supply:* The auriculotemporal nerve (branch of the mandibular nerve, CN V3) innervates both the TMJ and parts of the external and middle ear.

iii. *Muscle tension/referral:* Spasm or tension in masticatory muscles (especially the medial pterygoid and tensor veli palatini) may refer sensations to the ear (**Table 1**).

S/N	Symptoms	Proposed mechanisms	Clinical test	Treatment
1	Hearing loss	1. Eustachian tube dysfunction—muscle tension and hyperactivity 2. Inflammation, swelling, and compression—may affect middle ear due to proximity 3. Shared neural pathways (trigeminal nerve)—affecting the TMJ and auditory structures 4. Direct impact on the middle ear structure—through ligament and muscle attachment to the ossicles	1. Pure tone audiometry 2. Tympanometry 3. Computerized tomography scan	1. Conservative 2. Occlusal splint 3. Physical therapy 4. NSAIDs 5. Cognitive behavioral therapy 6. Myofunctional therapy
2	Otalgia	1. Shared neural pathways—Mandibular division of trigeminal nerve 2. Inflammation, swelling and compression 3. Myofascial pain referral	1. Pure tone audiometry 2. Tympanometry 3. Magnetic resonance image (MRI)	1. Conservative 2. Occlusal splint 3. Physical therapy 4. NSAID 5. Cognitive behavioral therapy 6. Myofunctional therapy 7. Dietary modifications
3	Tinnitus	1. Muscle hyperactivity 2. TMJ-middle ear direct contact 3. Stimulation of the somatosensory system	1. Pure tone audiometry 2. Tympanometry 3. Magnetic resonance image	
4	Vertigo	1. Anatomical proximity and direct contact 2. Auriculotemporal nerve irritation 3. Muscle dysfunction 4. Muscle hyperactive and spam 5. Cervicogenic components	1. Pure tone audiometry 2. Tympanometry 3. Magnetic resonance image	Conservative treatment i. Occlusal splints ii. Physical therapy for jaw and neck. iii. NSAIDs, muscle relaxants. iv. Stress management and behavioral therapy. *Vestibular therapy*: i. For persistent vertigo symptoms, vestibular rehabilitation exercises may help. *Multidisciplinary approach* (collaboration between dentists, ENT specialists, neurologists, and physical therapists is often needed).

S/N	Symptoms	Proposed mechanisms	Clinical test	Treatment
5	Ear fullness	i. *Anatomical proximity:* The TMJ lies to the external auditory canal. ii. *Shared nerve supply:* The auriculotemporal nerve (branch of the mandibular nerve) iii. *Muscle tension/referral:* Spasm or tension in masticatory muscles	1. Pure tone audiometry 2. Tympanometry	

Table 1.
Summary table showing mechanisms of TMD presentation, tests and treatment.

7. Conclusion

Temporomandibular disorders refers to a group of conditions affecting the temporomandibular joint (TMJ), masticatory muscles, and associated structures. The most frequent otological manifestations in relation to temporomandibular disorder (TMD) identified are: hearing loss, otalgia, tinnitus, ear fullness, and vertigo. Proposed theories that led to each of the symptoms were highlighted. Adequate history and proper clinical examination with appropriate investigations are very useful in the diagnosis of this condition and will assist in early recognition of ENT complaints. A multidisciplinary approach (ENT, Dentists, Physiotherapy and Oral and Maxillofacial) is therefore recommended in the management. Usually, most of the affected individuals normally respond to conservative treatment, physical therapy and analgesics. There is a need for more studies to further reveal the association between temporomandibular disorders and neuro-otologic manifestations.

Acknowledgements

I wish to thank my colleagues for the encouragement given during the preparation of this work.

Funding

This work is self-sponsored.

Conflict of interest

The authors declare no conflict of interest.

DOI: http://dx.doi.org/10.5772/intechopen.1012298

Author details

Toye Gabriel Olajide[1]*, Oyebanji Anthony Olajuyin[2], Atilade Waheed Adegbiji[1] and Segun Mathew Agboola[3]

1 Department of Otorhinolaryngology, Afe Babalola University, Ado Ekiti, Nigeria

2 Department of Otorhinolaryngology, Ekiti State University Teaching Hospital, Ado Ekiti, Nigeria

3 Department of Family Medicine, Federal Teaching Hospital, Ido Ekiti and Afe Babalola University, Ado Ekiti, Nigeria

*Address all correspondence to: olajiddetg@abuad.edu.ng

References

[1] Shaffer SM, Brismee JM, Sizer PS, Courtney CA. Temporomandibular disorders. Part 1: Anatomy and examination/diagnosis. The Journal of Manual & Manipulative Therapy. 2014;**22**(1):2-12

[2] Kusdra PM, Stechman-Neto J, Cavalcante-Leao BL, et al. Relationship between otological symptoms and TMD. The International Tinnitus Journal. 2018;**22**:30-34

[3] Skog C, Fjellner J, Ekberg E, et al. Tinnitus as a comorbidity to temporomandibular disorders—A systematic review. Journal of Oral Rehabilitation. 2019;**46**:87-99

[4] Farella MA, Michelotti A, Bocchino T, et al. Effects of orthognathic surgery for class III malocclusion on signs and symptoms of temporomandibular disorders and on pressure pain thresholds of the jaw muscles. International Journal of Oral and Maxillofacial Surgery. 2007;**2**:101-110

[5] Leeuw R. Orofacial Pain: Guideliness for Assessment Diagnosis and Management. USA: Quintessence Publishing; 2008. p. 5

[6] Sharma S, Gupta DS, Pal US, et al. Etiological factors of temporomandibular joint disorders. National Journal of Maxillofacial Surgery. 2011;**2**:116-119

[7] Caria PHF, Faria RJA, de Faria CRS, et al. Efficiency of occlusal splints on police officers with TMD. Brazilian Journal of Oral Sciences. 2014;**13**:292-296

[8] Stepan L, Shaw CKL, Oue S. Temporomandibular disorder in otolaryngology: Systematic review. The Journal of Laryngology and Otology. 2017;**131**:S50-S56

[9] Bagis B, Ayaz EA, Turgut S, Durkan R, Özcan M. Gender difference in prevalence of signs and symptoms of temporomandibular joint disorders: A retrospective study on 243 consecutive patients. International Journal of Medical Sciences. 2012;**9**(7):539-544

[10] Barreto DC, Barbosa ARC, Frizzo ACF. Relação entre disfunção temporomandibular e alterações auditivas. Revista CEFAC. 2010;**12**(6):1067-1076

[11] Pita MS, Ribeiro AB, Zuim PRJ, Garcia AR. Sintomas auditivose desordens temporomandibulares. Revista Odontológica de Araçatuba. 2010;**31**(1):38-45

[12] de Felício CM, Faria TG, da Silva MAMR, de Aquino AMCM, Junqueira CA. Desordem temporomandibular: Relações entre sintomas otológicos e orofaciais. Revista Brasileira de Oto-Rino-Laringologia. 2004;**70**(6):786-793

[13] Fernández-de-las-Peñas C, Ge HY, Cuadrado ML, Madeleine P, Pareja JA, Arendt-Nielsen L. Bilateral pressure pain sensitivity mapping of the temporalis muscle in chronic tension-type headache. Headache. 2008;**48**(7):1067-1075

[14] Ramírez LM, Ballesteros LE, Sandoval GP. Síntomas óticos referidos en desórdenes temporomandibulares. Relación con músculos masticatorios. Revista Médica de Chile. 2007;**135**(12): 1582-1590

[15] Tuz HH, Onder EM, Kisnisci RS. Prevalence of otogenic complaints

in patients with temporomandibular disorder. American Journal of Orthodontics and Dentofacial Orthopedics. 2003;**123**:620-623

[16] Keersmaekers K, De Boever JA, Van Den Berghe L. Otalgia in patients with temporomandibular disorders. The Journal of Prosthetic Dentistry. 1996;**75**:72-76

[17] Gonçalves DA, Camparis CM, Speciali JG, et al. Temporomandibular disorders are differentially associated with headache diagnoses: A controlled study. The Clinical Journal of Pain. 2011;**27**(7):611-615

[18] Lim PF, Smith S, Bhalang K, et al. Development of temporomandibular disorders is associated with greater bodily pain experience. The Clinical Journal of Pain. 2010;**26**(2):116-120

[19] Maixner W, Diatchenko L, Dubner R, et al. Orofacial pain prospective evaluation and risk assessment study—The OPPERA study. The Journal of Pain. 2011;**12**(11 suppl):T4-T11.e1-2

[20] Nichthauser B, Andrade F, Buarque WA, Rodrigues MFR, Buarque LL, Moura LG. Sintomas otológicos em pacientes com disfunção temporomandibular tratados com aparelhos oclusais lisos e planos. Revista Portuguesa de Estomatologia, Medicina Dentária e Cirurgia Maxilofacial. 2012;**53**(4):213-220

[21] Parker WS, Chole RA. Tinnitus, vertigo, and temporomandibular disorders. American Journal of Orthodontics and Dentofacial Orthopedics. 1995;**107**:153-158

[22] Wright EF. Otological symptom improvement through TMD therapy. Quintessence International. 2007;**38**(9):e564-e571

[23] Manfredini D, Bucci MB, Nardini LG. The diagnostic process for temporomandibular disorders. Stomatologija. 2007;**9**:35-39

[24] Mohammed RD. The otological manifestation of temporomandibular disorders. Mustansiriya Medical Journal. 2013;**12**(1):45-48

[25] Çebi AT. Presence of tinnitus and tinnitus-related hearing loss in temporomandibular disorders. Cranio: the Journal of Craniomandibular Practice. 2020;**41**(2):173-177

[26] Kitsoulis P, Marini A, Iliou K, et al. Signs and symptoms of temporomandibular joint disorders related to the degree of mouth opening and hearing loss. BMC Ear, Nose and Throat Disorders. 2011;**11**:5

[27] Effat KG. Otological symptoms and audiometric findings in patients with temporomandibular disorders: Costen's syndrome revisited. The Journal of Laryngology and Otology. 2016;**130**(12):1137-1141

[28] Berke J. TMJ-Related Hearing Loss. Available from: https://www.verywellhealth.com/temporomandibular-joint-disorder-1046500#toc-treatment-for-tmj-and-hearing-loss [Accessed: June 26, 2025]

[29] Ash MM, Ash CM, Ash JL, Ash GM. Current concepts of the relationship and management of temporomandibular disorders and auditory symproms. The Journal of the Michigan Dental Association. 1990;**72**(11-12):550-555

[30] Schames J, Schames M, King E, Ulansey S, Boyd J, Schames E. Trigeminal pharyngioplasty: Treatment of the forgotten accessory muscles of mastication which are associated with orofacial pain and ear symptomatology.

American Journal of Pain Management. 2002;**12**:102-112

[31] Malkin DP. The role of TMD dysfunction in the etiology of middle ear diseases. International Journal of Orthodontics. 1987;**25**:20-21

[32] Porto De Toledo I, Stefani FM, Porporatti AL, et al. Prevalence of otologic signs and symptoms in adult patientswith temporomandibular disorders: A systematic review and meta-analysis. Clinical Oral Investigations. 2017;**21**:597-605

[33] Vass Z, Shore SE, Nuttall AL, Miller JM. Direct evidence of trigeminal innervation of the cochlear blood vessels. Neuroscience. 1998;**84**(2):559-567

[34] Temporomandibular Joint (TMJ) Disorder and Hearing Loss. Available from: https://www.miracle-ear.com/blog-news/tmj-and-hearing-lossloss#:~:text=How%20can%20TMJ%20disorder%20affect%20your%20hearing?,and%20make%20it%20more%20difficult%20to%20hear [Accessed: June 26, 2025]

[35] Tinnitus and TMD: The Link between the Two Disorders. Available from: https://www.midwestheadaches.com/patient-education/tinnitus-and-tmd-the-linkbetween-the-two-disorders/ [Accessed: June 26, 2025]

[36] Tuz HH, Onder EM, Kisnisci RS. Prevalence of otologic complaints in patients with temporomandibular disorder. American Journal of Orthodontics and Dentofacial Orthopedics. 2003;**123**(6):620-623

[37] Solano N, Gutierrez P, Peraza A, Rodriguez D, Barrios O, Gutierrez V. Otological symptoms and temporomandibular disorders: Is it possible? Acta Scientific Otolaryngology Special Issue. 2021;**1**:13-16

[38] Israel HA, Davila LJ. The essential role of the otolaryngologist in the diagnosis and management of temporomandibular joint and chronic oral, head, and facial pain disorders. Otolaryngologic Clinics of North America. 2014;**47**(2):301-331

[39] Morais AA, Gil D. Tinnitus in individuals without hearing loss and its relationship with temporomandibular dysfunction. Brazilian Journal of Otorhinolaryngology. 2012;**78**(2):59-65

[40] Miller DA, Wyrwa EB. Ear pain: A dental dilemma. Compendium. 1992;**13**(8):676-684

[41] Salvetti G, Manfredini D, Barsotti S, Bosco M. Otologic symptoms in temporomandibular disorders patients: Is there evidence of an association-relationship? Minerva Stomatologica. 2006;**55**:627-637

[42] Wright EF, North SL. Management and treatment of temporomandibular disorders: A clinical perspective. Journal of Manual & Manipulative Therapy. 2009;**17**(4):247-254

[43] Klasser GD, Reyes MR. Orofacial Pain: Guidelines for Assessment, Diagnosis, and Management (AAOP The American Academy of Orofacial Pain). 6th ed. [Accessed June 26, 2025]

[44] Dalla-Bona D, Shackleton T, Clark G, Ram S. Unilateral ear fullness and temporary hearing loss diagnosed and successfully managed as a temporomandibular disorder: A case report. Journal of the American Dental Association (1939). 2015;**146**(3):192-194

[45] Cox KW. Temporomandibular disorder and new oral symptoms.

Archives of Otolaryngology – Head & Neck Surgery. 2008;**134**(4):389-393

[46] Youngxin P. Temporomandibular joint disorders as a cause of aural fullness. Clinical and Experimental Otorhinolaryngology. 2017;**10**(3):236-240

Chapter 5

Temporomandibular Joint Disorders in Otology: The Anatomical Ear-TMJ Connection

Bilal Hasan

Abstract

The temporomandibular joint (TMJ) and the ear exhibit a close anatomical and functional relationship, often complicating the diagnosis of otalgia (ear pain). A substantial number of patients reporting ear pain in clinical settings are found to have temporomandibular (TMJ) disorders as the underlying cause. This chapter examines the interplay between TMJ dysfunction and otalgia, focusing on shared embryological development, neurovascular pathways, and biomechanical connections that facilitate referred pain between these regions. Clinically, otalgia without primary otological pathology necessitates a systematic evaluation of the TMJ. Key diagnostic steps include assessing joint mobility, palpating trigger points, and excluding dental or musculoskeletal origins. The overlapping innervation by the trigeminal (CN V), facial (CN VII), glossopharyngeal (CN IX), and greater auricular (C2–C3) nerves provides a physiological basis for pain referral. Imaging studies further demonstrate the proximity of the TMJ to the external auditory canal and middle ear structures, reinforcing their clinical association. Understanding these mechanisms is critical for accurate diagnosis and management. Ear, nose, and throat (ENT) specialists must integrate TMJ assessment into otalgia workups to avoid unnecessary interventions, while collaboration with dental professionals can optimize treatment for TMJ-related ear symptoms. This synthesis of anatomical, neurological, and clinical perspectives aims to enhance diagnostic precision and therapeutic outcomes for patients with otalgia of non-otogenic origin.

Keywords: TMJ, otology, ear, temporal, otosurgery, otalgia

1. Introduction

The temporomandibular joint (TMJ) is a bilateral synovial joint located between the temporal bone of the skull above and the mandible below. The joint derives from these two bones. This joint is unique in being a bilateral joint functioning as a single unit, with the right and left joints working together and not operating as a single functional unit.

Diagnosing otalgia remains a frequent challenge in ENT clinics. One of the major challenges facing ear, nose, and throat (ENT) doctors in clinics is diagnosing the causes of pain, especially otalgia. To uncover these causes, the doctor relies on investigations, including otoscopy of the external auditory canal, tympanic membrane, and middle ear, searching for trauma, abrasions, tumors, inflammation, redness, or foreign bodies in the apparent hearing tract, as well as perforations, inflammation, otorrhea, redness, or congestion in the tympanic membrane. This is termed primary otalgia, indicating that the source of the pain is otologic. However, when no pathological indications are found during endoscopy, the ENT specialist is then challenged to identify the source of secondary otalgia, where the pain originates outside the ear.

Therefore, one of the essential tasks of the ENT doctor during the examination is to conduct a thorough examination of the ear, nose, pharynx, and neck, as the pain in the ear may be referred from another anatomical area. For instance, pharyngitis and tonsillitis can cause this type of pain, especially about a week after surgeries to remove the tonsils or to scrape oropharyngeal tumors, as well as inflammation and lesions of the sinuses and their surgeries, and diseases and lesions of the neck and esophagus. However, the most common causes of otalgia are maxillary and dental lesions, as most patients visiting ENT clinics due to ear pain are those with TMJ disorders, constituting over 50% of patients who complain of otalgia. This highlights the critical need for a detailed clinical examination in the otology clinic to differentiate between primary ear pathology and referred TMJ-related pain. We will discuss ear diseases and both benign and malignant tumors that affect the function of the temporomandibular joint and cause pain in the two organs, as well as discuss surgical procedures on the ear and their complications that cause disturbances in the function of the temporomandibular joint [1].

2. TMJ patient examination in the otology clinic

Most otalgia is referred pain from outside the ear. To contextualize, this ear pain resulting from an internal source is more acute and pronounced, especially in cases of external auditory canal problems such as inflammation, swelling, narrowing, foreign bodies in the canal, wounds, or irritation caused by excessive stress on the nerves in the external auditory canal.

A key diagnostic differentiator is pain severity. Middle ear injuries, such as a ruptured eardrum due to trauma, and acute otitis media, especially in children, are often intolerable, in addition to ear injuries resulting from falls, traffic accidents, or penetrating injuries to the ear. Whereas, chronic conditions like purulent otitis media, cholesteatoma, and benign or malignant tumors in their early and middle stages present milder discomfort. In all simple and complex otosurgeries, otalgia caused by otosurgery, from cosmetic surgery of the auricle to ossiculoplasty to mastoid surgery to inner ear surgery such as cochlear implantation, requires pain relief that can sometimes reach central pain relievers in larger surgeries. Studies indicate that patients with temporomandibular joint disorder suffer from ear infirmary, with 85% complaining of ear symptoms, including otalgia (64%), dizziness (42%), and muffling (30%) [2]. Most patients suffering from problems of malocclusion, issues with molars, and even gum problems, as well as temporomandibular joint problems, visit an otology clinic due to severe ear pain. Patients often describe the pain as sharp, needle-like sensations within the ear, and they may hear popping or buzzing sounds. Patients often do not realize that the complaint is related to the TMJ and not the ear, to the extent that they often present with a hand over the ear due to perceived ear pain. The first procedure that an ENT doctor must perform is to examine the ear with an endoscope and check the integrity of the external auditory canal and the eardrum, as well as try to look for any density (**Figure 1**), whether liquid or solid, in the middle ear through the transparency of the eardrum. The examiner also moves the auricle with their hand to ensure that the patient does not experience any pain (**Figure 2**). When the examining doctor does not find any pathological findings in the patient, this indicates that the ear pain is not primary but rather secondary, reflecting from a nearby anatomical area. The examining doctor then proceeds to examine the nose with an endoscope to look for any signs of sinusitis or issues in the nasopharynx, and when there are no pathological signs, the examiner moves on to inspect the oral pharynx, mouth, and tonsils, checking for any ulcers present in the mucous membrane in the oral cavity. When there are no pathological signs, the doctor then examines the neck through palpation to search for any palpable masses. When an ENT doctor examines the ear, nose, sinuses, pharynx, oral cavity, and neck and finds no indicators, he should look for dental issues and ask the patient about their previous history of dental treatment at the dentist's office. The doctor examines the jaw joint by pressing on the anatomical point in front of and below the ear on both sides of the face using his index finger symmetrically. He asks the patient to move the temporomandibular joint by opening and closing their mouth forcefully several times. The patient will experience ear pain upon joint movement, confirming TMJ dysfunction as the source. Before ordering advanced tests such as computed tomography and auditory tests like audiometry and tympanometry, the ENT doctor must first assess TMJ's health to avoid unnecessary radiation exposure, costs, and inefficiency. These investigations can be requested when there is no issue with the temporomandibular joint to search for the source of the unknown problem. An otologist should be proficient in oral and jaw examination to distinguish TMJ-related otalgia from primary ear conditions, ensuring accurate diagnosis.

To better understand why TMJ disorders so often manifest with otologic symptoms, it is essential to explore the anatomical and physiological basis of the close relationship between the TMJ and the ear, as discussed below.

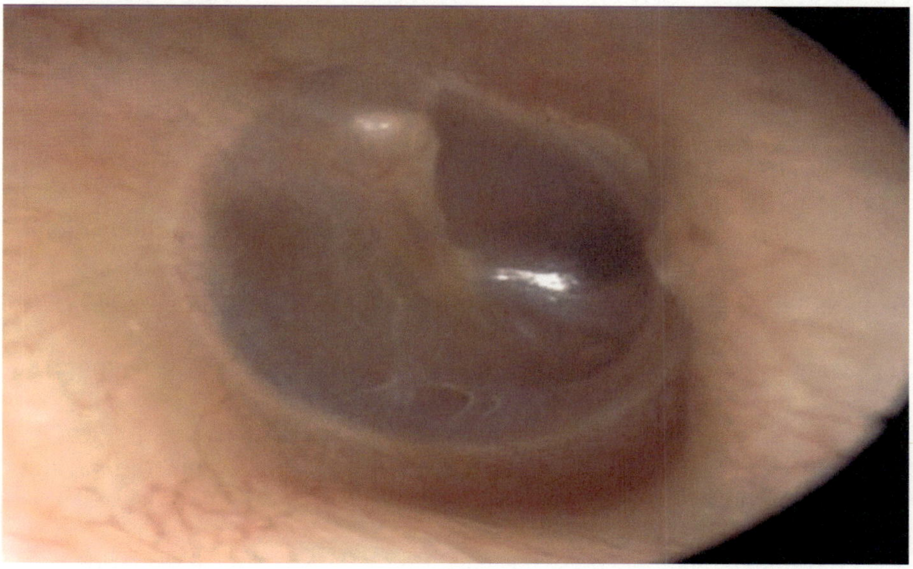

Figure 1.
Normal otoscopic view of the tympanic membrane, indicating no primary pathology.

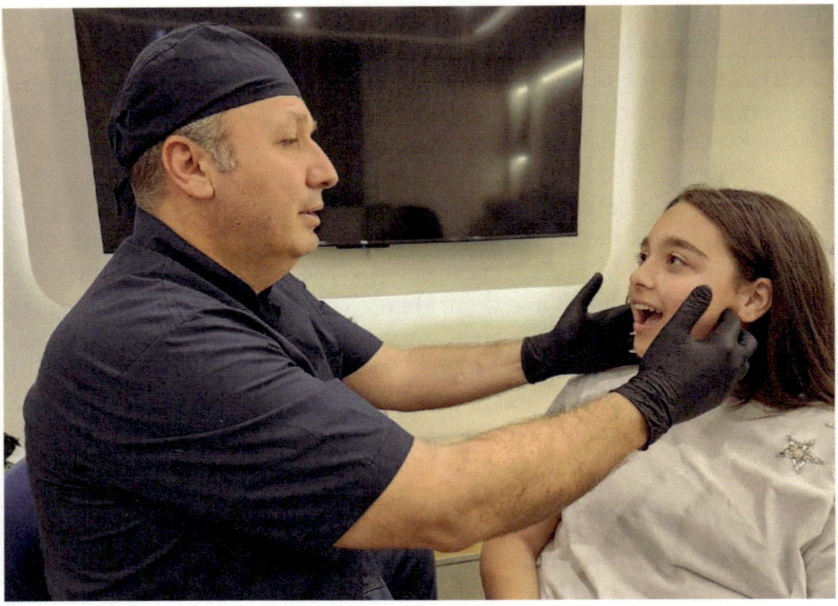

Figure 2.
Examination of the temporomandibular joint in the ENT clinic.

3. Causes of otalgia from TMJ

An important question and curiosity that comes to the minds of otology and dental doctors, as well as patients, is about the strange relationship between the jaw joint and the ear, to the point that the patient feels pain in their ear more than any other anatomical point. As a result of this recurring question, many researchers have conducted studies on this relationship and found answers [3]. Their findings highlight six key factors underpinning this relationship:

1. Embryonic development and morphological similarities of the ear and TMJ.

2. Positioning on a single bony surface very closely.

3. The common innervation between the ear and the temporomandibular joint.

4. The common blood supply between the ear and the temporomandibular joint.

5. The importance of the ligaments in the relationship between the temporal bone, the ear, and the temporomandibular joint.

6. The muscles covering and common between the temporal bone, the ear, and the temporomandibular joint.

To better understand how these mechanisms operate in clinical scenarios, it is helpful to examine each contributing factor individually.

3.1 Embryology

The first and most fundamental factor is embryonic development. During fetal growth, Meckel's cartilage forms in the mandibular process, with its tympanic and mandibular portions becoming fully developed by the 16th week. This cartilage gives rise to the auditory ossicles (malleus, incus, and stapes) and their supporting ligaments, playing a crucial role in facial structure organization during embryonic and fetal development. The mandibular primary growth center emerges in the 12th week within Meckel's cartilage, initiating intramembranous ossification of the mandible. After the 18th week, Meckel's cartilage gradually regresses and is eventually replaced by mandibular bone and secondary condylar cartilage during ossification. The temporal bone becomes visible by the 8–9th weeks, positioned superior to Meckel's cartilage distal end and the malleus-incus complex. Key developmental milestones include: zygomatic process ossification (8th week), medial disk thickening with concave contours (10th week), and articular fossa formation (11–12th weeks), which becomes consistently concave by the 12th week. The articular eminence and post-glenoid process develop after the 26th week [3]. As a remarkable hearing and balance organ, the ear develops from all three germ layers into three distinct anatomical regions: external, middle, and internal. Each section follows unique developmental pathways, with functional hearing beginning around 26 weeks of gestation. Developmental variations may lead to congenital anomalies [4]. This shared embryonic origin between middle ear components and the temporal bone may explain referred otalgia through the embryonic origin theory [3].

3.2 Anatomical proximity

While embryology explains their shared origins, the physical proximity of the TMJ and ear structures further amplifies this link.

Anatomically, the TMJ is shown in the box. The temporomandibular joint (TMJ), or jaw joint, is a synovial joint that allows the complex movements necessary for life. It is the joint between the condylar head of the mandible and the mandibular fossa of the temporal bone. This system is made up of the TMJ, teeth, and soft tissue, and it plays a role in breathing, eating, and speech [4].

The mandibular fossa (or glenoid fossa of the temporal bone) is a smooth, deep depression located on the inferolateral aspect of the temporal bone and consists of:

1. *Anterior articular portion*: Formed by the squamous temporal bone, articulating with the TMJ disc.

2. *Posterior nonarticular portion*: Composed of the tympanic part of the temporal bone.

The mandibular fossa contributes to the formation of the temporomandibular joint, along with the condylar process of the mandible and an intervening articular disc of the temporomandibular joint.

The jaw joint is placed on the surface of the hard temporal bone, and its proximity to the tympanic bone, which contains components of the middle ear, may explain the transfer of pain to the middle ear and the transmission of the sounds of joint movement, popping, and chewing due to sound transmission through the bone and the walls of the bony ear. We observe this bony connection in tympanic plate fractures in temporal bone trauma, where this injury often extends to the accompanying temporomandibular joint and causes injury along with the ear due to anatomical proximity [5]. Even any traumatic injury to the temporal bone or a concussion can negatively affect the temporomandibular joint—or vice versa—due to the close connection of the jaw joint with the temporal bone [6]. The individual may experience to have difficulty or limited joint movement and pain when chewing and speaking (**Figure 3**). This close anatomical relationship lays the groundwork for the complex neural interactions that follow.

3.3 Innervention

Beyond bony adjacency, the neurological overlap between the TMJ and ear plays an equally critical role. The transmission of pain from the temporomandibular joint to the ear involves multiple shared nerves.

From these nerves:

3.3.1 Trigeminal nerve (CN V)

The temporomandibular joint and trigeminal nerves are among the most vital facial structures. The TMJ disorders can affect several other head and neck regions when misaligned or otherwise impaired. Because the trigeminal nerve, which affects the TMJ, also affects a large portion of the face, ear, and neck, any dysfunction in this vital structure may result in head and face pain. The superior lateral surface of the auricle and most of the external auditory meatus (auriculotemporal branch), 70% of this 80% (cranial nerves), or more than half of the total input to our brain, is transmitted by the trigeminal nerve. With such a large amount of brain input, it must reach highly essential structures. The trigeminal nerve innervates: the teeth, the periodontal ligament, the joint that connects the teeth to the jaws, the muscles that move the jaw, and the muscle that tenses the eardrum. One of the branches of the trigeminal nerve

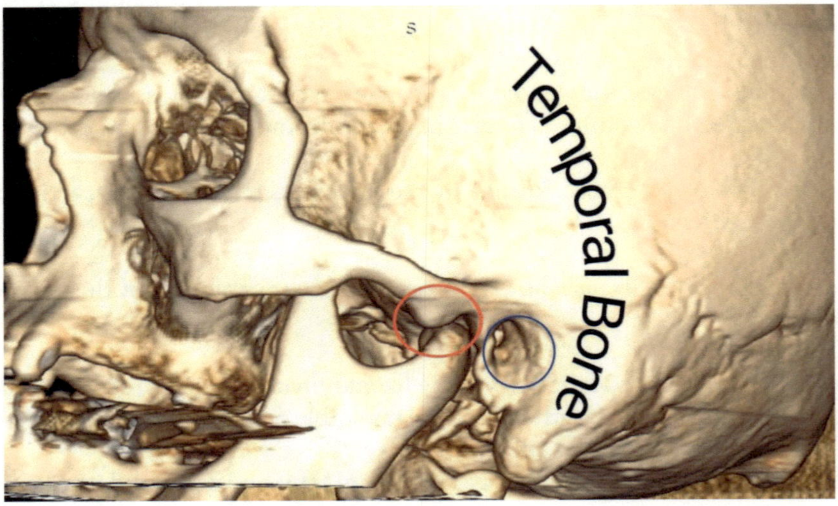

Figure 3.
3-dimensional computed tomography "3D CT" scan for the left side of the head. We see the large area of the temporal bone, and the temporomandibular joint (red circle) is located next to the external acoustic canal (blue circle).

DOI: http://dx.doi.org/10.5772/intechopen.1011695

is the third branch, which innervates the temporalis muscle and the digastric belly, closely associated with the ear. The mandibular nerve (CN V3) is the largest branch of the trigeminal nerve. The nerve exits the skull base through the foramen ovale. CN V3 is the only branch of the trigeminal nerve that has both sensory and motor components. The mandibular nerve receives sensory information from the lower third of the face, the floor of the mouth, the jaw, and the tongue. The motor root of CN V3 (portio minor) supplies the muscles of mastication (masseter, temporalis, pterygoids), the anterior digastric belly, and the mylohyoid [7].

3.3.2 Facial nerve (CN VII)

Marginal mandibular branch of the facial nerve: The facial nerve, also known as the seventh cranial nerve, plays a crucial role in controlling the muscles of the face. This nerve extends from the brain to the face, running within the ear and the temporal bone (**Figure 4**), reaching the jaw, and it provides motor commands to both the expressive muscles and sensory ability. The functions of the facial nerve include controlling a variety of functions, such as the movement of the muscles responsible for smiling, frowning, and other activities. Additionally, this nerve contributes to the sense of taste in the front part of the tongue.

3.3.2.1 Effects of facial nerve disorders on facial motor functions

When there is a disorder of the facial nerve, it can lead to weakness or paralysis of the facial muscles, negatively affecting facial expression and communication. Affected individuals may have difficulty smiling or performing other facial movements and may experience joint movement disturbances during chewing or speaking, impacting their daily lives. This means that any injury or disease affecting the nerve

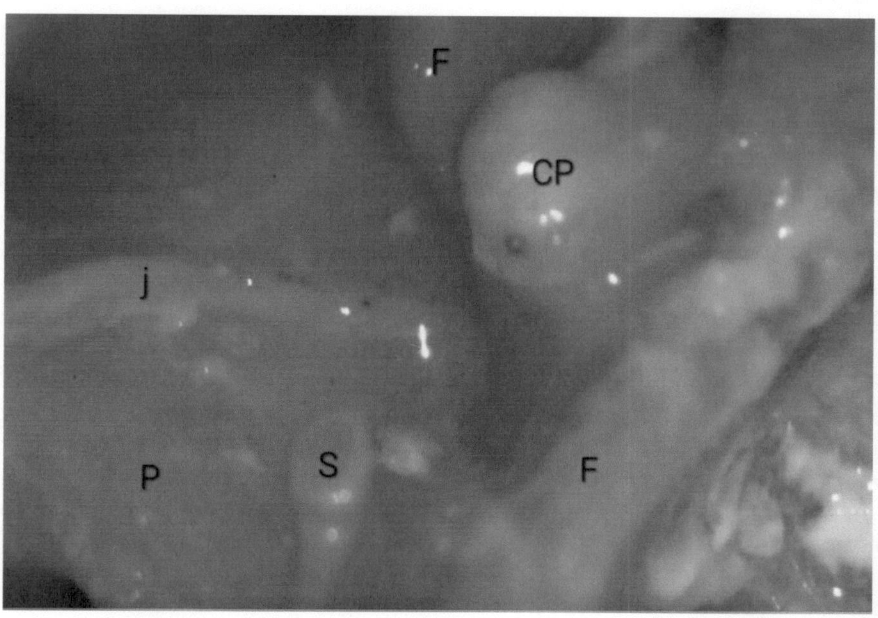

Figure 4.
A microscope view from the left middle ear shows the following: F: Facial nerve, S: Stapes, P: Promontory, CF: Cochleariform process, J: Jacobson nerve (Tympanic nerve).

structure in the ear will negatively affect the sensation or movement in the temporomandibular joint area [8]. The marginal mandibular branch of the facial nerve is closely related and strongly associated with the submandibular gland and the parotid gland. Therefore, any underlying For example, cholesteatoma tumors that penetrate the sheath of the facial nerve or facial nerve tumors in the internal auditory canal or the tympanic or temporal part, or chronic suppurative otitis media, transfer from the ear to these anatomical components, or their surgical intervention, can lead to damage in this branch and problems in the temporomandibular joint [9].

3.3.3 Glossopharyngeal nerve (CN IX)

Glossopharyngeal neuralgia (GPN) is a condition that causes pain in the throat, ear, and neck. The International Association for the Study of Pain (IASP) defines it as sudden, severe, short-lasting, and recurrent pain in the anatomical distribution of the glossopharyngeal nerve. It is described as a sharp, transient stabbing pain experienced in the ear, the base of the tongue, the tonsillar fossa, or under the angle of the jaw. However, the location of the pain can vary significantly and may involve overlap between the nerves that supply the face (trigeminal, vagus, facial) [10]. This is attributed to the interconnection of nerves in these anatomical areas where the glossopharyngeal nerve gives rise to the tympanic branch: Tympanic nerve (aka Jacobson's nerve)—carries parasympathetic fibers and eventually becomes the lesser petrosal nerve, exiting the skull via the foramen ovale and synapsing in the otic ganglion [11]. Many conditions can affect CN IX, some of which can impact the quality of life. These include—Glossopharyngeal Neuralgia (GPN)—sneezing, chewing, swallowing, and other activities that can trigger episodes of intense pain in your throat, the back of your tongue, or the middle ear. Concerns about future attacks can make eating difficult.

3.3.4 Greater auricular nerve (C2—C3)

The greater auricular nerve is a cutaneous branch of the cervical plexus that innervates the skin of the auricle as well as the skin over the parotid gland and mastoid process. The greater auricular nerve also supplies branches that innervate the deep layer of the parotid fascia. The great auricular nerve (GAN) originates from the cervical plexus at the levels of C2 and C3, supplying sensation to the skin overlying the lower aspect of the pinna and angle of the mandible. The GAN can be injured during many procedures in the head and neck, resulting in a significant negative impact on the patient's quality of life [12]. Some studies confirm the cases of communication between the greater auricular nerve and the marginal mandibular branch of the facial nerve, which explains the transmission of pain and sensation between the jaw and the ear as well [13].

Together, the intricate network of shared nerves between the TMJ and the ear provides a clear explanation for the referral of pain and sensory overlap, highlighting the complex neurological relationship underlying otalgia related to TMJ disorders. Beyond the intricate neural connections, the rich vascular supply to both the temporomandibular joint and the adjacent ear structures further emphasizes the close anatomical and functional relationship between these regions.

3.4 Blood supply

The temporomandibular joint is located in an anatomical area rich in blood vessels, and facial surgeons and otosurgeons need to have a good understanding of this anatomical region to avoid serious complications and excessive bleeding. The blood supply to the temporomandibular joint comes from the superficial temporal artery, the anterior tympanic artery, the deep temporal artery, the posterior auricular artery, the facial artery, the middle meningeal artery, and the maxillary artery along with their branches as the main sources of blood vessels for the lateral and medial temporomandibular joint [14]. Many of these vessels also contribute to the blood supply of the ear and the temporal region. The anterior tympanic artery, a branch of the maxillary artery, plays a vital role in supplying blood to the tympanic membrane, ear canal, and middle ear cavity. When this artery experiences compression, it can trigger a cascade of complex physiological consequences affecting ear health and function. During human fetal development, there is a wide connection across the tympanosquamosal fissure between the middle ear and the temporomandibular joint region. The anterior tympanic artery and its branches, as well as small venous vessels that are connected with the retrodiscal venous plexus, extend along the most lateral part of the fissure [15]. Compression of the maxillary artery can manifest through several distinctive symptoms:

- Ear pain (Otalgia): Reduced blood flow may cause discomfort ranging from mild aching to intense pain.

- Hearing loss: Compromised blood supply can lead to conductive hearing impairment.

- Tinnitus: Altered blood flow might produce phantom sounds like ringing or buzzing, discomfort in the temporomandibular joint area, and difficulty chewing.

The common conditions and disorders that affect the maxillary artery: Conditions that may affect your maxillary artery include:

- Temporal arteritis (giant cell arteritis), inflammation of your arteries.

- Aneurysm, a stretched-out artery wall.

- Pseudoaneurysm, an injured artery wall.

Signs or symptoms of conditions that affect the maxillary artery include:

A swollen area in front of the ear, a pulsing lump in front of the ear, fever, headaches, double vision, pain in the TMJ or jaw, and pain while chewing. One of the diseases of these arteries is called temporal arteritis. Common symptoms between the jaw and the temporal area in temporal arteritis include: headache and tenderness in both temples, jaw pain when chewing or opening the mouth widely, and ear pain and tenderness in the temporal area. In addition, other oral symptoms include: jaw claudication, trismus, odontogenic pain, dysphagia, dysarthria, submandibular mass, hypoesthesia of the chin (chin numbness), macroglossia, glossitis, lip necrosis, tongue necrosis, and facial swelling [16]. These clinical manifestations highlight the significant impact of TMJ-related vascular disorders, particularly when involving the maxillary or anterior tympanic arteries. However, vascular compromise is not the sole link between TMJ dysfunction to otologic symptoms. A deeper understanding of the ligamental and structural pathways that traverse this region further elucidates these complex interactions.

3.5 Ligamental linkages

In addition to its rich vascular network, the TMJ region is anatomically interlinked with several neurovascular and ligamentous structures *via* specialized bony fissures, which also serve as pathways for critical arteries and nerves. The temporomandibular joint (TMJ) is anatomically formed between the mandibular condyle and the glenoid fossa of the temporal bone. The mandibular fossa (also called the glenoid fossa of the temporal bone) consists of two distinct anatomical regions: an anterior articular area formed by the temporal squama and a posterior nonarticular area formed by the tympanic plate. The precise boundary between the medial aspect of the articular fossa and the tympanic plate corresponds to the squamotympanic fissure, which serves as the specific attachment site for the articular capsule of the TMJ. At the medial termination of the squamotympanic fissure, the thin anterolateral edge of the tegmen tympani (a specialized part of the petrous segment of the temporal bone that forms the precise roof of the mastoid antrum) divides this fissure into two distinct anatomical subdivisions: the petrotympanic fissure and the petrosquamous fissure. The petrosquamous fissure itself has two anatomical components: a descending portion that courses anteriorly in a nearly parallel orientation to the petrotympanic fissure, and an ascending portion that serves as the anatomical divider between the temporal and sphenoid bones. These three fissures (squamotympanic, petrotympanic, and petrosquamous) maintain an intimate anatomical relationship with the TMJ (**Figure 5**).

Three clinically significant anatomical structures pass through these fissures:

1. The anterior malleolar ligament.

2. The anterior tympanic artery.

3. The chorda tympani nerve.

The anterior ligament of the malleus represents one of the three supporting ligaments of the auditory ossicles (the other two being the lateral and superior ligaments). This ligament originates from both the neck and the anterior process of the malleus. Its main medial portion courses through the petrotympanic fissure to terminate either at the spine of the sphenoid bone or as a continuation into the sphenomandibular ligament. Some anatomical authorities classify the segment between the sphenoid spine and malleus as the tympanic portion of the sphenomandibular ligament. The ligament's thinner lateral portion also traverses the same fissure but undergoes a characteristic morphological transformation, gradually broadening into a triangular configuration before its final insertion at both the internal superior margin of the TMJ disc and the joint capsule. This complex anatomical structure has received multiple designations in the medical literature:

- Initially identified by Rees as the "disco-malleolar band" in fetal specimens.

- Later characterized by Pinto as a "tiny ligament" in adult anatomy.

- Currently termed the disco-malleolar ligament.

- Also referred to as the tympanomandibular ligament or mandibular malleolar ligament.

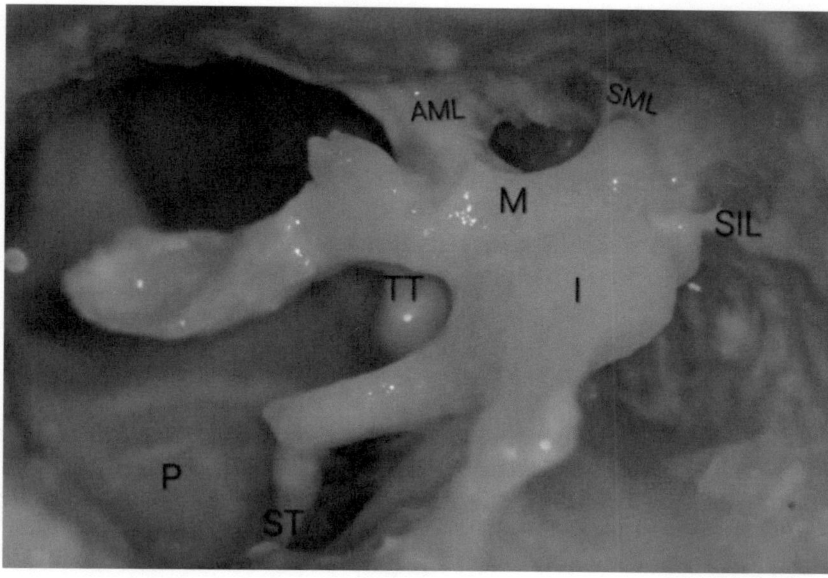

Figure 5.
A microscope view of the left middle ear showing the following: AML: anterior malleolar ligament, SML: superior malleolar ligament, SIL: superior incudal ligament, M: malleus, I: incus, TT: Tensor Tympani, ST: stapedius muscle, P: promontory.

This structure must be carefully distinguished from the tympanic portion of the sphenomandibular ligament. Research by Komori et al. has demonstrated that movement of the TMJ capsule and disc can mechanically influence the ossicular chain in the middle ear. Pathological changes in this ligament may contribute to various otologic symptoms, and iatrogenic displacement during TMJ surgery can potentially lead to serious otologic complications (though such occurrences are rare). The three temporal bone fissures (squamotympanic, petrotympanic, and petrosquamous) maintain close anatomical relationships with both the mandibular fossa and the TMJ. The important anatomical structures traversing these fissures include:

1. The anterior malleolar (or disco-malleolar) ligament.

2. The anterior tympanic artery.

3. The chorda tympani nerve.

The precise anatomical relationships between these structures and the fissures (particularly the petrotympanic fissure), as well as their connections to the TMJ, can give rise to various clinical symptoms affecting the ear, the tongue, and the adjacent anatomical regions. These symptoms may include: pain, tinnitus, hearing loss, and vertigo. When resulting from TMJ dysfunction, this symptom complex has been historically termed temporomandibular joint syndrome or Costen Syndrome. Costen originally attributed these symptoms specifically to dental malocclusion. Contemporary understanding recognizes a broader range of potential etiological factors:

- Degenerative changes related to aging.

- Traumatic injuries.

- Iatrogenic factors from therapeutic interventions.
- Other pathophysiological mechanisms affecting TMJ function.

While the term Costen's Syndrome has fallen out of clinical use due to the disproven nature of Costen's original anatomical explanations, it retains historical significance in the medical literature [17]. The anatomical fissures and ligamentous structures of the TMJ are closely interrelated with the muscular system that governs mandibular motion, further amplifying the impact of TMJ dysfunction on adjacent regions such as the ear and neck.

3.6 Temporal-ear-TMJ muscular interface

The muscles associated with the temporomandibular joint, also known as the masticatory muscles, are characterized by their connection to the jaw, the temporal bone, and the ear. The muscles of mastication can be divided into the primary muscles and secondary or accessory muscles.

- The primary muscles include: the masseter, temporalis, lateral pterygoid, and medial pterygoid.
- The secondary or accessory muscles are: the buccinator; suprahyoid muscles (digastric muscle, mylohyoid muscle, and geniohyoid muscle); and the infrahyoid muscles (the sternohyoid, sternothyroid, thyrohyoid, and omohyoid muscle) (**Figure 6**).

These muscles have a common blood supply and shared innervation. The temporalis muscle is a broad muscle that occupies most of the temporal fossa. Its origin point spans the entire surface of the fossa below the temporal line and the ear. Additionally, some fibers originate from the temporal fascia as well. The temporalis muscle is divided into the anterior and posterior parts. The anterior fibers run inferiorly, in an almost vertical direction, while its posterior fibers are directed almost horizontally. Both anterior and posterior fibers converge onto a narrow tendon that runs medial to the zygomatic arch. The tendon inserts onto the apex and medial surface of the coronoid process of the mandible. It is supplied by the deep temporal nerve, which is a branch from the anterior division of the mandibular nerve. The blood supply of the temporalis muscle is from the deep temporal part of the maxillary artery and the middle temporal branches of the superficial temporal artery.

- Masseter: It is a rectangular muscle that covers most of the lateral aspect of the ramus. It consists of three layers that blend anteriorly: the superficial layer, intermediate layer, and deep layer. The fibers of the muscle originate from the inferior zygomatic arch and the anterior two-thirds of the zygomatic arch, with a connection to the posterior aspect of the zygomatic bone. The fibers converge inferiorly, forming a tendon that inserts at the outer surface of the mandibular ramus and the coronoid process of the mandible. It is innervated by the mandibular division of the trigeminal nerve. Its blood supply is derived from the masseteric artery, which emerges from the maxillary artery.
- The digastric muscle is implicated as the source of pain in bruxism, or the habit of clenching teeth. Myofunctional physiotherapy or speech therapy can reduce

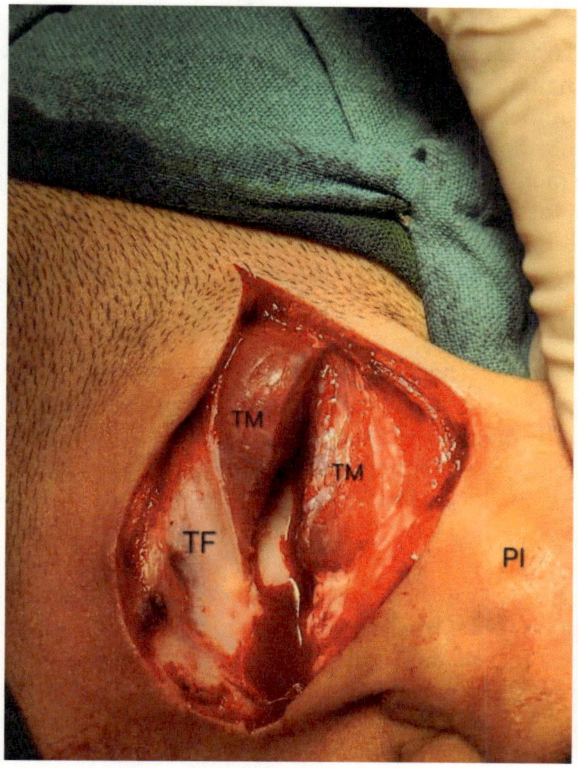

Figure 6.
Surgical incision created in the right ear pavilion: a section appears in the temporal muscle (TM) and the temporal fascia (TF), PI: Pinna.

the muscle's electrical activity and reduce pain during jaw movement. The digastric muscle's posterior portion is occasionally the site of a Citelli's abscess, a rare complication of otitis media. Management is surgical. Digastric muscle trigger points may cause referred pain in the teeth [18]. The blood supply and common innervation, as well as the proximity between these muscles and the ear, can lead to the transmission of some diseases from the ear or the jaw joint to the muscles, resulting in dysfunction, chewing disorders, pain, and limitations in the movement of the temporomandibular joint, as Citelli's abscess is an extra-temporal complication of otitis media. It occurs when pus from the mastoid tip trickles down along the posterior belly of the digastric muscle to the occipital and cervical region. It is a very unusual presenting complication of chronic otitis media. Citelli's abscess is a complication of otitis media. Urgent radiology, followed by drainage of pus, is performed to reduce pain and further progression of the infective process. The primary ear pathology is managed surgically after adequate treatment with intravenous antibiotics [19].

4. The relationship between TMJ disorders and hearing loss and tinnitus

Given the intricate anatomical and functional connections between the temporomandibular joint and the auditory system, particularly through shared muscles, nerves, and vascular supply, it becomes clinically relevant to explore the relationship between TMJ disorders and auditory manifestations such as hearing loss and tinnitus. Temporomandibular joint disorder signs and symptoms were more common and severe in females than males. TMJ severity is correlated with the degree of mouth opening and the number of aural symptoms. The absence or presence of mild TMJ is associated with normal audiograms, while moderate and severe TMJ are related to hearing loss in the median and low tones, respectively [20]. The reasons are attributed to several theories, including:

1. The repositioning of the joint disc during jaw movement increases pressure in the auditory tube and ear structures.

2. A tiny ligament called the disco-malleolar or Pinto's ligament, which originates from the anterior malleolar process, passes through the petrotympanic fissure, and inserts in the medial and posterosuperior part of the articular capsule and the disk. In the displacement of the temporomandibular joint disk, the disco-malleolar ligament can lead to traction of the malleus, the ossicular chain, and the tympanic membrane.

3. Common innervation of the tensor veli palatini, tensor tympani, masseter, temporalis, and pterygoid muscles by the motor nucleus of the trigeminal nerve is the underlying cause of the aural symptomatology in TMJ patients. If the tensor tympani or stapedial muscle contracts inappropriately, then the perilymphatic and endolymphatic pressures in the inner ear are changed via the oval window, causing vestibular and cochlear symptoms. This mechanism explains the vertigo and tinnitus in patients with temporomandibular joint disorder. Objective tinnitus is caused by the palatine and middle ear myoclonus, producing rhythmic movement of the tympanic membrane due to the tension of the stapedial and tensor tympani muscles. Tinnitus related to TMJ is thought to be produced by the lateral pterygoid muscles and the disco-malleolar ligament.

4. If the movement of the temporomandibular joint puts pressure on the carotid sheath, it increases the internal pressure in the hair cells of the cochlea, causing tinnitus and vertigo.

5. Peripheral sensitivity of the cranial nerves (facial nerve and trigeminal nerve) in patients with TMJ disorders leads to muscular tension in the middle ear muscles. This results in hearing loss at low frequencies. Research has found that acute temporomandibular joint disorders were associated with hearing loss at low frequencies, while moderate disorders were linked to hearing loss at mid frequencies [20].

Many studies have pointed to a relatively strong relationship between temporomandibular disorders, tinnitus, and self-reported hearing loss. This relationship was independent of the degree of hearing loss that was assessed objectively. The prevalence of recurrent headache episodes and fatigue or even muscle tension in the jaw is higher among tinnitus patients than would be expected even if these conditions were not related. About one-third of individuals suffering from tinnitus reported that jaw movements or pressure on the temporomandibular joint affected their tinnitus. Daytime teeth grinding and jaw fatigue appeared to be associated with fluctuating tinnitus, vertigo, and increased sensitivity to noise [21].

5. Ear diseases and their adjacent conditions that transfer to the temporomandibular joint

While numerous studies have highlighted how temporomandibular joint disorders can manifest with auditory symptoms, the relationship is bidirectional; certain ear pathologies may also extend their effects to the temporomandibular joint due to anatomical proximity and shared physiological pathways. In addition to the innervation, blood supply, and proximity between the temporomandibular joint and the ear, other theories attribute the transfer of certain diseases from the ear to the temporomandibular joint to some fissures between the two organs, such as the petrotympanic fissure, which is a soft tissue containing a connection between the middle ear and the temporomandibular joint [22]. Several articles have appeared in the medical literature regarding the transmission of chronic or acute suppurative otitis media or mastoiditis to the temporomandibular joint. This transmission may occur through these fissures directly or via the Eustachian tube. The disorder of the temporomandibular joint occurs due to the disturbance of the muscles connecting the Eustachian tube and the joint. Joint disorders can manifest as effusion, inflammation, or ankylosis. It is possible to reach a state of surgical treatment accompanied by antibiotics when the temporomandibular joint is involved in more complicated cases [23]. In children, the infection can spread from the ear or mastoid to the joint, where a case of septic arthritis of the temporomandibular joint was documented as a complication of acute otitis media [24]. In addition, the infection can also transfer from the joint to the middle ear. The current literature supports malocclusion with mandibular malposition and TMJ dysfunction as a predisposing factor to Eustachian tube dysfunction. This persisting condition could lead to otitis media, conservative treatments with removable oral appliances, Eustachian tube function, consenting middle ear ventilation, and preventing relapsing or persistent forms of otitis media [25]. Among the diseases that can affect the temporomandibular joint and the ear is the viral disease Ramsay Hunt. Herpes zoster oticus is caused by reactivation of latent herpes zoster infection from the geniculate ganglion (cranial nerve VII or facial nerve), but it can also involve cranial nerves V, IX, and X. Symptoms include ear pain and facial paralysis while the patient has vesicles in the external auditory canal, as well as pain resembling needle pricks in the cheek and jaw area, joint pain, and pain during chewing. Sometimes it can even lead to second or third-degree facial paralysis [26]. Frey syndrome is also one of the diseases that affect the temporomandibular joint and can be caused by inflammation of the parotid gland, its surgery, or injury or fracture of the mandible due to surgery or traumatic incidents. Frey syndrome arises from an unusual reinnervation process following damage to the auriculotemporal nerve. This nerve, a branch originating from the trigeminal nerve, consists of parasympathetic fibers that regulate saliva production in the parotid gland. Infections and traumas can lead to damage in the parasympathetic and sympathetic nerve fibers of the auriculotemporal nerve within the parotid region. Patients commonly exhibit indications such as facial warmth, flushing, and perspiration, particularly occurring during meals, within the region influenced by the auriculotemporal nerve. This encompassed area consists of the skin, the ear, the temporal region, the scalp, and the temporomandibular joint [27].

6. The otosurgical operations that affect the temporomandibular joint

Beyond naturally occurring disease transmission between the ear and the temporomandibular joint, surgical interventions in the otologic field can also exert significant impacts on the joint's function and integrity. Certain otologic procedures may influence TMJ function for the same reasons mentioned earlier regarding innervation, blood supply, proximity, and shared ligaments. Among the most important recommendations from the ear surgeon after ear surgeries is to cautiously limit jaw movement postoperatively and adhere to a liquid diet for the first 48 hours to minimize stress on middle ear structures, especially the middle ear and the ossicles. This chewing or excessive opening can also lead to the displacement of microscopic prosthetics in place, such as the stapes replacement or other small ossicles. When performing a tympanoplasty and placing a fascia graft instead of the tympanic membrane, it is very thin and not firmly attached, relying on its stability to not move. However, forcefully opening the temporomandibular joint or chewing hard food can shift the graft from its position, preventing it from healing and causing complications.

This caution is explained by the anatomical and functional aspects of the ligaments between the malleus and the temporomandibular joint [28]. On the other side, surgical procedures on the components of the temporomandibular joint can also cause damage to the middle ear and its components [29]. It was also observed about 6 months after otosurgeries, such as tympanoplasty or ossicular reconstruction, or mastoidectomy or facial nerve surgeries that require grafting to cover the nerve after exposing or connecting it, which necessitate a fascia graft from the temporal muscle fascia, that patients complain of a feeling of discomfort and dysfunction in the temporomandibular joint, especially during chewing. As mentioned, the temporalis muscle is one of the important muscles in the group of muscles of the temporomandibular joint. The otosurgeon may have to remove some tissue from this muscle while obtaining the graft from the temporal fascia and may have to use electric cautery to control bleeding in the area. This leads to changes in the composition, size, and fibers of the temporalis muscle, which can reflect on disturbances in the movement of the temporomandibular joint (**Figure 7**) [30].

A lot of tumor surgery in the temporal region, the tumor extension, or its surgery results in an impairment of the ear and the temporomandibular joint. Such as diffuse-type tenosynovial giant cell tumor invading the temporal bone, which is a destructive benign tumor-like proliferative disease that occurs in synovial tissue characterized by villous nodular hyperplasia of joints, tendon sheaths, and synovium. D-TSGCT invades

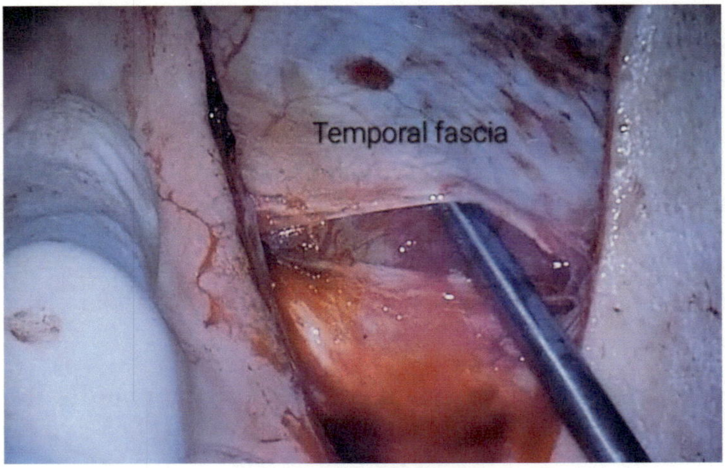

Figure 7.
View of a surgical incision behind the right ear and harvesting a graft from the temporal fascia.

the temporal bone originating from the temporomandibular joint (TMJ) [31]. Also, malignant tumors such as squamous cell carcinoma of the temporal bone or parotid gland squamous cell carcinoma invading the temporomandibular joint (**Figure 8**) [32].

In many cases of middle ear surgery, the chorda tympanic nerve, which supplies the sense of taste to two-thirds of the anterior tongue, may be at risk of injury, forcing the affected person to push food to the posterior third of the tongue, which leads to difficulties in chewing and temporomandibular joint disorders over time. Among the operations, ENT that can lead to disorders of the temporomandibular joint due to their complications are surgeries on the submandibular gland. When surgically removed in the case of a stone within or inflammation, it is closely located to the joint and shares many anatomical structures with it, such as the facial artery, and it is possible to injure Anastomoses of the marginal mandibular branch of the facial nerve with the buccal branch of the facial nerve during its surgery, which leads to a disorder in the joint [33]. Also, parotid gland surgery carries important complications, including facial nerve injury, which affects the function of its branches on the jaw joint. Additionally, one of the complications of parotid surgery is Frey syndrome, also known as Baillarger's syndrome, auriculotemporal syndrome, Dupuy syndrome, or gustatory hyperhidrosis. This syndrome represents aberrant reinnervation following injury to the auriculotemporal nerve, which is a branch of the trigeminal nerve. It consists of parasympathetic fibers that signal the parotid gland to produce saliva and sympathetic fibers that innervate the sweat glands of the face and scalp. Patients with Frey syndrome often present with facial warmth, flushing, and sweating in the territory of the auriculotemporal nerve overlying the parotid gland, which may include the preauricular skin, the temporal skin, the scalp, and the temporomandibular joint region. Symptoms occur during meals, especially with spicy and sour foods [34].

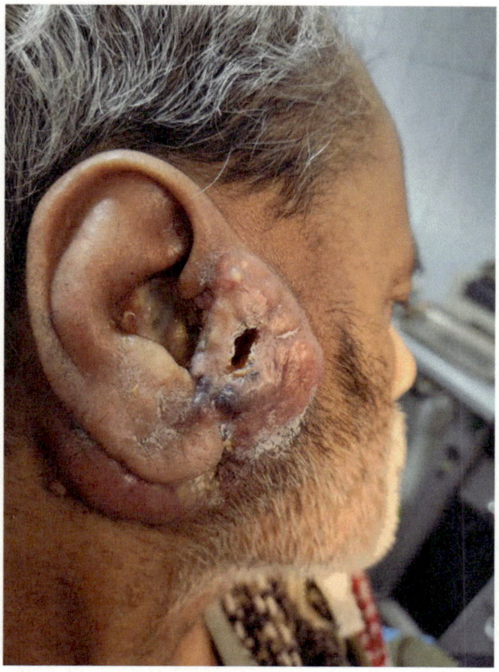

Figure 8.
Squamous cell carcinoma spread to the components of the right ear, the parotid gland, and the temporomandibular joint in a 65-year-old male patient.

7. Conclusion

The connection between the temporomandibular joint (TMJ) and the auditory system is more than just anatomical proximity; it reflects a complex neurophysiological relationship. This interdependence means that TMJ evaluation should not be overlooked when assessing ear-related symptoms, just as masticatory dysfunction should not be examined in isolation from potential otologic influences. A bidirectional link exists: TMJ disorders can manifest as auditory issues like tinnitus or hearing loss, while ear pathologies or surgeries may, in turn, affect TMJ function. This reciprocity underscores the necessity for a unified diagnostic and treatment strategy.

Acknowledging the TMJ as both a potential source and a target of otologic complications emphasizes the value of interdisciplinary cooperation among otolaryngologists, audiologists, radiologists, and dental professionals. Such teamwork not only improves diagnostic precision but may also mitigate long-term complications that diminish patient well-being. Moving forward, integrating TMJ assessment into clinical protocols for atypical ear symptoms or post-surgical auditory complaints could lead to more comprehensive patient care.

Author details

Bilal Hasan
Department of Otolaryngology, Yusuf al-Azma Hospital, Damascus, Syria

*Address all correspondence to: bilalhas78@gmail.com

References

[1] Petrides GA, Fadhil M, Meller C. Otalgia from temporomandibular disorder in ear, nose and throat surgery: A literature review and diagnostic algorithm. Australian Journal of Otolaryngology. 15 Mar 2024;7:7

[2] Cooper BC, Cooper DL. Recognizing otolaryngologic symptoms in patients with temporomandibular disorders. Cranio. 1993;**11**(4):260-267. DOI: 10.1080/08869634.1993.11677977

[3] Badel T et al. Temporomandibular joint development and functional disorders related to clinical otologic symptomatology. Acta Clinica Croatica. 2011;**50**(1):51-60

[4] Di Fabio RP. Physical therapy for patients with TMD: A descriptive study of treatment, disability, and health status. Journal of Orofacial Pain. 1998;**12**(2):124-135

[5] Wood CP et al. Tympanic plate fractures in temporal bone trauma: Prevalence and associated injuries. AJNR. American Journal of Neuroradiology. 2014;**35**(1):186-190. DOI: 10.3174/ajnr.A3609

[6] Williams, E.D. Concussions: Everyone Should Know the Missing Link. Newly Discovered Fractured Bones in the Temporal Mandibular Joint (TMJ) Will Produce the Same Symptoms that are used to Diagnose Concussions. Suburban Life Magazine. 2025. Available from: https://www.suburbanlifemagazine.com/article/2604/Concussions-the-Missing-Link [Accessed: May 28, 2025]

[7] Huff T, Weisbrod LJ, Daly DT. Neuroanatomy, cranial nerve 5 (trigeminal). In: StatPearls. Treasure Island (FL): StatPearls Publishing Copyright © 2025, StatPearls Publishing LLC; 2025

[8] Dingman RO, Grabb WC. Surgical anatomy of the mandibular ramus of the facial nerve based on the dissection of 100 facial halves. Plastic and Reconstructive Surgery and the Transplantation Bulletin. 1962;**29**:266-272. DOI: 10.1097/00006534-196203000-00005

[9] Liu AT et al. Anatomy of buccal and marginal mandibular branches of facial nerve and its clinical significance. Zhonghua Zheng Xing Wai Ke Za Zhi. 2007;**23**(5):434-437

[10] Singh PM, Kaur M, Trikha A. An uncommonly common: Glossopharyngeal neuralgia. Annals of Indian Academy of Neurology. 2013;**16**(1):1-8. DOI: 10.4103/0972-2327.107662

[11] Thomas K, Minutello K, Das JM. Neuroanatomy, cranial nerve 9 (glossopharyngeal). In: StatPearls. Treasure Island (FL): StatPearls Publishing Copyright © 2025, StatPearls Publishing LLC; 2025

[12] Murphy R et al. The great auricular nerve: An anatomic and surgical study. Journal of Otolaryngology - Head & Neck Surgery. 2012;**41**(Suppl 1):S75-S77

[13] Brennan PA et al. Communication of the anterior branch of the great auricular nerve with the marginal mandibular nerve: A prospective study of 25 neck dissections. The British Journal of Oral & Maxillofacial Surgery. 2010;**48**(6):431-433. DOI: 10.1016/j.bjoms.2009.07.015

[14] Cuccia AM et al. The arterial blood supply of the temporomandibular

joint: An anatomical study and clinical implications. Imaging Science in Dentistry. 2013;**43**(1):37-44. DOI: 10.5624/isd.2013.43.1.37

[15] Mérida-Velasco JR et al. The vascular relationship between the temporomandibular joint and the middle ear in the human fetus. Journal of Oral and Maxillofacial Surgery. 1999;**57**(2):146-153. DOI: 10.1016/s0278-2391(99)90229-x

[16] Paraskevas KI et al. Oral and ocular/orbital manifestations of temporal arteritis: A disease with deceptive clinical symptoms and devastating consequences. Clinical Rheumatology. 2007;**26**(7):1044-1048. DOI: 10.1007/s10067-006-0493-x

[17] Anagnostopoulou S, Venieratos D, Antonopoulou M. Temporomandibular joint and correlated fissures: Anatomical and clinical consideration. Cranio. 2008;**26**(2):88-95. DOI: 10.1179/crn.2008.013

[18] Tranchito EN, Bordoni B. Anatomy, head and neck, digastric muscle. In: StatPearls. Treasure Island (FL): StatPearls Publishing Copyright © 2025, StatPearls Publishing LLC; 2025

[19] Sahoo AK et al. Citelli's abscess following otitis media: A case report. Iranian Journal of Otorhinolaryngology. 2017;**29**(92):161-163

[20] Kitsoulis P et al. Signs and symptoms of temporomandibular joint disorders related to the degree of mouth opening and hearing loss. BMC Ear, Nose and Throat Disorders. 2011;**11**:5. DOI: 10.1186/1472-6815-11-5

[21] Gelb H, Gelb ML, Wagner ML. The relationship of tinnitus to craniocervical mandibular disorders. Cranio. 1997;**15**(2):136-143. DOI: 10.1080/08869634.1997.11746004

[22] Eckerdal O. The petrotympanic fissure: A link connecting the tympanic cavity and the temporomandibular joint. Cranio. 1991;**9**(1):15-22. DOI: 10.1080/08869634.1991.11678343

[23] Faerber TH, Ennis RL, Allen GA. Temporomandibular joint ankylosis following mastoiditis: Report of a case. Journal of Oral and Maxillofacial Surgery. 1990;**48**(8):866-870. DOI: 10.1016/0278-2391(90)90348-6

[24] Bast F et al. Septic arthritis of the temporomandibular joint as a complication of acute otitis media in a child: A rare case and the importance of real-time PCR for diagnosis. International Journal of Pediatric Otorhinolaryngology. 2015;**79**(11):1942-1945. DOI: 10.1016/j.ijporl.2015.08.014

[25] Bernkopf E et al. Temporomandibular Joint and Otitis Media: A Narrative Review of Implications in Etiopathogenesis and Treatment. Medicina (Kaunas). 2022;**58**(12). DOI: 10.3390/medicina58121806

[26] Yin M et al. Ramsay hunt syndrome and mandibular alveolar bone necrosis following herpes zoster: A case report and literature review. Frontiers in Neurology. 2022;**13**:1073607. DOI: 10.3389/fneur.2022.1073607

[27] Kostares E et al. Prevalence of Frey syndrome following extraoral surgical treatment for mandibular fractures: A systematic review and meta-analysis. F1000Res. 2023;**12**:1153. DOI: 10.12688/f1000research.140994.2

[28] Sencimen M et al. Anatomical and functional aspects of ligaments between the malleus and the temporomandibular

joint. International Journal of Oral and Maxillofacial Surgery. 2008;**37**(10):943-947. DOI: 10.1016/j.ijom.2008.07.003

[29] Loughner BA, Larkin LH, Mahan PE. Discomalleolar and anterior malleolar ligaments: Possible causes of middle ear damage during temporomandibular joint surgery. Oral Surgery, Oral Medicine, and Oral Pathology. 1989;**68**(1):14-22. DOI: 10.1016/0030-4220(89)90108-4

[30] Effat KG. A clinical study on the incidence of internal derangement of the temporomandibular joint following harvesting of temporalis fascia. Cranio. 2025;**43**(1):52-59. DOI: 10.1080/08869634.2022.2072452

[31] Huang Q et al. Diffuse-type tenosynovial giant cell tumor invading the temporal bone: Three cases. Ear, Nose, & Throat Journal. 2022;**104**(7):1455613221127578. DOI: 10.1177/01455613221127578

[32] Lovin BD, Gidley PW. Squamous cell carcinoma of the temporal bone: A current review. Laryngoscope Investigative Otolaryngology. 2019;**4**(6):684-692. DOI: 10.1002/lio2.330

[33] Batra AP, Mahajan A, Gupta K. Marginal mandibular branch of the facial nerve: An anatomical study. The Indian Journal of Plastic Surgery. 2010;**43**(1):60-64. DOI: 10.4103/0970-0358.63968

[34] Young A, Okuyemi OT. Frey syndrome. In: StatPearls. Treasure Island (FL): StatPearls Publishing Copyright © 2025, StatPearls Publishing LLC; 2025

Chapter 6

The Endocrine Link: Estrogen's Influence on Temporomandibular Disorders

Hima John and Jiss Mary George

Abstract

The disproportionate increase of temporomandibular disorders (TMD) in women strongly suggest a hormonal influence primarily rooted in estrogen activity. Inflammation mediated by estrogen may be through various mechanisms of action in the immune system, expression of estrogen receptors, and upregulation of voltage-gated sodium channels, or due to genetic variations called polymorphism. The temporomandibular joint (TMJ) contains estrogen receptors, which control how the joint experiences pain together with its ability to maintain a stable state. Estrogen levels decrease in post-menopause and menstrual periods and these states relate to higher pain intensity and decreased joint health through both inflammatory mechanisms and changes in sodium channel activity within trigeminal ganglia. The trigeminal ganglion is a cluster of nerve cell bodies located near the trigeminal nerve, within the skull that plays a crucial role in processing sensory information from the face. While the ganglion itself is not the source of pain in all cases, direct trigger to the ganglion produces unpleasant pain sensations. Women of reproductive age show susceptibility to disc displacement together with arthralgia effects that correlate with genetic variations in the estrogen receptor genes ESR1 and ESR2. The incidence of TMD increases among women who have polycystic ovary syndrome (PCOD) as it causes estrogen to remodel the extracellular matrix. Hormonal abnormalities, such as increased androgen levels and possibly decreased progesterone levels, are common in women with PCOS and can have an impact on the temporomandibular joint (TMJ) and surrounding tissues. TMD can develop and worsen as a result of these hormonal changes as well as possible inflammatory reactions. Therefore, hormonal status together with life stages of reproduction function as essential factors for managing TMD.

Keywords: temporomandibular joint, temporomandibular disorders in women, estrogen, hormonal fluctuations, orofacial pain, inflammation

1. Introduction

The term "temporomandibular disorders" (TMD) refers to a broad category of clinical illnesses marked by masticatory system dysfunction and discomfort.

Temporomandibular joint (TMJ) noises, jaw dysfunction, masticatory muscle pain, TMJ pain, and associated soft and hard tissues are common symptoms [1, 2].

Chronic pain conditions affecting women and their hormonal connections were identified by several previous researches. According to reports, the majority of patients presenting with TMD and receiving treatment for TMD are women. Based on several conflicting studies, there exists no significant variation statistically in the actual occurrence of modifications in joint structure by gender. However, considerable research indicates that women represent 80% of patients with TMD are predominantly women, who are 1.5–2 times more likely to suffer from the condition than men [3–6].

2. Epidemiology

The intensity of the symptoms in patients varies based on their age. Discomfort usually starts after puberty and rises over the years of adulthood and reproductive age. The frequency is minimal in children, teenagers, older adults, and most prevalent among females aged 20–40. The allocation of TMD by age and gender indicate a potential connection between the disease's pathogenesis and female hormonal pathway [7–10].

3. Hormones in temporomandibular disorders

3.1 Estrogen

The age and gender distribution of TMD proposes a possible link with the female hormonal system and the condition's underlying mechanisms. The connection between TMD and hormones, particularly estrogen, is intricate. Hormonal fluctuations, especially during the menstrual cycle, menopause, as well as when utilizing hormone-based contraceptives, could influence the symptoms of temporomandibular disorders (TMD) occur more frequently in women than in men. The temporomandibular joint (TMJ) and adjacent tissues have estrogen receptors present. Estrogen may affect inflammation and the perception of pain, potentially contributing to TMD [11, 12].

3.2 Progesterone

Progesterone influences Voltage-Gated Sodium Channel 1.7 in the trigeminal ganglion, decreasing allodynia (which is a type of neuropathic pain in which pain is experienced from stimuli that are not normally painful) of infected temporomandibular joint. Progesterone may inhibit neuronal excitability by modifying voltage-gated sodium currents (INa) in TG neurons. The presence of INa is essential for the reception of input from peripheral pain stimuli, and inflammation of the TMJ could increase the excitability of its afferents.

Increased threshold depolarization may occur due to this progesterone-driven rightward shift in activation, potentially reducing activation speed and decreasing neuronal excitability. As a result, progesterone might lower INa to produce its pain-relieving effect. These results bolster the idea that progesterone directly blocks voltage-gated sodium, calcium, and potassium channels to diminish excitotoxicity.

Although this study indicated that the complete array of sodium channels plays a role in progesterone-induced INa reduction, further investigation is needed to identify which sodium channels are the most significant [12].

3.3 Relaxin

Relaxin H2, a 6-kDa polypeptide 13, is the main form of relaxin that is stored and circulated in humans that appears to exert long-term effects on connective tissues by altering the turnover of collagen and proteoglycans. Relaxin induces alterations in the composition and organization of matrix in tissues such as the uterus, ovary, cervix, breast, and deciduas by altering the synthesis of matrix macromolecules and/or modifying the expression of matrix-degrading enymes [10–13]. It seems that increased degradative processes, rather than alterations in matrix production, lead to changes in matrix composition in the fibocartilaginous tissues of the TMJ and also pubic symphysis. Relaxin seems to aid in tissue breakdown by primarily activating various MMPs, including MMP-1, MMP-3, MMP-9, and MMP-13, in both reproductive and non-reproductive cells, such as skin and lung alveolar fibroblasts, as well as TMJ fibrocartilage [12, 13].

4. Estrogen in temporomandibular disorders

4.1 Presence and distribution of estrogen receptors in TMJ components

Estrogen receptors (ERs) are found abundantly in the temporomandibular joint tissue [6, 7]. This distribution illustrates how the joint reacts to hormone signals. The receptors specifically are Erα, Erβ, and GPER. The receptor ERα is seen in articular cartilage and subchondral bone and is also found in the synovial membrane, which implies estrogen can directly affect cell function and gene expression in these critical load-bearing tissues. ERβ follows a similar distribution in these tissues. GPER (GPR30) is also expressed in chondrocytes, and its distribution in other human tissues indicates it is involved in other components of the TMJ as well. The diversity of receptor types between TMJ tissues is central to the understanding of how estrogen influences the joint [5, 7, 10, 12]. **Table 1** provides a summary of the key estrogen receptors found in TMJ tissues and their primary mechanisms of action.

4.2 The effect of estrogen on TMJ tissue remodeling and metabolism

Estrogen has a significant influence on remodeling activities of the TMJ and on the extracellular matrix (ECM) and bone volume. It is an intricate effect involving a balance between tissue deconstruction and tissue construction [11, 13].

4.2.1 Articular cartilage

17β-estradiol (E2) has also shown to stimulate the expression of certain Matrix. Metalloproteinases (MMPs) include MMP-9 and MMP-13, in fibrochondrocytes of the TMJ. This is primarily through ERα activation, and the result is extracellular matrix breakdown and loss, a feature found in degenerative joint diseases. Elevated MMP levels have been identified as known causators of TMJ osteoarthritis (TMJ-OA) [10, 13]. Animal models confirm this, demonstrating that mechanical tension and

Receptor type	Primary location in TMJ tissues	Key signaling mechanisms	Known effects on TMJ
ERα	Articular cartilage, subchondral bone, synovial membrane (fibroblast-like type B cells), TMJ disc	Genomic (gene transcription *via* EREs), non-genomic (e.g., MAPK activation)	MMP-9/MMP-13 induction leading to ECM degradation, modulation of inflammation, bone remodeling, influence on cellular physiology
ERβ	Articular cartilage, subchondral bone, TMJ disc	Genomic (gene transcription *via* EREs), non-genomic (e.g., kinase interactions)	Modulation of cartilage turnover, bone metabolism, influence on immune responses, often with effects divergent from ERα
GPER	Chondrocytes, likely other TMJ components (e.g., synovial membrane, disc)	Rapid non-genomic (e.g., ERK1/2 transactivation, cAMP upregulation, cytosolic Ca^{2+} increase)	Potential role in jawbone regeneration, involvement in pain processing (spinal nociception *via* Ca^{2+} and ROS)

Table 1.
Key estrogen receptors in TMJ tissues and their primary mechanisms of action.

elevated estrogen levels can reduce TMJ cartilage thickness. Conversely, in TMJ-OA models, 17β-estradiol supplementation has been found to restore thickness of cartilage and reduce osteoclast activity, indicating a protective role under some conditions. This ambivalent role demonstrates that the action of estrogen on cartilage is a fine balance, concentration, and particular medical context [10–13].

4.2.2 Subchondral bone

Estrogen is essential for healthy bone metabolism and bone density. Estrogen deficiency, which often follows menopause, markedly increases the risk of osteoporosis and has been implicated in TMJ-OA, a disorder which is characterized by abnormal bone loss and growth. Studies indicate that reduced levels of dihydrotestosterone (DHT) and 17β-estradiol cause systemic bone loss, reflected by reduced bone volume/tissue volume (BV/TV) and decreased trabecular thickness, accompanied by greater trabecular spacing [7, 8, 10]. In contrast, 17β-estradiol supplementation decreases inflammatory markers (NFκB, Gremlin 1, RelA) and increases BMP7 expression, both of which are beneficial for bone integrity and also protect against TMJ-OA. Additionally, GPER1 has been noted as a critical gene that facilitates jawbone repair, particularly in the case of estrogen deficiency. The gene GPER1, sometimes referred to as GPR30, is essential for the healing of jawbones, especially in situations where estrogen levels are insufficient, as in the case of an estrogen deficit. By promoting osteogenesis and cell proliferation, it aids in the regeneration of jawbones [7, 9].

4.2.3 Articular disc

The organization and remodeling of the TMJ disc are also affected by estrogen. This heightened enzymatic activity caused by estrogen can diminish key extracellular matrix elements required for disc integrity. Biomechanical examinations of aging human TMJ discs reveal that female discs are more stiff overall and more resistant to relaxation after strain compared with male discs, providing evidence of a gender-based effect on disc properties [7–9, 11].

4.3 Estrogen's function in synovial fluid composition and joint lubrication

The synovial membrane surrounding the TMJ secretes synovial fluid, which keeps the inner surfaces of the joint well-nourished and lubricated. Studies indicate that estrogen has a negative influence by reducing the expression and activity of the proteoglycan 4 (PRG4) gene, also referred to as lubricin, in TMJ disc cells. PRG4 mainly offers lubrication, minimizing wear on joint tissues. The inhibitory effect of estrogen on PRG4 can result in reduced lubrication hence increased friction and subsequent breakdown of joint components, accounting for the observed gender differences among TMD patients. Also, the level of estrogen in synovial fluid is associated with the severity of arthritis in postmenopausal women, thus demonstrating its local effect on joint health. Estrogen also influences craniofacial anatomy, which results in variation in mandibular size and angle, affecting bite forces and chewing mechanisms [12–14]. When this anatomical predisposition is coupled with estrogen's direct influence on TMJ tissue—such as increasing disc stiffness and impacting lubrication negatively by PRG4 regulation—a particularly important interplay is in effect. These changes are not merely molecular; they have actual mechanical consequences. In addition to its direct effects on cells, estrogen could render women susceptible to TMD by modifying the TMJ's mechanical conditions and strength in subtle ways. Greater disc stiffness and reduced lubrication may predispose the joint to mechanical strain and wear, significantly contributing to the rising frequency of internal issues and degenerative change in females. This emphasizes the interrelationship of hormonal, structural, and mechanical factors and implies that the treatment of TMD must consider the impact of the hormonal effects on tissue properties [7, 13–17].

5. Estrogen and pain modulation in the temporomandibular joint

5.1 Gender differences in pain perception and TMJ pain sensitivity

Numerous researches show that the intensity and duration of the pain experience in women is more than men when it comes to orofacial pain, including TMD pain. Studies also confirm that women tend to have higher sensitivity to pain [15–17]. Estrogen receptors exist in primary sensory neurons, such as those located in the dorsal root ganglion (DRG) and the trigeminal ganglion (TG), which provides sensory nerve supply to the Jaw joint and masticatory muscles. Estrogen can directly affect trigeminal ganglion neurons, increasing their excitability and expanding their receptive fields. This effect helps explain the increased pain sensitivity seen in women [11, 14, 16, 18].

5.2 Estrogen's modulation of central pain pathways and descending modulatory systems

Estrogen impacts the neuroendocrine and nervous systems, enabling it to influence pain regulation. It directly affects the transmission of central pain. Estrogen boosts NMDA receptor-mediated communication and spinal long-term potentiation (LTP) *via* quick signaling that begins with estrogen receptors on membranes. This indicates how estrogen may amplify pain signals at the vertebral level [13, 14, 16, 19]. Estrogen also influences other important neural pathways that play a role in pain modulation, including serotonin, norepinephrine, dopamine, and natural opioid pathways. Reduced estrogen levels are associated with decreased opioid activity, which may result in increased pain sensations. Activation of GPER in the central nervous system has been demonstrated to result in spinal pain, driven through elevations in cytosolic calcium and accumulation of reactive oxygen species (ROS) [17–19].

5.3 Interaction of estrogen with inflammatory mediators

Estrogen significantly influences the control of inflammation in the TMJ. The monocytes and macrophages that are immune like cells generate pro-inflammatory cytokines like interleukin-1 (IL-1), interleukin-6 (IL-6), and tumor necrosis factor-alpha (TNF-α) under the regulatory effects of estrogen, which is notably high in the synovial fluid of TMD patients and is known to worsen TMJ osteoarthritis. Estrogen has been discovered to amplify pain reaction in TMJ tissues by the secretion of inflammatory substances, prostaglandins, and substance P [7, 9, 11, 16, 17].

Conversely, estrogen may also suppress the synthesis of specific cytokines (IL-1 IL-6, TNF-α), diminish microglial toxicity, and lower acute inflammation in models such as carrageenan-induced pleurisy. Prostaglandins and leukotrienes, originating from arachidonic acid, are crucial agents of acute inflammation. Non-steroidal anti-inflammatory drugs (NSAIDs) act by inhibiting the production of prostaglandins. This indicates that the role of estrogen in TMJ inflammation is intricate; it is

Estrogen effect (pro−/ anti-nociceptive/inflammatory)	Specific mechanism/mediator involved	Context/condition
Pro-nociceptive/ pro-inflammatory	Trigeminal ganglion sensitization (increased excitability, expanded receptive fields)	Mild localized TMJ inflammation, elevated estrogen
	Lowering pain threshold, modulating Nav1.7 in trigeminal ganglion	Inflamed TMJ
	Upregulation of NMDAR1 in DRG	Chronic sciatic nerve injury model
	Amplification of TRPV-1 channel function	Estrogen-treated animals
	Increased release of inflammatory mediators (cytokines, prostaglandins, substance P)	TMJ tissues
	Enhanced inflammatory nociception	Acute estrogen surge
	Increased monocytic release of cytokines after inflammatory insult	TMD patients with high estrogen levels
	Facilitation of NMDA receptor-mediated synaptic transmission and spinal LTP	Spinal cord
Anti-nociceptive/ anti-inflammatory	Suppression of cytokine induction (IL-1, IL-6, TNF-α)	Various inflammatory models
	Prevention of microglial toxicity	LPS-induced inflammation
	Reduction of acute inflammation (e.g., carrageenan-induced pleurisy)	Animal models
	Decreased pain in physiological pain	General physiological pain
	Protective mechanism against nociception	Stable hormone levels

Table 2.
Estrogen's dual role in TMJ inflammation and nociception.

influenced by several factors, such as the type of inflammation, estrogen levels, exposure time, and the particular cellular context. This intricacy is significant for therapeutic approaches. It suggests that a blanket strategy for anti-inflammatory treatment in TMD might not yield positive results. Interventions must consider the patient's hormonal condition and the inflammatory mediators and pathways involved, favoring a more tailored treatment approach [11, 12, 16, 17, 19]. **Table 2** illustrates estrogen's dual role in TMJ inflammation and nociception.

5.4 Dose-dependent and context-dependent effects of estrogen on pain

The impact of estrogen on pain is intricate and differs. It can both facilitate and reduce pain depending on the situation. For normal pain, estrogen usually seems to lower pain levels. However, its effects can change depending on the type and duration of inflammation. An acute rise in estrogen can increase pain associated with inflammation, while in cases of chronic inflammatory pain (like those using complete Freund's adjuvant), estrogen shows a pain-facilitating effect [11, 16, 19–22]. Clinical observations reveal that low or fluctuating estrogen levels, especially during the perimenstrual phase, connect to increased pain and severity. In contrast, stable hormone levels may help protect against pain. The dose and method of estrogen delivery are critical, where normal levels might provide protection, but higher doses could be harmful [20, 22, 23].

6. Clinical implications of estrogen's action on TMD

6.1 Impact of hormonal fluctuations on TMD prevalence and severity

The pattern of TMD prevalence indicates that it is most frequent during reproductive years (ages 20–40) and least frequent prior to puberty and post-menopause. This pattern corresponds with fluctuations in estrogen levels, indicating that estrogen significantly contributes to the development of TMD. The severity of TMD pain often fluctuates during the menstrual cycle. It frequently reaches its highest point during menstruation and the late luteal phase when estradiol levels are low or rapidly decreasing. This steady pattern suggests a distinct link between hormonal fluctuations and pain perceptions [20–24].

The relationship between the use of external hormones, such as oral contraceptives (OCs) and hormone replacement therapy (HRT), and TMD remains a topic of debate. Certain studies indicate a higher risk, yet recent reviews fail to conclusively demonstrate that estrogen replacement therapy elevates TMD risk. This discrepancy highlights the necessity for additional studies to grasp the actual impacts of external hormones. Pregnancy, characterized by elevated estrogen levels, presents varied outcomes related to TMD. Certain research suggests reduced orofacial pain during the third trimester, whereas other studies observe no meaningful connection between pregnancy and TMD functions. Hormonal imbalance conditions, like polycystic ovary syndrome (PCOS), are associated with a significantly increased prevalence of TMD, frequently accompanied by heightened inflammatory factors. These clinical findings emphasize that estrogen's involvement in TMD is intricate and situation-dependent, rather than just a straightforward issue of increased or decreased hormone levels [22–25]. **Table 3** summarizes the influence of various hormonal states on TMD prevalence and pain severity.

Hormonal state/intervention	Observed effect on TMD prevalence/severity/pain
Pre-puberty	Low prevalence, similar in boys and girls
Reproductive years (20–40 years)	Highest prevalence, peak pain intensity
Menstrual cycle phases	Pain peaks during low/rapidly falling estrogen (late luteal phase, menstruation)
Pregnancy	Inconsistent: some report reduced orofacial pain (3rd trimester); others find no clear association
Perimenopause/menopause	Lower prevalence than reproductive years
Oral contraceptive use	Inconsistent: Some suggest increased risk; others find no significant difference
Hormone replacement therapy (HRT/ERT)	Inconsistent: Some suggest increased risk; recent reviews find no conclusive evidence for increased risk
Polycystic ovary syndrome (PCOS)	Elevated inflammatory factors with significantly higher incidence of TMD.

Table 3.
Influence of hormonal states on TMD prevalence and pain severity.

6.2 Genetic predisposition: Estrogen receptor gene polymorphisms and estrogen metabolism enzymes

Genetic influences play a significant role in identifying individuals who are at greater risk for TMD. Particularly, variations in genes for estrogen receptors, such as estrogen receptor alpha (ESR1, e.g., XbaI/PvuII single-nucleotide polymorphisms (SNPs) and the estrogen receptor beta (ESR2)) are associated with an increased likelihood of TMJ disorders in females. For instance, the [GC] haplotype at the XbaI site in ERα is prominently present in females with TMJ disorders, indicating a genetic predisposition. These genetic differences can significantly alter the way estrogen functions in the TMJ and influence the emergence of TMJ issues [11, 13, 23, 24].

In addition to receptors, enzymes that metabolize estrogen also affect susceptibility. For the production of estrogen and conversion of androgens into estrogens, the role of the enzyme Aromatase (CYP19A1) is a crucial. Catechol-O-methyltransferase (COMT) helps break down catecholamines, which are neurotransmitters influenced by estrogen and involved in pain pathways. Variants of the COMT gene that lead to lower enzyme activity correlate with increased pain sensitivity and a higher incidence of TMD [7, 10, 11, 23, 25] . Certain polymorphisms in estrogen receptor genes and variations in estrogen metabolism enzymes show that an individual's risk for TMD and their response to estrogen are strongly influenced by their genetics. This explains why not all women with similar hormone levels experience TMD the same way or with equal severity, highlighting the need for personalized approaches in TMD treatment [22–24].

6.3 Biopsychosocial model and comorbidities in estrogen-related TMD

TMD's multifactorial nature is well-known, with significant biopsychosocial factors, including psychological issues like depression and anxiety, and behaviors like pain catastrophizing and fear-avoidance. TMD often coexists with other chronic overlapping pain conditions by IASP fact sheet 2024, such as migraines, fibromyalgia, and cervical spondylitis and cervical pain conditions, pointing to a shared underlying mechanisms. The interplay between psychological distress and chronic pain can form a "vicious circle," where each aspect worsens the other [4, 7, 23, 25].

Estrogen directly affects mental health and mood, with significant changes in estrogen levels raising the chances of occurrence of depression, anxiety, and post-traumatic stress disorder. This shows a direct link between hormonal state and the psychological factors that can worsen TMD. Hormonal fluctuations not only affect TMJ tissues and pain perception directly but also indirectly worsen TMD by harming psychological well-being. This psychological distress can exacerbate and possibly centralize the pain, making TMD more severe and chronic. Therefore, managing estrogen-related TMD requires a thorough approach that addresses both the biological influence of estrogen on the TMJ and the psychological impacts of hormonal changes, reinforcing the important role of the biopsychosocial model and integrated care [8, 10, 11, 23–30].

7. Diagnostic and management considerations for estrogen-related TMDs

7.1 Comprehensive patient history: Emphasizing hormonal status

Begin with a thorough history to explore estrogen's role.

7.1.1 Menstrual history, contraceptives and HRT

- Ask about menstrual regularity, cycle-related jaw pain, and use of hormonal contraceptives/HRT.
- Exogenous estrogen (*via* OCs or HRT) has been linked to a 20–30% increased odds of TMD symptoms

7.1.2 Pregnancy history and menopausal status

- Pregnancy often brings high estrogen levels; TMD pain typically decreases in the third trimester
- Low-estrogen states—postpartum and post-menopause—often exacerbate pain

7.2 Clinical examination: Identifying specific TMD subtypes

- Evaluate for myogenous vs. arthrogenous TMD, disc displacement, joint sounds, range-of-motion, and palpate TMJ/masticatory muscles.
- Track symptom fluctuation relative to menstrual cycle or hormonal changes.

7.3 Adjunctive diagnostic tools

- *Imaging*: MRI with contrast optimized by menstrual phase can clarify joint pathology
- *Inflammatory biomarkers*: Emerging research highlights systemic inflammation *via* estrogen-mediated pathways (e.g., IL-6, MCP-1)

7.4 Therapeutic strategies tailored to hormonal status

7.4.1 Pharmacological management

- *NSAIDs*, muscle relaxants, and neuromodulators are staples.
- In perimenopausal or hypoestrogenic women, consider low-dose *HRT* patches—some case reports document TMJ symptom relief.
- Be cautious: HRT may have conflicting effects—postmenopausal women on HRT sometimes show TMD worsened, other times no change

7.4.2 Non-pharmacological interventions

- *Physical therapy*: Exercises, jaw relaxation, posture correction (especially around low-estrogen phases). Some individuals often report relief via physical therapy.
- *Splint therapy*: Effective for muscle-related TMD and bruxism
- *Behavioral management*: Stress reduction can mitigate estrogen-amplified pain responses.

7.4.3 Nutritional and lifestyle modifications

- Anti-inflammatory diets, omega-3 supplementation (under clinician supervision).
- Regular exercise and good sleep hygiene to stabilize hormones and reduce inflammatory tone.

7.4.4 Multidisciplinary approach

- Collaborate with *gynecologists/endocrinologists* to assess estrogen status (e.g., menopausal transition, HRT suitability).
- In hypoestrogenic cases, HRT might reduce TMD pain—but must carefully weigh risks such as thromboembolism and breast cancer
- Integrating *mental health* and *physiotherapy* referrals ensures a biopsychosocial approach.

7.5 Estrogen plays a dual role in TMD

- *High/fluctuating levels* trigger inflammation and heightened pain perception (*via* ERα, TLRs, cytokines)
- *Low levels* (postpartum, menopause) may worsen chronic joint degeneration and pain.

Tailored management—factoring in menstrual phase, pregnancy, HRT, and lifestyle—leads to better outcomes. A *team approach* engages medical, physical, psychological, and lifestyle expertise [7, 12, 14, 27–34].

Recent systematic reviews on linking estrogen replacement therapy and temperomandibular disorders indicate that there is no definitive proof backing a higher likelihood of TMDs in women undergoing ERT.

8. Conclusion

The intricate relationship between hormones and the temporomandibular joint (TMJ), particularly concerning temporomandibular disorders (TMD), is a significant area of focus for our era. Of the numerous endocrine players, estrogen appears to be a potent hormone in the pathogenesis and course of TMD. Widespread receptors in the articular cartilage, synovium, and musculature of the TMJ indicate a direct effect on tissue remodeling, inflammation, and sensory perception. The greater prevalence of TMD in females, particularly during times of heightened hormonal changes such as puberty, menstruation, pregnancy, and menopause, makes this association a strong one. The diverse effects of estrogen, like its role in the metabolism of collagen, inflammatory mechanisms, and nociception, offer a rational biological explanation for its involvement in TMJ dysfunction and pain.

In addition, the effects of estrogen replacement therapy (ERT) in alleviating menopausal symptoms also reach the TMJ. Although ERT has the potential to provide systemic benefits, its effects on TMD symptoms are multifaceted and must be given careful thought. For some women, ERT may relieve pain and discomfort by stabilizing endogenous hormonal levels, which may limit inflammatory reactions or enhance joint tissue integrity. Yet, for others with pre-existing susceptibilities in TMJ or certain hormonal sensitivities, ERT may provide no relief or even worsen symptoms. This once again underscores the importance of individual evaluation and a sophisticated awareness of every patient's hormonal status and TMD presentation. As clinicians, we need to keep in mind the larger endocrine scenario when assessing and treating TMD patients, especially women, and consider the role of interventions such as ERT with informed prudence and individualized care. It is critical to conduct further studies to fully understand the complex molecular mechanisms involved and direct subsequent therapeutic advances in this multifaceted and frequently incapacitating disease.

Author details

Hima John* and Jiss Mary George
Department of Oral Medicine and Radiology, Annoor Dental College and Hospital, Muvattupuzha, Kerala, India

*Address all correspondence to: himajohn@gmail.com

References

[1] Zielinski G, Pajak-Zielinska B. Association between estrogen levels and temporo mandibular disorders: An updated systematic review. International Journal of Molecular Sciences. 2024;**25**:9867

[2] Berger M, Szalewski L, Bakalczuk M, Bakalczuk G, Bakalczuk S, Jacek SJ. Association between estrogen levels and temporomandibular disorders: A systematic literature review. Prz Menopauzalny. 2015;**14**(4):260-270

[3] Manfredini D, Winocur E, Piccotti F, Ahlberg J, Lobbezoo F. Research diagnostic criteria for temporomandibular disorders: A systematic review of axis I epidemiologic findings. Oral Surgery, Oral Medicine, Oral Pathology, Oral Radiology, and Endodontics. 2011;**112**:453-462

[4] Oleszek-Listopad J, Robak B, Szyma'nska J. Etiology and epidemiology of temporomandibular disorders. Hygiene and Environmental Health Advances. 2019;**54**:92-96

[5] Rollman GB, Lautenbacher S. Sex differences in musculoskeletal pain. The Clinical Journal of Pain. 2001;**17**:20-24

[6] Michalak M, J W'n-M, Wilczak M, Paulo M, A B˙z, Borowicz J. Correlation between eye and ear symptoms and lack of teeth, bruxism and other parafunctions in a population of 1006 patients in 2003-2008. Archives of Medical Science. 2012;**8**:104-110

[7] Athnaiel O, Cantillo S, Paredes S, Knezevic NN. The role of sex hormones in pain-related conditions. International Journal of Molecular Sciences. 1866;**2023**:24

[8] Tsang A, Von Korff M, Lee S, Alonso J, Karam E, Angermeyer MC, et al. Common chronic pain conditions in developed and developing countries: Gender and age differences and comorbidity with depression-anxiety disorders. The Journal of Pain. 2008;**9**:883-891

[9] Jedynak B, Jaworska-Zaremba M, B G ´n, Chmurska M, Janicka J, Kostrzewa Janicka J. TMD in females with menstrual disorders. International Journal of Environmental Research and Public Health. 2021;**18**:7263

[10] Wright GJ, Coombs MC, Wu Y, Damon BJ, Bacro TH, Kern MJ, et al. Electrical conductivity method to determine sexual dimorphisms in human temporomandibular disc fixed charge density. Annals of Biomedical Engineering. 2018;**46**:310-317

[11] Robinson JL, Johnson PM, Kister K, Yin MT, Chen J, Wadhwa S. Estrogen signaling impacts temporomandibular joint and periodontal disease pathology. Odontology. 2020;**108**:153-165

[12] Patil SR, Yadav N, Mousa MA, et al. Role of female reproductive hormones estrogen and progesterone in temporomandibular disorder in female patients. Journal of Oral Research and Review. 2015;**7**:41-43

[13] Puri J, Hutchins B, Bellinger LL, Kramer PR. Estrogen and inflammation modulate estrogen receptor alpha expression in specific tissues of the temporomandibular joint. Reproductive Biology and Endocrinology. 2009;**7**:155

[14] Dong XD, Mann MK, Kumar U, et al. Sex-related differences in NMDA-evoked rat masseter muscle afferent discharge result from estrogen-mediated modulation of peripheral

NMDA receptor activity. Neuroscience. 2007;**146**:822-832

[15] Isselée H, De Laat A, De Mot B, Lysens R. Pressure-pain threshold variation in temporomandibular disorder myalgia over the course of the menstrual cycle. Journal of Orofacial Pain. 2002;**16**:105-117

[16] Papka RE, Srinivasan B, Miller KE, Hayashi S. Localization of estrogen receptor protein and estrogen receptor messenger RNA in peripheral autonomic and sensory neurons. Neuroscience. 1997;**79**:1153-1163

[17] LeResche L, Sherman JJ, Huggins K, et al. Musculoskeletal orofacial pain and other signs and symptoms of temporomandibular disorders during pregnancy: A prospective study. Journal of Orofacial Pain. 2005;**19**:193-201

[18] LeResche L, Mancl L, Sherman JJ, Gandara B, Dworkin SF. Changes in temporomandibular pain and other symptoms across the menstrual cycle. Pain. 2003;**106**:253-261

[19] Hassan S, Muere A, Einstein G. Ovarian hormones and chronic pain: A comprehensive review. Pain. 2014;**155**:2448-2460

[20] Vilanova LS, Gonçalves TM, Meirelles L, Garcia RC. Hormonal fluctuations intensify temporomandibular disorder pain without impairing masticatory function. The International Journal of Prosthodontics. 2015;**28**:72-74

[21] Bay-Jensen C, Slagboom E, Chen-An P, Alexandersen P, Qvist P, Christiansen C, et al. Role of hormones in cartilage and joint metabolism: Understanding an unhealthy metabolic phenotype in osteoarthritis. Menopause. 2013;**20**:578-586

[22] Fischer L, Torres-Chavez KE, Clemente-Napimoga JT, Jorge D, Arsati F, de Arruda Veiga MC, et al. The influence of sex and ovarian hormones on temporomandibular joint nociception in rats. The Journal of Pain. 2008;**9**:630-638

[23] Madani AS, Shamsian AA, Hedayati-Moghaddam MR, Fathi-Moghadam F, Sabooni MR, Mirmortazavi A, et al. A crosssectional study of the relationship between serum sexual hormone levels and internal derangement of temporomandibular joint. Journal of Oral Rehabilitation. 2013;**40**:569-573

[24] Landi N, Manfredini D, Lombardi I, Casarosa E, Boseo M. 17-beta estradiol and progesterone serum levels in temporomandibular disorder patients. Minerva Stomatologica. 2004;**53**:651-660

[25] Kang SC, Lee DG, Choi JH, Kim ST, Kim YK, Ahn HJ. Association between estrogen receptor polymorphism and pain susceptibility in female temporomandibular joint osteoarthritis patients. International Journal of Oral and Maxillofacial Surgery. 2007;**36**:391-394

[26] Marino M, Galluzzo P, Ascenzi P. Estrogen signaling multiple pathways to impact gene transcription. Current Genomics. 2006;**7**:497-508

[27] Alam MK, Ibrahim MA, Almaslamani MJ, Saeed MH, Siurkel Y, Ronsivalle V, et al. Correlating estrogen replacement therapy and temporomandibular disorders: A comprehensive review following PRISMA principles and cochrane handbook for systematic reviews of interventions. BMC Oral Health. 2024;**24**:93

[28] Nekora-Azak A, Evlioglu G, Ceyhan A, Keskin H, Berkman S, Issever H. Estrogen replacement therapy

among post-menopausal women and its effects on signs and symptoms of temporomandibular disorders. Cranio. 2008;**26**:211-215

[29] Leucuta D-C, Anton D, Almasan O. Estrogen hormones implications on the physiopathology of temporomandibular dysfunction. Journal of Clinical Medicine. 2024;**13**:4406

[30] Farzin M, Taghva M, Babooie M. Comparison of temporomandibular disorders between menopausal and non-menopausal women. Journal of the Korean Association of Oral and Maxillofacial Surgeons. 2018;**44**:232

[31] Hornung RS, Benton WL, Tongkhuya S, Uphouse L, Kramer PR, Averitt DL. Progesterone and allopregnanolone rapidly attenuate estrogen-associated mechanical allodynia in rats with persistent temporomandibular joint inflammation. Frontiers in Integrative Neuroscience. 2020;**14**:26

[32] Abdrabuh A, Baljon K, Alyami Y. Impact of estrogen therapy on temporomandibular joints of rats: Histological and hormone analytical study. Saudi Dental Journal. 2021;**33**:608-613

[33] Ye T, Sun D, Mu T, Chu Y, Miao H, Zhang M, et al. Differential effects of high-physiological oestrogen on the degeneration of mandibular condylar cartilage and subchondral bone. Bone. 2018;**111**:9-22

[34] Kroeff GPH, de Castro JM, Braga HB, Bosco TD, de Oliveira TC, de Sousa Morais IT, et al. Hormone replacement therapy did not alleviate temporomandibular joint inflammatory pain in ovariectomized rats. Odontology. Jan 2025;**113**(1):232-244

Section 2

Temporomandibular Joint Disorders – New Perspectives in Therapy

Chapter 7

Non-Steroidal Anti-Inflammatory Drugs (NSAIDs) in Pain Management Caused by Temporomandibular Joint (TMJ) Disorders

Elahe Aleebrahim-Dehkordi, Mahmoud Bahrami Dashtaki and Sina Ahmadi

Abstract

In temporomandibular joint (TMJ) disorders, inflammation is accompanied by pain and cartilage degeneration. This pain may be caused by temporomandibular disorders due to muscular or joint conditions, or both. However, it is not clear which non-invasive treatments work best. In the treatment of this disorder, there are two main options for pharmacological management of pain, one of which is the use of nonsteroidal anti-inflammatory drugs (NSAIDs). These drugs stop the production of prostaglandins, which is why NSAIDs, by inhibiting the enzyme, reduce the production of prostaglandins and reduce inflammation. NSAIDs are now one of the first-line treatments for mild-to-moderate inflammatory pain in patients with TMJ because of their strong analgesic and anti-inflammatory properties, including the capacity to inhibit cyclooxygenase and hence prevent prostaglandin formation. This chapter provides a comprehensive classification of TMJ and then goes on to discuss the NSAIDs' mechanism of action, administration, side effects, contraindications, management, and monitoring. It also covers crucial information for healthcare professionals. Since topical NSAIDs have minimal gastrointestinal effects, they might be safe for treating TMJ. Considering their risk-benefit ratio in relation to alternative anti-TMJ therapies, topical NSAIDs should be considered for TMJ. Effective treatment for TMD requires a multidisciplinary approach between dentists, pain specialists, physiotherapists, psychologists and neurologists. NSAIDs these drugs are among the successful treatment options in reducing pain and inflammation in TMJ disease. It is highly advised to use NSAIDs at the lowest effective dose for the shortest amount of time, and to reduce the gastrointestinal risk of associated with NSAIDs, should be supplementary gastroprotective agent's medications prescribed.

Keywords: temporomandibular disorders, NSAIDs, inflammation, orofacial pain, cyclooxygenase inhibitors, topical therapy, gastrointestinal risks

1. Introduction

Temporomandibular disorders (TMD) are usually associated with significant pain and inflammation, which can be characterized as pain in the temporomandibular joint (TMJ), masticatory muscles, or both. In fact, the main cause of pain in TMD patients is joint inflammation, which causes stiffness and limitation of jaw movement. The trigeminal ganglion (TG) or (Gasserian or semilunar ganglionis) a nerve node located at the base of the skull and is part of the trigeminal nerve (the fifth cranial nerve). This ganglion contains sensory neurons that transmit sensory information from the face, including touch, pain, and temperature, to the brain. The TG is the most important factor in the transmission of pain sensation in the TMJ, which plays a very important role in the regulation of TMJ pain. Inflammation in the TMJ increases the excitability of neurons in the TG and also affects the expression of some genes that are related to pain in the TG [1]. Mechanical overload of the TMJ is a major contributing factor to the development of TMJ OA, also known as temporomandibular joint osteoarthritis. This causes the TMJ's intra-articular pressure to rise, which in turn results in transient hypoxia (low oxygen levels). This hypoxia in the TMJ can trigger the expression of vascular endothelial growth factor (VEGF) by activating hypoxia-induced transcription factor 1 (TCF1) [2]. Pain, joint noises, locking, reduced mouth opening, and difficulty eating are among the predominant symptoms and, if left untreated, can be disabling for the individual and affect the quality of life. Pain caused by the TMJ or related masticatory muscles is manifested by tenderness to touch in the respective anatomical area. To measure the degree of mouth opening, the distance between the tips of the upper and lower incisors at maximum opening (interincisal distance) is considered and if it is less than (35 mm), it is considered abnormal. Locking and joint noises, are caused by internal derangement of the joint mechanism which includes the mandibular condyle, intra-articular disc, and the glenoid fossa. Locking and joint noises can sometimes be caused by inflammatory debris that is deposited as part of the disease process. All of this, along with pain and restricted opening, can lead to eating problems [3]. TMJ dysfunction treatment necessitates a multidisciplinary approach. This implies that the therapy of this illness may require a number of professionals, such as dentists, physiotherapists, pain specialists, etc. The three primary objectives of TMJ treatment are symptom reduction, which includes pain management, disease inactivation, and the restoration of normal joint function in order to lessen pain and the capacity to carry out everyday tasks. TMJ treatment options fall into a number of categories, ranging from the least invasive to the most intrusive. These include: 1-conservative care, which includes physical therapy; 2-pharmaceutical and occlusal splinting therapy; 3-less invasive surgery, which includes arthrocentesis and joint injections; and 4-invasive surgery, which includes open joint surgery and arthroscopy, also known as arthroscopic or keyhole surgery [4, 5]. Nonsteroidal anti-inflammatory drugs (NSAIDs) are a large group of drugs that inhibit the formation of prostaglandins by inhibiting cyclooxygenases. The cyclooxygenase (COX) enzyme is a key structural enzyme in the production of the body's inflammatory mediators, or prostanoids, including (prostaglandins F2α, E2, D2, I2 and thromboxane A2). NSAIDs are among the most widely used medical medication prescribed for pain in the orofacial region [6]. This chapter provides a comprehensive classification of TMJ and then describes the mechanism of action, administration, adverse effects, contraindications, management, and monitoring, as well as important points for providers regarding NSAIDs.

2. A review of temporomandibular joint (TMJ) disorders

Temporomandibular joint disorders (TMDs) are a heterogeneous group of musculoskeletal and neuromuscular issues affecting the temporomandibular joint (TMJ), masticatory muscles, and related structures [7]. TMDs are among the most common causes of non-dental orofacial pain and has a global prevalence of 5–12% [8]. TMDs are a leading cause of chronic pain due to long-term underdiagnosis or misdiagnosis, resulting in chronic pain, distress, and poor quality of life [9]. TMDs are multifactorial in origin, stemming from biological, psychological, environmental, and behavioral influences, such as parafunctional activities including bruxism, emotional stress, trauma, inflammatory joint disease, and congenital/acquired anatomical issues [10]. TMD is defined by the American Academy of Orofacial Pain as a group of conditions involving the TMJ, masticatory muscles and related structures [11]. The Diagnostic Criteria for Temporomandibular Disorders (DC/TMD) divides TMD into muscle-related and joint-related categories, with the latter encompassing internal derangements (e.g., disc displacement, with and without reduction) as well as arthralgia, degenerative joint disease (DJD), and osteoarthritic changes in hard tissues of the joint [12, 13].

The clinical presentation of TMDs can differ widely and may include jaw pain or tenderness, limited mandibular movement, jaw sounds (i.e., clicking or popping), headaches, earaches, changes in occlusion, etc. [13]. With chronic cases, there can be recurrent pain patterns which may manifest together with depression, anxiety, and sleep problems [14, 15]. Symptoms often overlap with other comorbid orofacial conditions, which lead to diagnostic and management challenges [14]. TMDs occur more frequently in females undergoing hormonal fluctuations, and the peak prevalence occurs in the 20 to 40 age range [16].

According to epidemiological data from a recent systematic review and meta-analysis, the prevalence of TMJ disorders is 11.3% in children and young adolescents and about 31.1% in adults and geriatric age groups. Disc displacement with reduction (DDwR) is the most common subtype and occurs in approximately 26% of adults and 7.4% in younger populations [17, 18]. Degenerative joint conditions, such as osteoarthritis (OA), is less common in children but prevalence rises significantly as children reach adulthood or older age, reaching almost 17% in the older generation. Information described from meta-analysis highlights the need for early identification and modulation for appropriate management in individual age groups [17, 19].

The diagnosis of TMDs is based on clinical assessment and various imaging approaches. Conventional imaging methods such as panoramic radiography are typically the first line of imaging for TMDs [7]. However, magnetic resonance imaging (MRI) is the modality of choice for the evaluation of soft tissue structures (i.e., articular disc, synovium, and joint effusion), and should be considered the gold standard method of imaging [20]. MRI provides high-resolution, multiplanar imaging and is needed to assess subtle pathologies that occur intra-particularly, such as disc displacement, synovitis, and osseous degeneration. Although MRI is the best method of diagnostic imaging, it has a reduced diagnostic access due to cost, patient availability, and other contraindications in certain patient populations [21].

Ultrasonography (US) has been recently considered as an adjunctive imaging modality, and used to assess TMDs unique characteristics, because of its non-invasive procedure, reduced costs and dynamic imaging capabilities [22]. The advantage of US is that it can visualize TMJ movement and demonstrate where the disc is relative to the bony components of the TMJ during jaw functions, which is advantageous for screening purposes and also for point of care evaluation [23, 24]. Overall, meta-analytic data suggested that MRI correlates highly with the definition of a true positive and false negative (it has a pooled odds ratio (OR) of 0.64 and a relative risk (RR) of 0.80), or an improved accuracy compared to ultrasound [25]. Nevertheless, US is still a reasonable first imaging modality, in the case that MRI cannot be performed or is not accessible to the patient. However, US diagnostic performance is heavily reliant on US operator experience, US imaging protocol used, and patient-dependent factors [26].

TMD management should be individualized, and most patients are treated conservatively and non-invasively at first. Conservation and non-invasive treatment include patient education, behavior modification, pharmacologic agents (NSAIDs, muscle relaxants), physical therapy and the use of occlusal splints or stabilization appliances [27]. Most cases of TMD resolve using conservative treatment and only a few of the cases progress to completing more invasive procedures. Consensus guidelines from the appropriate international body recommend for refractory or significantly anatomically impaired cases of TMD, procedures such as arthrocentesis and arthroscopy can be considered and open joint surgical procedure reserved for conditions such as ankylosis, joint fusion, or severe disc derangement that failed conservative treatment [28, 29]. Evidence shows better surgical outcomes when surgical procedures are preceded by thorough imaging conventions, MRI being preferred [25].

2.1 Classification of TMJ disorders

Over the past few decades, the classification of temporomandibular joint (TMJ) disorders has progressed immensely, and continues to progress, which is a reflection of the increasing knowledge surrounding the anatomical, physiological, and psychosocial complexities involved with these disorders [13]. TMJ disorders, broadly termed TMDs, are a heterogeneous group of musculoskeletal and neuromuscular disorders that involve the TMJ, masticatory muscles, and related structures [13, 15, 16]. Classification is not simply an academic endeavor; it is necessary for accurate diagnosis, treatment planning, and consistency among researchers and in clinical practice [30]. However, we currently have no universally accepted system, and various attempts at parallel classifications exist in research and clinical practice. One of the most commonly used classifications is the AAOP (American Academy of Orofacial Pain) classification, which categorizes TMDs primarily by anatomical and pathophysiological characteristics into two categories: (1) joint disorders, and (2) masticatory muscle disorders [This disease affecting the muscles involved in chewing (mastication)] [31]. Joint disorders contain arthralgias, disc displacements, hypomobilities and hypermobilities, degenerative joint diseases (such as osteoarthritis and osteoarthrosis), fractures, and congenital disorders. Masticatory muscle disorders include varieties of myalgia (including localized myalgia, myofascial pain, and myalgia with referral), tendonitis, myositis, and centrally mediated pain disorders, such as fibromyalgia [32]. The AAOP classification is the most complex of those available, with over 50 clinical entities noted in the 6th edition, making it the most extensive, and most complicated for routine practice [31]. Another significant parallel framework is the Diagnostic Criteria for Temporomandibular Disorders (DC/TMD), developed through the International Network for Orofacial Pain and Related Disorders Methodology (INfORM) [12, 33]. The DC/TMD adapted the previous Research Diagnostic Criteria for Temporomandibular Disorders (RDC/TMD) by further splitting Axis I disorders into pain-related groups, e.g., myalgia, arthralgia, and headache attributed to TMD, and intra-articular TMDs, e.g., simple disc dislocation in varying forms and degenerative diseases of the joint. In addition, the DC/TMD model prepped Axis II measures to cross-reference and assess psychosocial components which include pain-related disability, depression, and anxiety, and thus offered a biopsychosocial view [12]. One more classification model, Okeson's classification, is not used by a single association or organization as a framework, however, it is said to have influenced contemporary thought. Okeson has categorized his disorders into masticatory muscle disorders, TMJ disorders, chronic mandibular hypomobility, and disorders of growth [34]. The value of this classification is the clinician's logic; however, it does not account for many disease processes such as systemic arthritides and movement disorders of the orofacial region [34].

As an additional refinement to classifying pain-related TMDs, the ICOP (International Classification of Orofacial Pain) was developed through the partnership of the International Headache Society and the IASP [35, 36]. It delineates primary from secondary temporomandibular pain by recognizing the acute and chronic presentation of myofascial or TMJ-related pain [34]. This distinction is clinically important, because the management strategies for chronic TMD pain would be quite different from acute TMD pain, which may include central sensitization [37]. In terms of epidemiology and health system classification, the WHO ICD-11 classification provides yet another level of classification [38]. TMDs are classified in so many chapters of the ICD-11 description, it's evidence of the complexity of TMDs [39]. The ICD-11 system can aid to track diseases globally, however, it does not have the clinical detail that would allow for nuanced diagnoses and intervention [39]. In contrast, the multifaceted ACTTION-American Pain Society Pain Taxonomy (AAPT) paradigm encompasses not only diagnostic criteria but also comparable characteristics, shared comorbidities, functional implications, and underlying biopsychosocial mechanisms [40]. The AAPT was originally designed for chronic pain syndromes such as fibromyalgia, but it is amenable to TMD and endorses individual-based classification and treatment [40]. Furthermore, the American Academy of Craniofacial Pain (AACP) has offered a model similar to the earlier work of Pertes and Gross in separating TMD as related to the joint, muscle, and congenital/developmental conditions [41]. The AACP model is limited as it is an earlier model that has not been updated recently, and is still using ICD-9 codes [41]. Classification is increasingly discussing genetics, neurobiology, and artificial intelligence (AI). Newer evidence also suggests that genetic variants, including those that predispose individuals to potential chronic TMD pain (e.g., genetic alterations associated with opioid receptors and the body's response to stress) [8]. Imaging studies have indicated a change in structural brain volumes in chronic TMD individuals indicating a need for clinical classification systems that heed central sensitization and pain chronification [23, 24]. Future classification systems including biomarkers and AI-based diagnostic tools will offer a new foundation for individualized diagnosis and treatment. It will enable data-driven and individualized diagnosis and management in the future.

3. Pathophysiology of pain

Pain in temporomandibular joint (TMJ) disorders has a complex nature, which encompasses peripheral tissue damage but goes far beyond simple direct inflammation and mechanistic events, emphasizing intricate neurophysiological processes in both the spinal and supraspinal nervous systems [13, 31]. The pathophysiology of

TMJ pain cannot simply be explained in terms of nociceptive stimulation of local inflammation or mechanical stress, and TMJ pain predicts a dynamic response, with repeated interactions and influences of biomechanical events and insults, neuroimmune responses, and central pain processing and modulation events [42]. Understanding the multifactorial nature of pain is important, especially when considering the diagnosis and treatment of TMJ disorders [42]. The TMJ nociceptors are primarily found in peripheral TMJ tissues such as the synovium, joint capsule, ligaments, and articular cartilage where there is an extensive network of nociceptors that are primarily activated by inflammatory mediators, mechanical strain, or injury [13, 43]. The nociceptors include A-delta and C fibers which transduce noxious stimuli to electrical signals relayed from the trigeminal nerve to the central nervous system [44]. When the joint is overloaded beyond its adaptive capacity either from the usual functional demands or when joints do not adapt due to various dynamics, there is excess input in the mechanoreceptors and nociceptors, triggering biochemical and degenerative processes [45]. TMJ overload is classified as either absolute, which occurs when normal tissues are overloaded with excessive forces (i.e., trauma or bruxism), or relative, an acute normal loading of normal tissues, but against tissues that have lost their physiologic resilience (e.g., aging, systemic inflammatory disorders, and hormonal changes) [46]. The overloading unloads the homeostasis of connective tissues, resulting in maladaptive remodeling, cartilage degeneration, and inflammation of the synovial. Matrix metalloproteinases (MMPs-particularly MMP-1 and MMP-13) degrade components of the extracellular matrix which include collagen and proteoglycans [46–49]. MMPs activity is typically increased by pro-inflammatory cytokines or growth factors (such as IL-1β, TNF-α, and VEGF), which result in an imbalance in synthesis or degradation of the matrix, which results in degenerative joint disease [49]. Neurogenic inflammation is another contributor to TMJ pain. Sensory neurons release neuropeptides (substance P and CGRP) that increase vascular permeability, promote leukocyte migration, and potentiate the inflammatory environment [50]. The neuropeptides sensitize peripheral nociceptors by lowering the threshold for activation, which results in peripheral sensitization [51]. This is a clearly defined characteristic of chronic inflammatory pain. As the disease progresses to chronic, central sensitization can occur, through the process of repeated nociceptive input that affect changes in the spinal trigeminal nucleus and higher brain centers, resulting in altered long-term functional properties [31]. Central sensitization involves an increase in excitability and spontaneous activity within second-order neurons, a decreased inhibitory modulation, and alterations to the somatosensory maps [32]. Clinically, those changes have been shown to manifest through hyperalgesia, and allodynia, and persistent pain that is not explained through the presence of peripheral pathology [8, 10]. There have been recent functional neuroimaging evidence looking exclusively at TMD chronic pain patients, demonstrating changes in brain activity while chronic TMD patients are imaging their pain states, especially notable in the anterior cingulate cortex, insula and, prefrontal cortex which suggest the contributions of a central component in regard to chronic TMJ pain [52]. Emerging evidence is suggesting that glial cell activation and neuroinflammation within the central nervous system is also an important contributor to TMJ pain persistence [53]. When astrocytes and microglia activate, they produce cytokines and reactive oxygen species while also modifying synaptic activity effects nociceptive signaling and modulating that pain experience. This modified physiological mechanism may also explain the transition from acute to chronic pain states for some predisposed individuals [53, 54]. The recognition of psychosocial factors as a contributor to chronic pain perception is growing. Psychological stress and behavioral-physiological changes can activate hypothalamic-pituitary-adrenal and sympathetic nervous system mechanisms that may lead to increased muscle tension, changes in autonomic change and fresh modulator on inflammatory pathways [55, 56]. Finally, there are lots of comorbid conditions with TMD patients and it is important as sleeping, anxiety, and depression can occur together with clinical conditions and contribute to TMD chronic pain gracefully [55]. In addition to inflammatory and neuropathic processes, mechanical derangements such as disc displacement and/or joint hypomobility may mechanically irritate intra-articular structures and generate nociceptive responses [50, 51]. While these changes often represent painful states, they do not adequately explain the severity or persistence of symptoms [53]. It has been reported that pain intensity is more closely related to psychosocial impairment and alterations in central processing than to joint changes on imaging [52]. At the end, TMJ-related pain reflects a confluence of peripheral nociception, neurogenic inflammation, central sensitization, and psychosocial modulation. Such complexity and multifactorial influence means that a strictly structural or anatomical approach to diagnosis is insufficient. Effective management will need to consider local joint pathology and systemic and behavioral factors contributing to chronicity. A biopsychosocial model incorporating elements of molecular biology and neurophysiology and psychology appears to provide the most comprehensive understanding of TMJ pain and most effective management.

3.1 Causes and signs of temporomandibular joint pain

Pain in the temporomandibular joint (TMJ) is a common symptom of temporomandibular disorders (TMDs) that are the result of an interplay of structural, functional, neuro muscular and psychosocial factors [10, 34]. The cause of TMJ pain is multifactorial and patient specific, comprising both peripheral pathologies and central modulation of pain perception [13]. Furthermore, signs and symptoms that may correlate with TMJ pain are often multi-dimensional and can make diagnosis and treatment approach difficult for clinicians. A common cause of TMJ pain is dysfunction or hyperactivity of the masticatory muscles, particularly the masseter and temporalis [57, 58]. Electromyographic (EMG) studies have shown that patients diagnosed with TMD have higher baseline and stimulus-induced activity of the masticatory muscles compared to healthy controls [59, 60]. The pathological activity may occur at baseline or as the result of psychological or environmental stressors. A landmark electromyographical study demonstrated that patients with TMJ dysfunction had substantially greater masseter activation both at rest and with visual and/or auditory stress, supporting the hypothesis that hyperfunction of the masticatory muscles are a key generator of TMJ pain [61]. Of interest, about 20% of patients demonstrated simultaneous activation of non-masticatory musculature including the trapezius—indicating a global increase in muscular tension in addition to area associated with the orofacial region [62]. In addition to muscle possible sources, intra-articular pathologies can also generate nociceptive input from the joint structures (displacement of disc, joint effusion, and degenerative joint disease) [10]. These intra-articular pathologies also alter the biomechanics, generate mechanical stress and measurable inflammation [13]. The actual inflammation process is mediated by cytokines like interleukin 1β and TNF-α, as well as various prostaglandins that sensitize the joint nociceptors and lead to both acute and chronic pain states [50]. Vascular endothelial growth factor (VEGF), matrix metalloproteinases (MMPs) also contribute to joint degradation as well as inflammatory pain [47]. Maladaptive loadings of the joint through bruxism, physiologic and/or traumatic joint loading, malocclusion are reasons for increased stress to the joint and influence microtrauma to the joint leading toward pain and dysfunction [63]. The impact of psychosocial stress on TMJ pain is also being studied [55]. Emotional stressors such as anxiety and depression may lead to increased muscle contraction and alter the central processing of pain, causing mechanical sensitivity to be increased among these patients [55]. Studies using surface EMG for patients with TMD and higher scores on an anxiety scale demonstrated greater masseter muscle activity and also more subjective distress during experimental stimulation [60, 61]. This increased exposure/stress it appears can be minimized through psychosocial methods. In terms of chronic pain, it also has its own mood issues contributing, which leads to a cycle of pain and dysfunction that can be both painful to the patient and burdensome in clinical practice [55, 64]. Clinically, TMJ pain may exhibit localized tenderness in the joint and surrounding musculature, referred pain to the temple, ear, or neck, and pain with jaw movements [15]. Plenty of patients with TMJ pain will report clicking or popping, difficulties in mandibular movements such as deviations or a restricted range of motion, muscle tension headaches, and consistent exacerbation of pain with chewing, speaking, or yawning [15, 65]. Interestingly, the symptomology of TMJ pain does not always match objective findings in structural abnormalities patients may report nearly unbearable pain with minimal imaging findings, while others with clear evidence of intra-articular pathology remain asymptomatic [13]. The issue of TMJ pain emphasizes the need to incorporate individual pain tolerance, central sensitization, and psychological overlay into clinical considerations [10]. A striking clinical observation is the lack of consistency between the amount of structural joint pathology and the amount of pain reported [13]. Many individuals who demonstrate radiographic evidence of both disc displacement and/or osteoarthritis are symptomatic, while others who show only minor changes may express severe pain with a lower degree of pain tolerance. Such phenomena would seem to suggest an influence of central sensitization and psychological influence on the pain experience [55, 66]. There are gender differences evident in TMJ pain occurrence as TMJ pain predominates in female populations, especially in the ages of 20 to 40 years [16]. There are likely hormonal influences that account for the chance of TMJ pain, especially the varying effects of estrogen on pain threshold and the varying coping strategies for pain [16]. Findings from the OPPERA cohort confirm that female patients with TMD had greater pain sensitivity and greater pain-related disability than males before treatment [67]. Further complicating diagnosis is the typical nature of TMJ pain to represent unilateral presentation even if the use of EMG does not clearly demonstrate differences in muscular activity between symptomatic and asymptomatic sides [60, 61]. These differences may reflect asymmetries in sensory thresholds, affected coordination of regional muscle units, or variations in attention rather than differences in motor output. Moreover, referred pain from TMJ involvement, including headache, earache, and cervical tightness patterns of nociception, can obscure the true source of nociception and delay diagnosis [10, 14, 15].

3.2 Pain mechanisms in TMJ

TMJ disorders involve pain that is highly dynamic, multifactorial neurobiological phenomenon involving peripheral and central mechanisms [42]. The traditional assumption that pain intensity is proportional to the amount of local tissue damage is inadequate to account for the clinical variability seen in TMJ pain [68]. For example, some patients with disabling pain report little or no comprehension of tissue-level injury or peripheral pathology, whereas others with clear joint injury/disease appear asymptomatic [42]. This mismatch alludes to the ongoing peripheral activation of nociceptive inputs versus central nervous system modulation [51]. This discrepancy is increasingly being represented and conceptualized as "centralized pain." [68]. At the peripheral level, nociceptive pain in TMJ originates primarily as a result of inflammation, tissue damage, or mechanical dysfunction of the joint and/or associated musculature [50, 51]. Nociceptors (pain sensing receptors) embedded in the synovium, joint capsule, ligaments, and masticatory muscles respond to noxious stimuli and send signals via the trigeminal nerve [44, 50, 69, 70]. In TMJ dysfunction, repetitive micro trauma, or parafunctional habits (e.g., bruxism), or internal derangements are often associated with persistent nociceptive activation and the development of peripheral sensitization. In this condition, there is enhanced responsiveness to both noxious and innocuous stimuli within the affected region [44, 70]. However, pain mechanisms in TMJ disorders extend beyond peripheral nociception. In many patients with chronic TMD, central sensitization, or abnormal pain amplification by the central nervous system, is significant. Central sensitization includes increased excitability of spinal and supraspinal neurons, decreased inhibition, and greater synaptic efficacy in pain pathways [42, 68]. Functional neuroimaging studies indicated increased pain-evoked activity in the anterior cingulate cortex, insula, and prefrontal cortex of individuals with TMD, indicating an altered central pain processing [70]. The central pain component is further corroborated by OPPERA's findings of differentiated clusters of TMD patients that sorted according to levels of experimental pain sensitivity and levels of psychological distress [67]. A significant percentage of the sample exhibited widespread hyperalgesia, sensory amplification, and even comorbid conditions, including fibromyalgia and irritable bowel syndrome; some of these are in TMDs more considered to some common pathophysiologic mechanisms. For patients exhibiting the preceding, the peripheral source and/or maintenance for the pain is predominantly a function of central mechanisms than local pathology [28, 46, 67]. Quantitative sensory testing (QST) has shown that many TMD patients exhibit generalized pain hypersensitivity, including heightened pressure and thermal sensitivity of different symptomatic and remote locations [71, 72]. Modest evidence of deficits in conditioned pain modulation (i.e., endogenous pain inhibitory capacity) are common occurrences in TMD due to some impairment in the central regulation of pain [72]. These findings are compounded by a cluster of psychological distress measures (anxiety, depression, and somatic symptom burden). This cluster of variables suggests a significant affective component to centralized pain [68, 72]. Genetic and neuroimmune factors are also involved in pain mechanisms in TMJ [73, 74]. Genes that encode specific proteins for the metabolism of monoamines (e.g., COMT, DRD4), genes regulating pro-inflammatory and anti-inflammatory cytokines (e.g., IL-10, IL-6), and voltage-gated ion channels have been correlated to increased susceptibility to pain and the likelihood of developing chronic pain. In the absence of TMJ pain, higher systemic levels of pro-inflammatory cytokines (e.g., IL-8, TNF-α) demonstrate lower pressure pain thresholds and greater time summation of pain [13, 68, 74]. These findings fit a model of a "pain-prone" phenotype that is characterized by central neuroinflammation and compromised pain perception [75]. Both the genetic phenotype and exposure to environmental stimuli such as adverse childhood events or trauma appear to converge to result in the "pain-prone" phenotype [75]. Another primary component of centralized pain includes the imbalance of neurotransmitters [51]. Specifically, greater excitability in pronociceptive systems (e.g., glutamatergic) and greater inhibition of antinociceptive systems (e.g., serotonin, norepinephrine, GABA) are important contributors to dysregulated sensory processing, sleep disturbances, fatigue, and cognitive dysfunction [51]. The overlap of neurotransmitters involved in pain, mood, and sensory integration highlights the complexity of TMD pain [51]. The overlap allows justification for the use of centrally acting pharmacologic agents (e.g., serotonin-norepinephrine reuptake inhibitors (SNRIs)). and anticonvulsants (e.g., pregabalin) for clinical patients who demonstrate centralized features of pain [51, 64, 66, 68]. In conclusion, the difference between peripheral and centralized pain has important treatment implications. While patients with peripheral nociceptive pain may show positive treatment effects from localized interventions (like occlusal splints, NSAIDs, or physical therapy), those whose pain is primarily centralized are more likely to benefit from a biopsychosocial approach [42]. This can include pharmacologic modulation of central mechanisms, cognitive-behavioral therapy, and treatment of comorbid mood and sleep disorders [42, 68]. Patient-centered treatment via mechanistic profiling not solely from anatomical diagnosis will provide the best outcomes in TMD and other similar pain conditions.

3.3 Management of pain caused by temporomandibular joint (TMJ) disorders

TMD is a term used generically to describe a variety of clinical problems involving the masticatory muscles and the temporomandibular joint (TMJ) [76]. Pain from this disorder may often radiate to various areas, including the dental arches, temples, ears, occiput, forehead, cervical region of spine or shoulder girdle. However, despite the fact that TMJ can cause severe and sometimes unbearable pain, relatively few patients seek treatment [77]. Intra-articular diseases involve the TMJ and are managed aggressively based on clinical, laboratory, and imaging evidence. In this disorder, misdiagnosis can often lead to ineffective management, and ultimately the consequences can be more serious and cause the patient to feel hopeless, anxious, and depressed [76]. Based on the results of research Bae and Park, it has been shown that performing active and relaxation exercises can improve the limited range of motion, deviation, and pain in the masticatory muscles. They recommend that to relaxation the muscle, the patient should putt the front one-third of the tongue on the anterior palate and apply a light force to the tip of the tongue, so that it does not touch the teeth and continue this position as long as he can tolerate. These exercises should be performed three times over a 4-week period, each time for 10 minutes [78]. Other recommendations for reducing pain in patients with TMJ include sulfur and iodine baths. Cryotherapy is another type of temperature-related treatment, but in this method, cold is used instead of heat. Among the analgesic agents used in this treatment method are cold packs, cold spray or air, and ice compresses as analgesic agents. Immediately before kinesiotherapy, cold is used, which combats hypertension in the muscles and tendinopathies. Of course, in this method, it should be remembered that the risk of frostbite (skin damage due to low temperatures) is high. As a result, cold compresses should be applied for (10 to 15 minutes). Cryotherapy can lead to pain, reduced stiffness of the TMJ, and increased mobility of the mandibular [79]. In managing pain and also increasing the overall quality of life in patients with TMJ, also medication options can play a very important role. According to published reports, it has been found that 50% of patients with TMJ disorders who suffered from severe pain used medication for management [80]. Also, several studies have examined the effectiveness of various drug treatments in painful orofacial pain conditions, including temporomandibular joint disorders the results have shown that drug therapy has been able to effectively reduce severe pain in patients [81].

4. Pharmacological therapy for temporomandibular joint disorders

The disorders caused by Temporomandibular Joint (TMJ) disease affect the surrounding tissues, Therefore, the treatment for this disease varies depending on its stage and severity. The treatment classification for this disease includes (1) non-invasive methods; (2) minimally invasive; or (3) invasive methods. Non-invasive methods are the first treatment option for patients with TMJ, which include medications such as anti-inflammatory drugs and muscle relaxants, physical therapy, and acupuncture [82]. The most important thing that can help the physician in recommending initial therapy is to accurately diagnose the origin of pain, whether it is intra-articular or muscular. Still unknown, though, is which non-invasive treatments are most effective. Damage or structural alterations in the TMJ are linked to the development and progression of TMD. Patients with TMD most frequently complain of pain, malocclusion, irregular and restricted jaw action, and joint sounds. Also, the development of concomitant headaches and disruption of the normal sleep pattern led to a severe decrease in the quality of life of patients. Fortunately, in the past 25 years, pharmaceutic therapies have been widely used to relieve TMD syndrome. NSAIDs, corticosteroids, opioids, muscle relaxants, anxiolytics drugs, antidepressants, and anticonvulsants are among the most effective pharmacological agents used to treat TMD [6]. For pharmacological management of pain, there are two main options, non-steroidal anti-inflammatory drugs (NSAIDs) and opiate/opioid analgesics. NSAIDs, which are among the most widely used medications worldwide, are often preferred for several reasons, including their low potential for abuse, robust efficacy, and long history of clinical use [83]. Inflammation is frequently linked to discomfort and cartilage degradation in TMD. Therefore, it is advised to treat TMD using medications such NSAIDs that block the release of inflammatory cytokines. NSAIDs are the first-choice medications for mild to moderate inflammatory pain in patients with TMD due to their potent analgesic and anti-inflammatory properties, which stem from their mechanism of inhibiting cyclooxygenase to block prostaglandin formation. However, the majority of NSAIDs, such as ibuprofen and naproxen, which are taken orally to treat TMJ pain, may have some adverse effects that need to be taken into account [84].

5. The mechanism of action of NSAIDs

Nonsteroidal anti-inflammatory medications (NSAIDs) are among the most widely used analgesics for treating pain in the oral and orofacial region. Five subgroups of NSAIDs can be distinguished based on their chemical structures. Derivatives of aryl(heteroaryl)acetic acids or aryl(heteroaryl) methanes [naproxen and ibuprofen], derivatives of indole and indene acetic acid [etodolac, indomethacin], anthranilates [mefenamic acid, diclofenac], derivatives of salicylic acid (SA) [acetylsalicylic acid (ASA), sodium salicylate], and derivatives of enolic acid [meloxicam, piroxicam]. Because NSAIDs have varying plasma half-lives, they are separated into two subgroups: short-acting NSAIDs (like ibuprofen, aspirin, and diclofenac) with a plasma half-life of up to 6 hours and long-acting NSAIDs (like naproxen and celecoxib) with a plasma half-life of more than 10 hours [6, 85, 86]. NSAIDs can inhibit the activity of "COXs" (cyclooxygenases), enzymes located in the endoplasmic reticulum. Three isoforms of cyclooxygenases-(COX-1), (COX-2), and (COX-3)-are primarily found in the central nervous system. A structural constitutive isoenzyme that is continuously found in a variety of tissues, COX-1 takes part in a number of physiological functions. The kidneys, brain, and uterus are among the few organs that constitutively express COX-2, in contrast to COX-1. COX-2 is mainly an inducible cyclooxygenase isoform. Although the shape of the active sites varies, both isoforms play the same role in the same metabolic activities. It has been discovered that the COX-1 active site is smaller than the COX-2 active site. Growth factors and proinflammatory cytokines are associated with COX-2 expression [87–89]. Since the majority of NSAIDs are non-selective cyclooxygenase inhibitors, they can inhibit both COX-1 and COX-2 isoforms. This class of drugs comprises ibuprofen, ketoprofen, naproxen, and aspirin [90]. Researchers who examined non-selective NSAID doses [which inhibit 50% of cyclooxygenase activity (IC_{50})] discovered that the most inhibitory potencies for COX-2 in blood were diclofenac, valeryl salicylate, dexamethasone, mefenamic acid, and nimesulide, while the highest inhibitory potencies for COX-1 were flurbiprofen, ketoprofen, indomethacin, and diclofenac. According to these researchers' findings, diclofenac appears to be the most powerful and selective inhibitor of COX-2. Despite having a 20-fold higher selectivity for COX-2 than for COX-1, diclofenac is still a useful inhibitor of COX-1 [90]. Consequently, diclofenac has a significantly decreased risk of gastrointestinal events linked to NSAIDs, but it also significantly raises the risk of cardiovascular events linked to NSAIDs [88]. A summary of TMJ disorder and the mechanism of action of nonsteroidal anti-inflammatory drugs (NSAIDs) is shown in **Figure 1**.

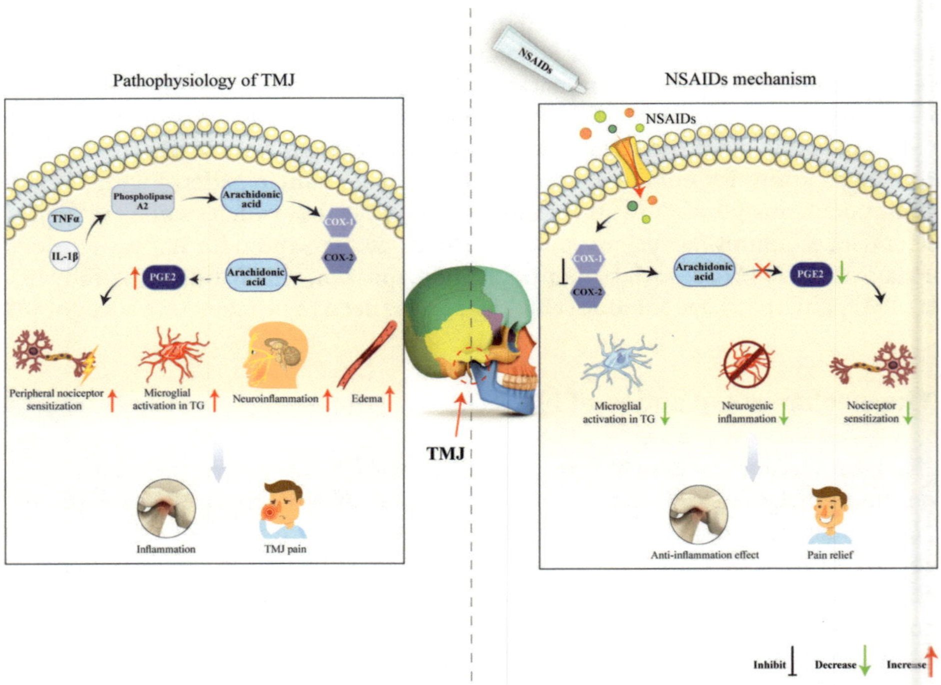

Figure 1.

Pathophysiology of disorders temporomandibular joint (TMJ)-related pain and its treatment with non-steroidal anti-inflammatory drugs: The temporomandibular joint (TMJ) is a small joint compared to other joints in the body. Symptoms of TMJ usually, resolve without medication. However, sometimes the pain can be severe enough to interfere with daily activities, which can be very uncomfortable if not treated promptly. In cases where pain and inflammation are present, the most effective medications used to treat TMJ are NSAIDs. NSAIDs can inhibit the activity of "cyclooxygenases," enzymes located in the endoplasmic reticulum. Three isoforms of cyclooxygenases-COX-1, COX-2, and COX-3-are primarily found in the central nervous system. As the text fully mentions this disorder and the mechanism of action of NSAIDs.

5.1 Adverse effects, and contraindications NSAIDs

5.1.1 Adverse effects

NSAIDs are used to relieve various pains. This class of drugs, in addition to relieving pain and reducing fever, has another important property including reducing inflammation [85]. Among various drugs, NSAIDs are among the most common and widely used classes of drugs prescribed for the treatment of craniofacial pain and have proven effectiveness in relieving pain in Temporomandibular disorders (TMD). As a painkiller, a small amount of any of the NSAIDs may be sufficient, but for their anti-inflammatory effects to appear in some diseases, a larger amount of the drug is required. Also, in diseases that require long-term treatment, the use of these drugs lasts longer. However, the use of NSAIDs can lead to the development of several side effects that may occur at any time during the course of treatment [37, 89, 90]. The most common adverse effects include cardiovascular, gastrointestinal (GI), and hepatic complications, as well as impaired renal function, respiratory disorders (aspirin-exacerbated respiratory disease (AERD) also called Samter's triad), clotting problems, and prolonged pregnancy or labor [6, 90–92]. Based on reported results, it has been found that in up to 60% of patients taking NSAIDs for a long term, gastrointestinal complications may occur [88, 93, 94].

Both topical and systemic NSAIDs can harm the gastrointestinal tract. The majority of NSAIDs have acidic qualities. Consequently, the topical mechanism is the direct harm that NSAIDs induce to the stomach mucosa. NSAIDs' systemic adverse effects can be explained by the fact that non-selective NSAIDs can inhibit the structural forms of cyclooxygenase (COX) and reduce prostaglandin formation, which can impact mucus secretion and hydrochloric acid [6, 91, 92, 95, 96]. There are four types of NSAID side effects that impact the upper gastrointestinal system, per Sostres et al. (1) gastroduodenal damage (associated with NSAIDs that have unclear clinical significance); (2) the presence of ulcers with symptoms and other gastrointestinal complications like perforation, obstruction, and gastrointestinal bleeding; (3) mortality; and (4) symptoms such as dyspepsia, nausea, vomiting, abdominal pain, and heartburn. NSAID users are at risk for gastrointestinal issues due to a number of factors [92]. A history of complicated ulcers, concurrent use of anticoagulants, concurrent use of multiple nonsteroidal NSAIDs, including low-dose aspirin, a history of uncomplicated ulcers, the use of high-dose NSAIDs (or ketorolac, marketed under the brand name Toradol, or piroxicam, which belongs to the oxicam class), and individuals over 60 are some of these risk factors. Severe sickness, *Helicobacter pylori* infection, and concomitant corticosteroid use [88, 92, 97]. There is a correlation between a higher risk of acute cardiovascular events with both selective and non-selective COX inhibitors (apart from aspirin) [98, 99]. Two possible pathways have been proposed to explain the development of coronary events: renal effects during long-term renal disease and COX-1/COX-2 selectivity. Inhibition of COX-2 might result in water retention and impaired salt excretion, which raise blood pressure [100]. Both mechanisms rely on duration and dose. Although it has not been verified, the theory that myocardial infarction risk and COX-2 selectivity are related is supported by two NSAIDs: rofecoxib [(MK 966, Vioxx®)], a selective COX-2 inhibitor, and diclofenac, a non-selective COX inhibitor, which have been associated with an increased risk of myocardial infarction (MI) when used long-term and at high doses [100]. The partnership between Coxib and researchers in the field of CNT (conventional NSAID trialists) demonstrated that diclofenac and Coxibs can significantly increase the risk of vascular complications. Furthermore, they found that while naproxen, the safest NSAID, appeared to be unable to increase either vascular or coronary events, whereas ibuprofen can significantly increase large coronary (not vascular) events [101].

5.1.2 Contraindications

Simultaneous use of NSAIDs and antihypertensives can lead to increased blood pressure levels and in some patients can cause various problems, including ineffectiveness of antihypertensive treatments [102]. Therefore, if NSAIDs are used for more than 5 days, the effects of antihypertensive drugs [such as diuretics] may be increased. Since NSAIDs have an antiplatelet effect by inhibiting thromboxane synthesis, these drugs should be used with caution in patients who are being treated with anticoagulant therapy [such as, warfarin (Coumadin)] [103, 104]. Given that NSAIDs are available over the counter (OTC) and without medical prescription, data on the prevalence of their use during pregnancy are not easy estimable available. Limited records of NSAID use have led to an underestimation of actual use. Since 1975, the United States Food and Drug Administration (FDA) has established a pregnancy risk classification for various drugs used during the first trimesters. According to this classification, NSAIDs are classified as category B in the three trimesters of pregnancy. This means that there is no evidence of risk to the fetal risk on animal reproduction studies or in women in the first trimester. They are classified as category D in the second trimester, this means that there is evidence of risk to the human fetal [105]. In all during trimester of pregnancy, doses of aspirin >150 mg/day are classified as considered category D, while aspirin (to low-dose) is classified to the category C. However, several studies have reported that exposure to NSAIDs during pregnancy can cause fetal and neonatal adverse effects. People exposed to NSAIDs in the first trimester have been linked to an increased risk of miscarriage and malformation. In contrast, third-trimester exposed to these drugs was associated with premature closure of the fetal ductus arteriosus and oligohydramnios. There have also been reports of fetal and neonatal adverse effects (after exposure to NSAIDs during pregnancy) affecting the kidney, lung, brain, skeleton, gastrointestinal tract, and cardiovascular system. In the past, FDA has advised pregnant women to stop taking NSAIDs and aspirin during the last 3 months of pregnancy, from 28th week until the end of pregnancy. The FDA also announced on 15 October 2020, that pregnant women should avoid taking NSAIDs around 20 weeks of pregnancy because they may lead to the onset of oligohydramnios and kidney problems in the newborns [105–107]. Since many women are likely to be taken NSAIDs during the periconceptional period, if NSAID use during pregnancy, particularly around the time of conception, is linked to miscarriage, it may have wide-ranging therapeutic implications. Even though more research is required to confirm the link between NSAID use and the risk of miscarriage, doctors should exercise caution when prescribing this class of medications, and pregnant women should be aware of this possible risk and refrain from taking NSAIDs around the time of conception [108]. Although there are different methods to reduce pain in TMJ patients, but the focus of this chapter is on pharmacotherapy. The names of nonsteroidal anti-inflammatory drugs along with their dosages as well as effective doses used in clinical studies related to TMJ disorders are presented in **Table 1**. However, for the treatment of pain and inflammation caused by TMJ, the type and dosage of the drug may vary depending on the patient's condition, age, underlying diseases, etc.

NSAID type	Dosage	Indications in TMD
Diclofenac	75 mg two times a day or 50 mg three times a day 100 mg once/day sustained-release	75 mg once daily or 75 mg every 12 hours (oral dosage only for adults)/maximum daily dose: 150 mg/not recommended for children.
Flurbiprofen	300–600 mg four times a day (oral dosage), maximum recommended daily dose: 300 mg.	No information
Ibuprofen	400–800 mg four times a day	400 mg every 6–8 hours (oral dosage only for adults) [maximum daily dose: 2400 mg]. 20 mg/kg/day 3–4 doses for children
Fenoprofen	300–600 mg four times a day (oral dosage)	No information
Mefenamic acid	250 mg PO q6hr PRN usually not to exceed 7 days, 500 (mg)	No information
Diflunisal	500 mg oral tablets	No information
Meloxicam	7.5 mg once/day (oral dosage).	7.5 mg once daily (oral dosage only for adults)/maximum daily dose: 15 mg.
Indomethacin	25 mg three to four times a day 75 mg two times a day sustained-release (oral dosage).	No information
Etodolac	300–500 mg two times a day (oral dosage).	No information
Nabumetone	1000–2000 mg/day in 1 dosage or in divided dosages (500–1000 mg two times a day/oral dosage).	No information
Ketorolac	30 mg single dose or 30 mg every 6 hours (IV and IM dosing for adults)/not exceeding 120 mg in 24 hours. (20 mg) single-dose after [IV or IM therapy], then 10 mg every 4–6 hours, not exceeding 40 mg in 24 hours (for adults)/dosage of ketorolac in children is 0.5 mg/kg (maximum duration of treatment:48 hours), oral dosage is 0.25 mg/kg to a maximum of 1.0 mg/kg/day, with a maximum duration of 7 days.	20 mg as a starting dosage plus 10–30 mg intramuscularly or intravenously over 4–6 hours; not advised for children less than 16
Tolmetin	400 mg three times a day (oral dosage).	No information
Ketoprofen	50–75 mg four times a day 200 mg once/day sustained-release (oral dosage).	100 mg every 12 hours (oral dosage only for adults)/maximum daily dose: 200 mg.
Dexketoprofenthro metamol	50 mg 8–12 hourly	50 mg intramuscularly or intravenously every 8–12 hours. It is not advised for kids.
Oxaprozin	1200 mg once/day (oral dosage). Maximum dose per day: 1200 or 1800 mg depending on body weight	No information
Nimesulide	100 mg twice daily (for adults) for no more than 15 days	100 mg every 12 hours (oral dosage only for adults)/maximum daily dose: 200 mg.
Naproxen	250–500 mg two times a day (oral dosage).	250–500 mg every 12 hours (oral dosage only for adults)/maximum daily dose: 1250 mg/dose of children: 10 mg/kg/day 2 doses
Sulindac	150–200 mg two times a day (oral dosage).	

NSAID type	Dosage	Indications in TMD
Acetylsalicylic acid (Aspirin)	325 to 1000 mg every 4 to 6 hours (oral dosage), maximum dose per day: 4000 mg	500 mg/4–6 hours (oral dosage only for adults).
Piroxicam	20 mg once/day (oral dosage). Maximum dose per day: 20 mg	Adults should take 40 mg daily on the first day and 20 mg daily the next day. Dose of children: not recommended.
Celecoxib [COX-2 selective NSAIDs] (also known as coxibs)	200 mg once/day or two times a day (oral dosage).	200 mg once daily or 100 mg every 12 hours (oral dosage only for adults)/maximum daily dose: 400 mg. Not evaluated in children
Lornoxicam (member of the oxicam group)	Doses > or = 8 mg to control pain, oral doses of lornoxicam of 16–24 mg daily	No information
Tolfenamic acid	Two capsules of 100 mg three times daily	No information
Parecoxib	20 mg and 40 mg/the published information on this compound is inadequate to draw any conclusion about its tolerability.	No information

* *In 2004 and 2005, the drugs rofecoxib and valdecoxib were withdrawn from the market, respectively.*
* *NSAIDs are usually available as oral tablets. The dosage for the most common NSAIDs (some of which are also available over-the-counter) is listed on the package insert.*
* *Use of NSAIDs in children should be based on the "Drug Facts" label, which includes instructions for the child's age or weight, the dose, and how often to take the medication. Although, based on the reported results, some of these medications are not recommended for children, but a doctor should still be consulted.*
* *It is predicated on comparative dosages from clinical trials and approved ranges dosing ranges by the US Food and Drug Administration.*
* *Although Nimesulide it is not available in the US, is frequently used to treat acute pain in other countries.*
* *In children, Nimesulide is deemed contraindicated. Nimesulide comes in both generic and trade formulations versions (Sulide, Nimside, and others) and can be obtained with a prescription as 200 mg suppositories and 100 mg oral suspension capsules or granules.*
* *The drug parecoxib was banned by the FDA in 2005, and a letter of non-approval was issued.*

Table 1.
Clinical decision-making taking NSAIDs [88, 109–117].

6. Pharmacological treatment outcomes for temporomandibular joint (TMJ) disorders

In a study conducted by Ta et al., on the effectiveness of celecoxib (100 mg twice a day) and naproxen (500 mg twice a day) compared to placebo in patients with TMJ, the results showed that the greatest effect in reducing temporomandibular joint pain was related to naproxen. Celecoxib, however, performed marginally better than a placebo. Within 3 weeks of starting treatment, naproxen was able to considerably lessen the intensity of TMJ pain. According to these researchers' findings, inhibiting both COX isoforms-COX-1 and COX-2 is necessary to reduce TMJ pain to the greatest extent possible [88]. A study by Di Rienzo Businco et al., showed that all patients with TMJ who were treated with diclofenac sodium (50 mg/every 12 hours/orally) for (14 days) as well as topical diclofenac (16 mg/mL/topical diclofenac solution, 10 drops 4 times a day) for (14 days) had a significant reduction in pain. The authors showed that the topical approach is the only way to completely eliminate the possibility of systemic side effects that could arise from oral administration of diclofenac sodium, and that there is no difference in the effectiveness of topical application and oral administration of multiple doses of the medication. The findings demonstrated that shorter durations of oral diclofenac sodium administration at lower dosages produced significant pain alleviation [109]. de Carli and colleagues also showed, in a randomized, double-blinded trial, that the drug piroxicam, a cyclooxygenase-2 inhibitor, was able to show the least pain at 30-day follow-up compared to placebo [110]. According to Cryer and Feldman's analysis of non-selective NSAID concentrations that inhibit (50%) of cyclooxygenase activity (IC_{50}), the drugs ketoprofen, indomethacin (indomethacin), diclofenac, ketorolac, and flurbiprofen (derived from phenyl alkanoic acid derivatives) produced the highest inhibitory potency for COX-1 in blood. In contrast, diclofenac, valeryl salicylate, dexamethasone (a fluorinated glucocorticoid drug), mefenamic acid, and nimesulide had the strongest inhibitory potency in blood for COX-2. Thus, diclofenac appears to be the most effective and specific inhibitor of COX-2 [111]. In a study involving patients with TMD-J, the effect of NSAIDs was examined and the results showed that diclofenac sodium can have a significant effect in reducing pain, but if this drug is combined with bromelain (enzyme extract derived from the stems of pineapples), rutoside (flavonoid glycoside), trihydrate, and trypsin, it can produce a better effect and be more effective in reducing pain [112]. In another study, comparing the drug ibuprofen with the endocannabinoid-like lipid mediator Palmitoylethanolamide (PEA), the results showed that although ibuprofen could significantly reduce pain and increased MMO (Maximum Mouth Opening), but PEA was more effective [113]. Two studies that compared each other the effects of ibuprofen and glucosamine sulfate, the results showed that ibuprofen could lead to similar or less pain reduction than glucosamine [114]. Kurita Varoli et al., in their study, they studied a group of patients suffering from chronic masticatory muscles pain due to TMD with different drug groups and occlusal splints or night guard. A placebo was administered twice daily for 10 days, along with 50 mg of diclofenac sodium twice daily for 10 days, and 300 mg of acetaminophen, 50 mg of sodium diclofenac, 125 mg of carisoprodol, and 30 mg of caffeine twice daily for 10 days using panacea. Between the various medication treatments, there were 11-day washout periods. The patients did not utilize any medicine or occlusal splints throughout the washout periods. According to the researchers, occlusal splints with NSAIDs or panacea were able to reduce pain on the third day of treatment, while compared to placebo, occlusal splints with placebo were able to reduce pain on the eighth day of treatment. It was also found that there was no difference between the groups in terms of analgesic effect after 10-day treatment periods. Therefore, it can be concluded that the administration of diclofenac sodium with occlusal splints can reduce pain earlier [115].

7. Recommendations for improving, management, evaluating, and drug-drug interaction evidence

Because of the possibility of side effects, NSAID use is associated with 30% of hospital admissions. Consequently, a thorough understanding of how sensitive some major organs are to NSAIDs—which are frequently used in daily life—is vital and required. This will lead to increased awareness about the prudent use of these drugs. Nonetheless, more research is required to examine the different facets of organ damage brought on by NSAID use, including other organs and bodily systems. The use of these drugs should be evaluated from a mechanistic perspective, such as how mitochondria and other organelles contribute to the pathophysiology of NSAIDs and the examination of genetic variations that are likely linked to NSAID sensitivity. Population-based research may prove useful in addressing the intricate gene-driven effects on xenobiotic metabolism in the context of NSAIDs. A particular NSAID use plan should be created for older persons because they are more likely than others to experience cardiovascular, renal, gastrointestinal (GI), and hepatic problems [85]. NSAID medication therapy for TMJ patients typically lasts 2 to 4 weeks [6]. NSAIDs may occasionally be administered for a longer duration of time, contingent on the patient's condition and if required. The aforementioned adverse effects may become more likely if these medications are used for an extended period of time. Therefore, it is strongly recommended to use NSAIDs at the lowest effective dose for the shortest period of time in order to reduce the risk of side effects [90, 91, 116]. To reduce the gastrointestinal risk of associated with NSAIDs, should be supplementary gastro-protective agent's medications prescribed [90, 94]. Several medications, including high-dose H_2-receptor antagonists, PPIs (proton pump inhibitors), and misoprostol (is a synthetic prostaglandin medication), which serve as gastroprotective agents [92, 94]. Proton pump inhibitors, by inhibiting the H^+/K^+ ATPase enzyme in the gastric parietal cells, significantly reduce, and stop gastric acid secretion [117–119]. Therefore, they can lessen NSAID-related upper gastrointestinal complications, particularly ulcers and mucosal damage. The lower gastrointestinal issues linked to NSAID use cannot be prevented by PPIs. Additionally, it has been demonstrated that PPIs cause SIBO (small intestinal bacterial overgrowth), or dysbiosis, in the bacterial flora of the small intestine. As a result, it can be said that this side effect might make the little intestine damage brought on by NSAIDs worse [117–120]. In addition, it should be noted that long-term use of PPIs may lead to some other potential side effects, including micronutrient deficiencies (lack of essential vitamins and minerals), bone fractures, infections, dementia and kidney disease or renal disease. However, the evidence about PPI side effects is generally of low or extremely low quality [117, 121]. Thus, it is stressed that communication between various specialists, such as cardiologists, primary care physicians, and gastroenterologists, is crucial for patients, particularly those who are at high risk of gastrointestinal and cardiovascular issues [122].

Since NSAIDs may in some cases lead to kidney damage (ranging from a simple reversible inflammation of the kidneys to serious permanent damage) and also implicated in the rapid deterioration of kidney function, therefore, according to national guidelines, it is recommended that these drugs be used with caution and in a specific dosage, and it is also recommended that nephrotoxic drugs (including nonsteroidal NSAIDs) be avoided in people with chronic renal impairment [123, 124]. Studies have shown that in prescribing NSAIDs, increasing clinician knowledge, it has very minimal or no effect. In one study, based on the evidence provided It was found that there was no association between knowledge of NSAID therapy and suboptimal management. In another study found that targeted educational intervention, had only a small effect on prescriber's actions in the use of NSAIDs. Other explanations may relate to differences between physicians in their perceptions of the importance of the risks of treatment or also in the expected benefits of drug therapy, especially given the conflicting advertising around issues such as the cardiovascular risk associated with NSAIDs use. Physicians may not be aware of contraindications to the use of NSAIDs in individual patients for various reasons because patients may refer to a number of general practitioners and specialists for their care. Therefore, it can be concluded that patient attitude and knowledge, as well as willingness to ask questions of physicians, and physicians' knowledge of the patient's condition, can affect the use of NSAIDs. Some NSAID users, may be fully aware of the potential harms of these drugs, but use them to relieve pain that cannot be relieved by other means. However, many patients are unaware of the toxicity of NSAIDs, as it is per the published data from the US on the use of these drugs among patients, it is shown that they were unaware of the toxicity of NSAIDs and did not have sufficient knowledge in this field [124].

The safest strategy to prevent the risk of excessive bleeding is to, avoid taking NSAIDs with oral anticoagulants (OACs). However, if this is not possible, NSAIDs should be prescribed in the lowest possible doses and for the shortest possible duration to reduce potential risks. It is important to note that the choice of agent and route of can also be important. According to current guidelines for the use of NSAIDs, the place strong emphasis is on topical rather than systemic administration [125].

One of the most accessible OTC (over-the-counter) medications is NSAIDs. Even though these medications' adverse effects have been researched for a while, further investigation and more accurate findings are still required to ascertain whether NSAIDs and high blood pressure (HTN-C) are related. It is necessary for physicians to constantly warn their patients about the uncontrolled and unsupervised use of NSAIDs, and therefore it is necessary for physicians to be aware of the risks, and to be particularly careful when prescribing medications to patients who suffer from or have risk factors for hypertensive, and to schedule regular follow-ups to monitor drug use. In addition, in people taking aspirin, based on the higher risk of HTN-C, it has been suggested that from aspirin should not only be avoided as a primary atherosclerotic cardiovascular disease (ASCVD), rather, in people diagnosed with hypertension and ASCVD, after initial treatment, to reduce the risk of HTN-C, if medication is needed, monotherapy with clopidogrel (class of medications called antiplatelet medications) or concomitant use of rivaroxaban (Xarelto) with aspirin should be considered [126]. Effective treatment for TMD requires a multidisciplinary approach between dentists, pain specialists, physiotherapists, psychologists and neurologists. However, we sometimes see fragmented treatment approaches and conflicting management strategies this is because many healthcare systems lack integrated care models [127]. The selective COX-2 inhibitors celecoxib and etoricoxib preferentially block the COX-2 isoform. It is not advised to prescribe NSAIDs to patients with active gastrointestinal issues because these medications have a lower risk of gastrointestinal side effects when taken alone, but when taken in combination with aspirin (at low doses), the risk of upper gastrointestinal ulcer bleeding is comparable to that of non-selective COX inhibitors [128]. NSAIDs can also interact with other drugs, including lithium. For example, lithium clearance is reduced after administration of NSAIDs. Therefore, this can lead to increased serum lithium concentration and, consequently, increased toxicity [129].

To update the existing European Alliance of Associations for Rheumatology (EULAR) points for use of NSAIDs: [130].

- There is no indication of a higher risk of miscarriage or teratogenicity associated with early pregnancy exposure to NSAIDs.

- While there is little information available for COX-2 inhibitors, the most reassuring data is provided for ibuprofen and diclofenac.

- The majority of the data available for NSAID usage in the second trimester relates to ibuprofen, which suggests that short-term use (7–10 days) does not appear to offer significant hazards for the fetus.

- The use of nonselective NSAIDs with a short half-life, such as ibuprofen, at the lowest effective dose for a brief period of time (7–10 days), is preferred because safety data on NSAIDs in the second trimester show that fetal adverse effects depend on exposure time, treatment duration, dosage, and intensity of prostaglandin inhibition.

- Since the fetus becomes more susceptible to NSAID-related risks in late pregnancy, such as oligohydramnios or narrowing/occlusion of the foetal ductus arteriosus, NSAIDs should be limited to the first and second trimesters and stopped after gestational week (GW) 28 (the end of the second trimester).

- NSAIDs can interfere with ovulation, as this process depends on prostaglandins. NSAID exposure during the periovulatory period might cause luteinized unruptured follicle (LUF) syndrome, which lowers a woman's fecundability. Women who are having trouble getting pregnant are advised to think about stopping NSAIDs.

INfORM/IADR key points for good clinical practice based on standard of care: [131].

- The process of managing TMDs, which includes taking a patient's history, examining them, diagnosing them, and treating them, requires patient-centered decision-making in addition to patient involvement and viewpoint. Expectations should focus on learning to control and manage the symptoms and lessen their influence on the person's daily life.

- The diagnosis of temporomandibular joint disorders (TMD) should be based on compliance with some established protocols. In fact, the diagnosis of this disease should be based on taking a standard and valid history as well as a detailed clinical assessment by a trained examiner, taking into account the patient's perspective.

- While imaging has been shown to be useful in certain situations, it cannot take the place of a thorough history and clinical examination. The current standard of care for soft tissues is magnetic resonance imaging, and for bone, it is cone beam computerized tomography. Imaging should only be done if it could influence the diagnosis or course of treatment.

- The goal of TMD treatment should be to reduce the impact of pain and decrease functional limitation. Also, outcomes should be evaluated to in relation with the reduction of exacerbations, education in how to manage exacerbations, and improvement in quality of life.

- The mainstays of TMD treatment should include conservative methods including cognitive-behavioral therapy and physical therapy, as well as the promotion of supported self-management. Oral appliance use that is temporary, interim, and time-limited is considered a second-line treatment to assist self-management. Surgical interventions are recommended only very seldom and in very specific conditions.

- Complex clinical presentations with an unclear prognosis, such as comorbidities or concurrent widespread pain, central sensitization, chronic pain, or a history of unsuccessful interventions, should raise suspicions of TMD or non-TMD pain chronification. Therefore, it is advised to refer a patient to a suitable specialist; the specialty will be geographic-specific as not all countries have a specialty of orofacial pain.

8. Conclusion

TMJ disorder has many signs and symptoms, and because many of these symptoms overlap with those of other conditions, TMJ disorders are often difficult to diagnose. Effective treatment for TMD requires a multidisciplinary approach between dentists, pain specialists, physiotherapists, psychologists and neurologists. NSAIDs are a group of drugs with analgesic, anti-inflammatory, and antipyretic effects, whose main mechanism of action is to inhibit the activity of the COX enzyme and thereby reduce the level of prostaglandins. These drugs are among the successful treatment options in reducing pain and inflammation in TMJ disease. Many NSAIDs are available OTC. However, stronger doses of these medications can only be obtained with a doctor's prescription. These medications are safe and effective when used as directed doctors, but inappropriate use of NSAIDs can lead to a wide range of adverse effects, including gastrotoxicity, nephrotoxicity, cardiotoxicity, hepatoxicity, and even in some caused death. Although the available evidence, it supports the use NSAIDs in patients with TMJ for pain relief, but further studies with more precise and consistent diagnostic and therapeutic criteria are needed.

Conflict of interest

The authors declare no conflict of interest.

Author details

Elahe Aleebrahim-Dehkordi[1*], Mahmoud Bahrami Dashtaki[2] and Sina Ahmadi[3,4]

1 Systematic Review and Meta-Analysis Expert Group (SRMEG), Universal Scientific Education and Research Network (USERN), Tehran, Iran

2 Shahrekord University of Medical Sciences, Shahrekord, Iran

3 Key Laboratory of Shaanxi Province for Craniofacial Precision Medicine Research, College of Stomatology, Xi'an Jiaotong University, Xi'an, Shaanxi, China

4 Department of Oral and Maxillofacial Surgery, College of Stomatology, Xi'an Jiaotong University, Xi'an, Shaanxi, China

*Address all correspondence to: elahe.aleebrahim@gmail.com

References

[1] Rui Yun BI, Ding Y, Gan YH. Non-steroidal anti-inflammatory drugs attenuate hyperalgesia and block upregulation of trigeminal ganglionic sodium channel 1.7 after induction of temporomandibular joint inflammation in rats. Chin. Journal of Dental Research. 2016;**19**(1):35-42

[2] Tanaka E, Detamore MS, Mercuri LG. Degenerative disorders of the temporomandibular joint: Etiology, diagnosis, and treatment. Journal of Dental Research. 2008;**87**:296-307. DOI: 10.1177/154405910808700406

[3] O'Connor RC, Fawthrop F, Salha R, Sidebottom AJ. Management of the temporomandibular joint in inflammatory arthritis: Involvement of surgical procedures. European Journal of Rheumatology. 2017;**4**(2):151-156. DOI: 10.5152/eurjrheum.2016.035. Epub 2017 Feb 23

[4] Derwich M, Mitus-Kenig M, Pawlowska E. Interdisciplinary approach to the temporomandibular joint osteoarthritis-review of the literature. Medicina. 2020;**56**:225. DOI: 10.3390/medicina56050225

[5] Al-Moraissi EA, Wolford LM, Ellis E 3rd, Neff A. The hierarchy of different treatments for arthrogenous temporomandibular disorders: A network meta-analysis of randomized clinical trials. Journal of Cranio-Maxillo-Facial Surgery. 2020;**48**:9-23. DOI: 10.1016/j.jcms.2019.10.004

[6] Ouanounou A, Goldberg M, Haas DA. Pharmacotherapy in temporomandibular disorders: A review. Journal of the Canadian Dental Association. 2017;**83**(7):1-8

[7] Gauer RL, Semidey MJ. Diagnosis and treatment of temporomandibular disorders. American Family Physician. 2015;**91**(6):378-386

[8] Lee SH, Jo JH, Park JW. Temporomandibular disorders patients with migraine symptoms have increased disease burden due to psychological conditions. Journal of Oral & Facial Pain and Headache. 2025;**39**(1):70

[9] Jogna F, Graenicher AA, Rey-Millet Q, Groz A, De Grasset J, Stollar F, et al. Pharmacological and non-pharmacological approaches to temporomandibular disorder chronic pain: A narrative review. Pain Management. 4 May 2025;**15**(5):285-296

[10] Warzocha J, Gadomska-Krasny J, Mrowiec J. Etiologic factors of temporomandibular disorders: A systematic review of literature containing diagnostic criteria for temporomandibular disorders (DC/TMD) and research diagnostic criteria for temporomandibular disorders (RDC/TMD) from 2018 to 2022. Healthcare (Basel). 2024;**12**(5)

[11] Reiter S, Goldsmith C, Emodi-Perlman A, Friedman-Rubin P, Winocur E. Masticatory muscle disorders diagnostic criteria: The American Academy of Orofacial Pain versus the research diagnostic criteria/temporomandibular disorders (RDC/TMD). Journal of Oral Rehabilitation. 2012;**39**(12):941-947

[12] Schiffman E, Ohrbach R, Truelove E, Look J, Anderson G, Goulet JP, et al. Diagnostic criteria for temporomandibular disorders (DC/TMD) for clinical and research applications: Recommendations of the

international RDC/TMD consortium network and orofacial pain special interest group†. Journal of Oral & Facial Pain and Headache. 2014;**28**(1):6-27

[13] Ohrbach R, Sollecito T, Omolehinwa T, Greenberg MS. Temporomandibular disorders. In: Burket's Oral Medicine. 30 Aug 2021. pp. 349-417. DOI: 10.1002/9781119597797.ch10

[14] Krasińska-Mazur M, Homel P, Gala A, Stradomska J, Pihut M. Differential diagnosis of temporomandibular disorders-A review of the literature. Folia Medica Cracoviensia. 2022;**62**(2):121-137. DOI: 10.24425/fmc.2022.141703

[15] Demerjian GG, Sims AB, Patel M, Balatgek TL, Sabal EB Jr. Head and neck manifestations of temporomandibular joint disorders. In: Temporomandibular Joint and Airway Disorders: A Translational Perspective. Cham: Springer International Publishing; 2018. pp. 73-93

[16] Warren MP, Fried JL. Temporomandibular disorders and hormones in women. Cells, Tissues, Organs. 2001;**169**(3):187-192

[17] Valesan LF, Da-Cas CD, Réus JC, Denardin ACS, Garanhani RR, Bonotto D, et al. Prevalence of temporomandibular joint disorders: A systematic review and meta-analysis. Clinical Oral Investigations. 2021;**25**(2):441-453

[18] Silva MAG, Pantoja LLQ, Dutra-Horstmann KL, Valladares-Neto J, Wolff FL, Porporatti AL, et al. Prevalence of degenerative disease in temporomandibular disorder patients with disc displacement: A systematic review and meta-analysis. Journal of Cranio-Maxillofacial Surgery. 2020;**48**(10):942-955

[19] Lei J, Han J, Liu M, Zhang Y, Yap AU-J, Fu K-Y. Degenerative temporomandibular joint changes associated with recent-onset disc displacement without reduction in adolescents and young adults. Journal of Cranio-Maxillofacial Surgery. 2017;**45**(3):408-413

[20] Limchaichana N, Petersson A, Rohlin M. The efficacy of magnetic resonance imaging in the diagnosis of degenerative and inflammatory temporomandibular joint disorders: A systematic literature review. Oral Surgery, Oral Medicine, Oral Pathology, Oral Radiology, and Endodontology. 2006;**102**(4):521-536

[21] Wang Y, Wluka AE, Jones G, Ding C, Cicuttini FM. Use magnetic resonance imaging to assess articular cartilage. Therapeutic Advances in Musculoskeletal Disease. 2012;**4**(2):77-97

[22] Maranini B, Ciancio G, Mandrioli S, Galiè M, Govoni M. The role of ultrasound in temporomandibular joint disorders: An update and future perspectives. Frontiers in Medicine. 2022;**9**:926573

[23] Bag AK, Gaddikeri S, Singhal A, Hardin S, Tran BD, Medina JA, et al. Imaging of the temporomandibular joint: An update. World Journal of Radiology. 2014;**6**(8):567-582. DOI: 10.4329/wjr.v6.i8.567

[24] Friedman SN, Grushka M, Beituni HK, Rehman M, Bressler HB, Friedman L. Advanced ultrasound screening for temporomandibular joint (TMJ) internal derangement. Radiology Research and Practice. 2020;**2020**(1):1809690

[25] AbdelAziz S, El-Goly NA, Maged AM, Bassiouny N, El-Demiry N, Shamel A. Diagnostic accuracy of

magnetic resonance imaging in the diagnosis of placenta accreta spectrum: A systematic review and meta-analysis. Maternal-Fetal Medicine. 2025;7(01):15-21

[26] Hussain S, Mubeen I, Ullah N, Shah S, Khan BA, Zahoor M, et al. Modern diagnostic imaging technique applications and risk factors in the medical field: A review. BioMed Research International. 2022;**2022**:5164970

[27] Minervini G, Franco R, Crimi S, Di Blasio M, D'Amico C, Ronsivalle V, et al. Pharmacological therapy in the management of temporomandibular disorders and orofacial pain: A systematic review and meta-analysis. BMC Oral Health. 2024;**24**(1):78

[28] Tang YH, van Bakelen NB, Gareb B, Spijkervet FKL. Office-based arthroscopy versus arthrocentesis as treatment for temporomandibular joint pain and dysfunction: Preliminary results of a randomized controlled trial. Journal of Clinical Medicine. 2025;**14**(9):2929

[29] Bouloux GF, Chou J, DiFabio V, Ness G, Perez D, Mercuri L, et al. The contemporary management of temporomandibular joint intra-articular pain and dysfunction. Journal of Oral and Maxillofacial Surgery. 2024;**82**(6):623-631

[30] Stegenga B. Nomenclature and classification of temporomandibular joint disorders. Journal of Oral Rehabilitation. 2010;**37**(10):760-765

[31] Buescher JJ. Temporomandibular joint disorders. American Family Physician. 2007;**76**(10):1477-1482

[32] Peck CC, Goulet JP, Lobbezoo F, Schiffman EL, Alstergren P, Anderson GC, et al. Expanding the taxonomy of the diagnostic criteria for temporomandibular disorders. Journal of Oral Rehabilitation. 2014;**41**(1):2-23

[33] Manfredini D, Häggman-Henrikson B, Al Jaghsi A, Baad-Hansen L, Beecroft E, Bijelic T, et al. Temporomandibular disorders: INfORM/IADR key points for good clinical practice based on standard of care. Cranio. 2025;**43**(1):1-5

[34] Okeson JP. Temporomandibular disorders: Etiology and classification. In: TMD and Orthodontics: A Clinical Guide for the Orthodontist. Cham: Springer International Publishing; 2015. pp. 19-36

[35] Benoliel R, Svensson P, Evers S, Wang S-J, Barke A, Korwisi B, et al. The IASP classification of chronic pain for ICD-11: Chronic secondary headache or orofacial pain. Pain. 2019;**160**(1):60-68

[36] DM-uKeVid d. Internationale Klassifikation orofazialer Schmerzen (ICOP), 1. Auflage. Der Schmerz. 2021;**35**:73-152

[37] Ferrillo M, Giudice A, Marotta N, Fortunato F, Di Venere D, Ammendolia A, et al. Pain management and rehabilitation for central sensitization in temporomandibular disorders: A comprehensive review. International Journal of Molecular Sciences. 2022;**23**(20):12164

[38] Brämer GR. International statistical classification of diseases and related health problems. Tenth revision. World Health Statistics Quarterly. 1988;**41**(1):32-36

[39] Klasser GD, Goulet J-P, Moreno-Hay I. Classification and diagnosis of temporomandibular disorders and temporomandibular disorder pain. Dental Clinics of North America. 2023;**67**(2):211-225

[40] Fillingim RB, Bruehl S, Dworkin RH, Dworkin SF, Loeser JD, Turk DC, et al. The ACTTION-American Pain Society Pain Taxonomy (AAPT): An evidence-based and multidimensional approach to classifying chronic pain conditions. The Journal of Pain. 2014;**15**(3):241-249

[41] Jalal K, Charest A, Wu X, Quigg RJ, Chang S. The ICD-9 to ICD-10 transition has not improved identification of rapidly progressing stage 3 and stage 4 chronic kidney disease patients: A diagnostic test study. BMC Nephrology. 2024;**25**(1):55

[42] Cairns BE. Pathophysiology of TMD pain—Basic mechanisms and their implications for pharmacotherapy. Journal of Oral Rehabilitation. 2010;**37**(6):391-410

[43] Sperry MM, Ita ME, Kartha S, Zhang S, Yu YH, Winkelstein B. The interface of mechanics and nociception in joint pathophysiology: Insights from the facet and temporomandibular joints. Journal of Biomechanical Engineering. 2017;**139**(2):0210031-02100313

[44] Dubin AE, Patapoutian A. Nociceptors: The sensors of the pain pathway. The Journal of Clinical Investigation. 2010;**120**(11):3760-3772

[45] Jaumard NV, Welch WC, Winkelstein BA. Spinal facet joint biomechanics and mechanotransduction in normal, injury and degenerative conditions. Journal of Biomechanical Engineering. 2011;**133**(7):071010

[46] Vinayak V, Ram KA, Chandran J. Exploring the complexities of temporomandibular joint function and dysfunction: A contemporary review. Odovtos - International Journal of Dental Sciences. 2024;**26**(3):79-98

[47] Chow YY, Chin KY. The role of inflammation in the pathogenesis of osteoarthritis. Mediators of Inflammation. 2020;**2020**(1):8293921

[48] Mehana E-SE, Khafaga AF, El-Blehi SS. The role of matrix metalloproteinases in osteoarthritis pathogenesis: An updated review. Life Sciences. 2019;**234**:116786

[49] Mukherjee A, Das B. The role of inflammatory mediators and matrix metalloproteinases (MMPs) in the progression of osteoarthritis. Biomaterials and Biosystems. 2024;**13**:100090

[50] Chiu IM, von Hehn CA, Woolf CJ. Neurogenic inflammation and the peripheral nervous system in host defense and immunopathology. Nature Neuroscience. 2012;**15**(8):1063-1067

[51] Shi X, Wang L, Li X, Sahbaie P, Kingery WS, Clark JD. Neuropeptides contribute to peripheral nociceptive sensitization by regulating interleukin-1β production in keratinocytes. Anesthesia and Analgesia. 2011;**113**(1):175-183

[52] Shrivastava M, Ye L. Neuroimaging and artificial intelligence for assessment of chronic painful temporomandibular disorders-a comprehensive review. International Journal of Oral Science. 2023;**15**(1):58

[53] Villa G, Ceruti S, Zanardelli M, Magni G, Jasmin L, Ohara PT, et al. Temporomandibular joint inflammation activates glial and immune cells in both the trigeminal ganglia and in the spinal trigeminal nucleus. Molecular Pain. 2010;**6**:89

[54] Ji RR, Donnelly CR, Nedergaard M. Astrocytes in chronic pain and itch. Nature Reviews. Neuroscience. 2019;**20**(11):667-685

[55] Gritzner S, Jackson V, Strigo I, Spiegel D. Treating the TMD/chronic

pain patient: Psychiatry and psychology. In: Contemporary Management of Temporomandibular Disorders: Non-Surgical Treatment. Cham: Springer International Publishing; 2019. pp. 199-214

[56] Ahmed OAS. Relationship of TMD Diagnosis and Self-Reported Biopsychosocial Status of Patients Attending the TMD Clinic. University of the Western Cape; 2018. Available from: https://hdl.handle.net/10566/10890

[57] Franks AS. Masticatory muscle hyperactivity and temporomandibular joint dysfunction. The Journal of Prosthetic Dentistry. 1965;**15**(6):1122-1131. DOI: 10.1016/0022-3913(65)90188-5

[58] Pihut M, Ferendiuk E, Szewczyk M, Kasprzyk K, Wieckiewicz M. The efficiency of botulinum toxin type A for the treatment of masseter muscle pain in patients with temporomandibular joint dysfunction and tension-type headache. The Journal of Headache and Pain. 2016;**17**:1-6

[59] Pinho JC, Caldas FM, Mora MJ, Santana-Penín U. Electromyographic activity in patients with temporomandibular disorders. Journal of Oral Rehabilitation. 2000;**27**(11):985-990

[60] Schroeder H, Siegmund H, Santibáñez-H G, Kluge A. Causes and signs of temporomandibular joint pain and dysfunction: An electromyographical investigation. Journal of Oral Rehabilitation. 1991;**18**(4):301-310

[61] Ardizone I, Celemin A, Aneiros F, del Rio J, Sanchez T, Moreno I. Electromyographic study of activity of the masseter and anterior temporalis muscles in patients with temporomandibular joint (TMJ) dysfunction: Comparison with the clinical dysfunction index. Medicina Oral, Patología Oral y Cirugía Bucal. 2010;**15**(1):e14-e19

[62] Romero-Reyes M, Uyanik JM. Orofacial pain management: Current perspectives. Journal of Pain Research. 2014;7:99-115

[63] Barrientos E, Pelayo F, Tanaka E, Lamela-Rey MJ, Fernández-Canteli A, de Vicente JC. Effects of loading direction in prolonged clenching on stress distribution in the temporomandibular joint. Journal of the Mechanical Behavior of Biomedical Materials. 2020;**112**:104029

[64] Crofford LJ. Psychological aspects of chronic musculoskeletal pain. Best Practice & Research. Clinical Rheumatology. 2015;**29**(1):147-155

[65] Peterson C, The TMJ. Healing Plan: Ten Steps to Relieving Headaches, Neck Pain and Jaw Disorders. Turner Publishing Company; 2011. Available from: https://www.amazon.com/TMJ-Healing-Plan-Relieving-Headaches/dp/0897935241

[66] Finan PH, Buenaver LF, Bounds SC, Hussain S, Park RJ, Haque UJ, et al. Discordance between pain and radiographic severity in knee osteoarthritis: Findings from quantitative sensory testing of central sensitization. Arthritis and Rheumatism. 2013;**65**(2):363-372

[67] Maixner W, Diatchenko L, Dubner R, Fillingim RB, Greenspan JD, Knott C, et al. Orofacial pain prospective evaluation and risk assessment study—The OPPERA study. The Journal of Pain. 2011;**12**(11 Suppl):T4-11.e1-2

[68] Harper D, Schrepf A, Clauw D. Pain mechanisms and centralized pain in

temporomandibular disorders. Journal of Dental Research. 2016;**95**(10):1102-1108

[69] Perry SK, Emrick JJ. Trigeminal somatosensation in the temporomandibular joint and associated disorders. Frontiers in Pain Research. 2024;**5**:1374929

[70] Pinho-Ribeiro FA, Verri WA Jr, Chiu IM. Nociceptor sensory neuron-immune interactions in pain and inflammation. Trends in Immunology. 2017;**38**(1):5-19

[71] Meng H, Dai J, Li Y. Quantitative sensory testing in patients with the muscle pain subtype of temporomandibular disorder: A systemic review and meta-analysis. Clinical Oral Investigations. 2021;**25**(12):6547-6559

[72] Fernández-de-Las-Peñas C, Svensson P, Arendt-Nielsen L. Quantitative sensory testing in temporomandibular disorders. In: Temporomandibular Disorders: Manual Therapy, Exercise and Needling. Handspring Publishing; 2018. pp. 79-88

[73] Yi Y, Zhou X, Xiong X, Wang J. Neuroimmune interactions in painful TMD: Mechanisms and treatment implications. Journal of Leukocyte Biology. 2021;**110**(3):553-563

[74] Melis M, Di Giosia M. The role of genetic factors in the etiology of temporomandibular disorders: A review. Cranio. 2016;**34**(1):43-51

[75] Exposto F, Svensson P, Arendt-Nielsen L. Temporomandibular disorder comorbidity. In: Comorbidities in Headache Disorders. 2017. pp. 161-180

[76] Mercuri LG. Temporomandibular joint disorder management in oral and maxillofacial surgery. Journal of Oral and Maxillofacial Surgery. 2017;**75**(5):927-930

[77] Wieckiewicz M, Boening K, Wiland P, Shiau YY, Paradowska-Stolarz A. Reported concepts for the treatment modalities and pain management of temporomandibular disorders. The Journal of Headache and Pain. 2015;**16**:1-2

[78] Bae Y, Park Y. The effect of relaxation exercises for the masticator muscles on temporomandibular joint dysfunction (TMD). Journal of Physical Therapy Science. 2013;**25**:583-586

[79] Wozniak K, Piatkowska D, Lipski M, Mehr K. Surface electromyography in orthodontics—A literature review. Medical Science Monitor. 2013;**19**:416-423

[80] Häggman-Henrikson B, Alstergren P, Davidson T, Högestätt ED, Östlund P, Tranaeus S, et al. Pharmacological treatment of oro-facial pain-health technology assessment including a systematic review with network meta-analysis. Journal of Oral Rehabilitation. 2017;**44**(10):800-826. DOI: 10.1111/joor.12539

[81] Christidis N, Al-Moraissi EA, Barjandi G, Svedenlöf J, Jasim H, Christidis M, et al. Pharmacological treatments of temporomandibular disorders: A systematic review including a network meta-analysis. Drugs. 2024;**84**(1):59-81

[82] Trindade D, Cordeiro R, José HC, Ângelo DF, Alves N, Moura C. Biological treatments for temporomandibular joint disc disorders: Strategies in tissue engineering. Biomolecules. 2021;**11**(7):933. DOI: 10.3390/biom11070933

[83] Brune K, Patrignani P. New insights into the use of currently available non-steroidal anti-inflammatory drugs. Journal of Pain Research. 2015;**8**:105-118.

DOI: 10.2147/JPR.S75160. eCollection 2015

[84] Wu M, Cai J, Yu Y, Hu S, Wang Y, Wu M. Therapeutic agents for the treatment of temporomandibular joint disorders: Progress and perspective. Frontiers in Pharmacology. 2021;**11**:596099

[85] Bindu S, Mazumder S, Bandyopadhyay U. Non-steroidal anti-inflammatory drugs (NSAIDs) and organ damage: A current perspective. Biochemical Pharmacology. 2020;**180**:114147. DOI: 10.1016/j.bcp.2020.114147. Epub 2020 Jul 10

[86] Sobhani K, Li J, Cortes M. Nonsteroidal anti-inflammatory drugs (NSAIDs). In: First Aid Perioperative Ultrasound: Acute Pain Manual for Surgical Procedures. Cham: Springer International Publishing; 2023. pp. 127-138

[87] Cruz JV, Rosa JM, Kimani NM, Giuliatti S, dos Santos CB. The role of celecoxib as a potential inhibitor in the treatment of inflammatory diseases—A review. Current Medicinal Chemistry. 2022;**29**(17):3028-3049

[88] Derwich M, Mitus-Kenig M, Pawlowska E. Orally administered NSAIDs general characteristics and usage in the treatment of temporomandibular joint osteoarthritis a narrative review. Pharmaceuticals. 2021;**14**(3):219

[89] Faki Y, Er A. Different chemical structures and physiological/pathological roles of cyclooxygenases. Rambam Maimonides Medical Journal. 2021;**12**(1):e0003. DOI: 10.5041/RMMJ.10426

[90] Ho KY, Cardosa MS, Chaiamnuay S, Hidayat R, Ho HQT, Kamil O, et al. Practice advisory on the appropriate use of NSAIDs in primary care. Journal of Pain Research. 2020;**13**:1925-1939. DOI: 10.2147/JPR.S247781

[91] Kulkarni S, Thambar S, Arora H. Evaluating the effectiveness of nonsteroidal anti-inflammatory drug (s) for relief of pain associated with temporomandibular joint disorders: A systematic review. Clinical and Experimental Dental Research. 2020;**6**(1):134-146

[92] Harirforoosh S, Asghar W, Jamali F. Adverse effects of nonsteroidal antiinflammatory drugs: An update of gastrointestinal, cardiovascular and renal complications. Journal of Pharmaceutical Sciences. 2013;**16**(5):821-847. DOI: 10.18433/j3vw2f

[93] Rafaniello C, Ferrajolo C, Sullo MG, Sessa M, Sportiello L, Balzano A, et al. Risk of gastrointestinal complications associated to NSAIDs, low-dose aspirin and their combinations: Results of a pharmacovigilance reporting system. Pharmacological Research. 2016;**104**:108-114. DOI: 10.1016/j.phrs.2015.12.026

[94] Sostres C, Gargallo CJ, Arroyo MT, Lanas A. Adverse effects of non-steroidal anti-inflammatory drugs (NSAIDs, aspirin and coxibs) on upper gastrointestinal tract. Best Practice & Research. Clinical Gastroenterology. 2010;**24**:121-132. DOI: 10.1016/j.bpg.2009.11.005

[95] Sostres C, Gargallo CJ, Lanas A. Nonsteroidal anti-inflammatory drugs and upper and lower gastrointestinal mucosal damage. Arthritis Research & Therapy. 2013;**15**:S3

[96] Watanabe T, Fujiwara Y, Chan FKL. Current knowledge on non-steroidal anti-inflammatory drug-induced small-bowel damage: A comprehensive review. Journal of Gastroenterology.

2020;**55**:481-495. DOI: 10.1007/s00535-019-01657-8

[97] Bjarnason I, Scarpignato C, Holmgren E, Olszewski M, Rainsford KD, Lanas A. Mechanisms of damage to the gastrointestinal tract from nonsteroidal anti-inflammatory drugs. Gastroenterology. 2018;**154**:500-514

[98] Scarpignato C, Hunt RH. Nonsteroidal antiinflammatory drug-related injury to the gastrointestinal tract: Clinical picture, pathogenesis, and prevention. Gastroenterology Clinics of North America. 2010;**39**:433-464

[99] Goldstein JL, Cryer B. Gastrointestinal injury associated with NSAID use: A case study and review of risk factors and preventative strategies. Drug, Healthcare and Patient Safety. 2015;7:31-41. DOI: 10.2147/DHPS.S71976

[100] Schink T, Kollhorst B, Varas LC, Arfe A, Herings R, Lucchi S, et al. Risk of ischemic stroke and the use of individual non-steroidal anti-inflammatory drugs: A multi-country European database study within the SOS project. PLoS ONE. 2018;**13**:e0203362. DOI: 10.1371/journal.pone.0203362

[101] Strand V. Are COX-2 inhibitors preferable to non-selective non-steroidal anti-inflammatory drugs in patients with risk of cardiovascular events taking low-dose aspirin? Lancet. 2007;**370**:2138-2151. DOI: 10.1016/S0140-6736(07)61909-6

[102] Moore N. Coronary risks associated with diclofenac and other NSAIDs: An update. Drug Safety. 2020;**43**:301-318. DOI: 10.1007/s40264-019-00900-8

[103] Bhala N, Emberson J, Merhi A, Abramson S, Arber N, Baron JA, et al. Vascular and upper gastrointestinal effects of non-steroidal anti-inflammatory drugs: Meta-analyses of individual participant data from randomised trials. Lancet (London, England). 2013;**382**(9894):769-779

[104] Villa J, Cano A, Franco D, Monsalve M, Hincapié J, Amariles P. Clinical relevance of drug interactions between nonsteroidal antiinflammatory drugs (NSAIDs) and antihypertensives. Atencion Primaria. 2014;**46**:464-474. DOI: 10.1016/j.aprim.2013.11.010

[105] Montinaro F, Nucci L, d'Apuzzo F, Perillo L, Chiarenza MC, Grassia V. Oral nonsteroidal anti-inflammatory drugs as treatment of joint and muscle pain in temporomandibular disorders: A systematic review. CRANIO®. 2024;**42**(6):641-650

[106] Mujakperuo HR, Watson M, Morrison R, Macfarlane T, v. Pharmacological interventions for pain in patients with temporomandibular disorders. Cochrane Database of Systematic Reviews. 2010;(10):CD004715. DOI: 10.1002/14651858.CD004715.pub2

[107] D'Ambrosio V, Vena F, Scopelliti A, D'Aniello D, Savastano G, Brunelli R, et al. Use of non-steroidal anti-inflammatory drugs in pregnancy and oligohydramnios: A review. The Journal of Maternal-Fetal & Neonatal Medicine. 2023;**36**(2):2253956

[108] Antonucci R, Zaffanello M, Puxeddu E, et al. Use of non-steroidal anti-inflammatory drugs in pregnancy: Impact on the fetus and newborn. Current Drug Metabolism. 2012;**13**(4):474-490. DOI: 10.2174/138920012800166607

[109] Singgih MF, Achmad H, Sukmana BI, Carmelita AB, Putra AP, Ramadhany S, et al. A review of nonsteroidal anti-inflammatory drugs

(NSAIDs) medications in dentistry: Uses and side effects. Systematic Reviews in Pharmacy. 2020;**11**(5):293-298

[110] Barkin RL. Topical nonsteroidal anti-inflammatory drugs: The importance of drug, delivery, and therapeutic outcome. American Journal of Therapeutics. 2015;**22**(5):388-407

[111] Chou R, McDonagh MS, Nakamoto E, Griffin J. Analgesics for Osteoarthritis: An Update of the 2006 Comparative Effectiveness Review [Internet]. Rockville (MD): Agency for Healthcare Research and Quality (US); 2011. Report No.: 11(12)-EHC076-EF

[112] Hoofnagle JH, Serrano J, Knoben JE, Navarro VJ. LiverTox: A website on drug-induced liver injury. Hepatology. 2013;**57**(3):873-874. DOI: 10.1002/hep.26175

[113] Radhofer-Welte S, Rabasseda X. Lornoxicam, a new potent NSAID with an improved tolerability profile. Drugs Today (Barc). 2000;**36**(1):55-76. DOI: 10.1358/dot.2000.36.1.566627

[114] Sørensen K, Christiansen LV. Long-term therapy with tolfenamic acid pINN. A clinical and toxicological study with special reference to clinical and chemical laboratory parameters. Scandinavian Journal of Rheumatology. Supplement. 1977;(20):1-7. DOI: 10.3109/03009747709095484

[115] Barden J, Edwards JE, McQuay HJ, Moore RA. Oral valdecoxib and injected parecoxib for acute postoperative pain: A quantitative systematic review. BMC Anesthesiology. 2003;**3**(1):1. DOI: 10.1186/1471-2253-3-1

[116] Mahmoodi AN, Patel P, Kim PY. Ketorolac. 2024 Feb 28. In: StatPearls [Internet]. Treasure Island (FL): StatPearls Publishing; 2025

[117] Forrest JB, Heitlinger EL, Revell S. Ketorolac for postoperative pain management in children. Drug Safety. 1997;**16**(5):309-329. DOI: 10.2165/00002018-199716050-00003

[118] Ta LE, Dionne RA. Treatment of painful temporomandibular joints with a cyclooxygenase-2 inhibitor: A randomized placebo-controlled comparison of celecoxib to naproxen. Pain. 2004;**111**:13-21

[119] Di Rienzo Businco L, Di Rienzo Businco A, D'Emilia M, Lauriello M, Coen Tirelli G. Topical versus systemic diclofenac in the treatment of temporomandibular joint dysfunction symptoms. Acta Otorhinolaryngologica Italica. 2004;**24**:279-283

[120] de Carli ML, Guerra MB, Nunes TB, di Matteo RC, de Luca CE, Aranha AC, et al. Piroxicam and laser phototherapy in the treatment of TMJ arthralgia: A double-blind randomised controlled trial. Journal of Oral Rehabilitation. 2013;**40**:171-178

[121] Cryer B, Feldman M. Cyclooxygenase-1 and cyclooxygenase-2 selectivity of widely used nonsteroidal anti-inflammatory drugs. The American Journal of Medicine. 1998;**104**:413-421

[122] Jayachandran S, Khobre P. Efficacy of bromelain along with trypsin, rutoside trihydrate enzymes and diclofenac sodium combination therapy for the treatment of TMJ osteoarthritis—A randomised clinical trial. Journal of Clinical and Diagnostic Research: JCDR. 2017;**11**(6):ZC09-ZC111

[123] Marini I, Bartolucci ML, Bortolotti F, Gatto MR, Bonetti GA. Palmitoylethanolamide versus a nonsteroidal anti-inflammatory drug in the treatment of temporomandibular

joint inflammatory pain. Journal of Orofacial Pain. 2012;**26**(2):99-104

[124] Haghighat A, Behnia A, Kaviani N, Khorami B. Evaluation of glucosamine sulfate and ibuprofen effects in patients with temporomandibular joint osteoarthritis symptom. Journal of Research in Pharmacy Practice. 2013;**2**(1):34-39

[125] Kurita VF, Sucena PM, Sato S, Issa JP, do Nascimento C, Pedrazzi V. Analgesia evaluation of 2 NSAID drugs as adjuvant in management of chronic temporomandibular disorders. Scientific World Journal. 2015;**2015**:359152. DOI: 10.1155/2015/359152

[126] Abdu N, Mosazghi A, Teweldemedhin S, Asfaha L, Teshale M, Kibreab M, et al. Non-Steroidal Anti-Inflammatory Drugs (NSAIDs): Usage and co-prescription with other potentially interacting drugs in elderly: A cross-sectional study. PLoS ONE. 2020;**15**:e0238868. DOI: 10.1371/journal.pone.0238868

[127] Gwee KA, Goh V, Lima G, Setia S. Coprescribing proton-pump inhibitors with nonsteroidal anti-inflammatory drugs: Risks versus benefits. Journal of Pain Research. eCollection. 2018;**11**:361-374. DOI: 10.2147/JPR.S156938

[128] Scheiman JM. The use of proton pump inhibitors in treating and preventing NSAID-induced mucosal damage. Arthritis Research & Therapy. 2013;**15**:S5. DOI: 10.1186/ar4177

[129] Jackson MA, Goodrich JK, Maxan ME, Freedberg DE, Abrams JA, Poole AC, et al. Proton pump inhibitors alter the composition of the gut microbiota. Gut. 2016;**65**:749-756. DOI: 10.1136/gutjnl-2015-310861

[130] Fujimori S. What are the effects of proton pump inhibitors on the small intestine? World Journal of Gastroenterology. 2015;**21**:6817-6819. DOI: 10.3748/wjg. v21.i22.6817

[131] Freedberg DE, Kim LS, Yang YX. The risks and benefits of long-term use of proton pump inhibitors: Expert review and best practice advice from the American Gastroenterological Association. Gastroenterology. 2017;**152**:706-715. DOI: 10.1053/j.gastro.2017.01.031

Chapter 8

Temporomandibular Joint Osteoarthritis: Emerging Roles of Stem Cells, Nanocarriers, and Tissue Engineering

Tharanikumar Sivakumar, Chandrsekaran Krithika, U. Elaveyini, Chitathoor Sridhar, S. Nachiappan and Ashok Prasanna

Abstract

Temporomandibular joint osteoarthritis (TMJOA) is a progressive degenerative disorder characterized by cartilage breakdown, subchondral bone remodeling, and chronic inflammation. Conventional treatments are largely palliative, providing symptomatic relief without reversing structural pathology. Advances in regenerative medicine offer novel therapeutic opportunities, including mesenchyme stem cell (MSC) therapy, nanotechnology-based drug delivery, exosome applications, and biomimetic scaffold engineering. MSCs contribute to repair by differentiating into chondrocytes and modulating the immune microenvironment, while nano-carriers enable targeted delivery and sustained retention of bioactive agents. Exosome-based therapies provide cell-free, immune-compatible alternatives with regenerative potential. Concurrently, hydrogel and scaffold systems supply structural support, enhance cellular proliferation, and improve integration with host tissue. Emerging strategies that integrate these modalities often combined with platelet-rich plasma (PRP) or advanced 3D bio-printing hold promise for restoring joint architecture and function. Despite encouraging preclinical data, clinical translation remains limited by variability in cell sources, delivery protocols, and outcome measures. Continued multidisciplinary research is essential to standardize methods, ensure safety, and advance patient-specific regenerative therapies for TMJOA.

Keywords: temporomandibular joint, osteoarthritis, mesenchymal stem cell (MSC) therapy, nanotechnology-based drug delivery systems, exosome applications

1. Introduction

Temporomandibular joint osteoarthritis (TMJOA) is a chronic, progressive disorder marked by degradation of the articular cartilage, abnormal remodeling of the subchondral bone, and synovial inflammation. These structural changes manifest clinically as pain, restricted mandibular movement, joint sounds, and impaired quality of life [1]. TMJOA is particularly prevalent among middle-aged individuals and women. Despite its frequency, conventional management remains largely symptomatic. Non-steroidal anti-inflammatory drugs (NSAIDs), occlusal splints, physiotherapy, and, in severe cases, surgical interventions primarily aim to relieve discomfort, restore function, and correct mechanical imbalances; however, they do not address or reverse the underlying joint degeneration [2].

This therapeutic limitation has fueled increasing interest in regenerative medicine approaches that target the root causes of TMJOA. Regenerative strategies seek not only to mitigate symptoms but also to repair damaged tissues and restore joint integrity. Among the most promising modalities are mesenchymal stem cells (MSCs), nanotechnology-based drug delivery, exosome-mediated therapies, and bioengineered scaffolds. MSCs derived from bone marrow, adipose tissue, or synovial fluid demonstrate chondrogenic and osteogenic potential, in addition to potent immunomodulatory and anti-inflammatory properties. Through the secretion of bioactive factors, MSCs influence the joint microenvironment, accelerate tissue repair, and regulate immune responses.

Nanotechnology complements these approaches by enabling targeted and sustained delivery of therapeutic molecules, thereby enhancing local retention and reducing systemic side effects. Nanomaterials can also be engineered into scaffolds with extracellular matrix-like properties, further promoting cartilage and bone regeneration. Tissue-engineered scaffolds fabricated from natural, synthetic, or hybrid biomaterials provide a structural niche for cell attachment, proliferation, and differentiation. Advances in 3D printing and biomaterials science have enabled the design of patient-specific, biodegradable scaffolds that integrate seamlessly with host tissue.

Together, these regenerative modalities represent a paradigm shift from symptomatic management to biologically driven repair of TMJOA. As research advances, the integration of MSCs, nanotechnology, and scaffold engineering holds promise for durable, functional joint restoration.

2. Conservative treatment options for TMJOA that focus on oral appliances

Conservative, non-invasive interventions are considered first-line management for TMJOA, particularly in early or moderate stages. Among these, oral appliances (occlusal splints) are widely used due to their accessibility, safety, and efficacy in reducing symptoms without surgery [3]. Fabricated from acrylic, splints are designed to fit over the maxillary or mandibular arch, with therapeutic goals including redistribution of occlusal forces, reduction of parafunctional activities such as bruxism, and alleviation of excessive joint loading [4].

Different splint types are prescribed according to clinical presentation: stabilization splints (flat-plane), anterior repositioning splints, and soft splints. Stabilization splints are most commonly used in TMJOA, as they promote even occlusal contact, reduce mechanical stress on the joint, and serve as the protective night guards during episodes of increased masticatory muscle activity [5]. Mechanistically, oral appliances relieve symptoms by reducing micro-trauma associated with clenching and grinding, relaxing hyperactive masticatory muscles, and realigning the mandibular position.

Clinical evidence confirms their effectiveness in reducing joint pain, improving mandibular mobility, and diminishing joint noises such as clicking and crepitus [5].

Despite these benefits, oral appliances do not promote cartilage regeneration or halt disease progression. Their role is therefore best defined as palliative and preventative, contributing to symptom control and slowing degenerative changes [6]. Splints are most effective when used within a multimodal regimen that may include NSAIDs for pain and inflammation, muscle relaxants, non-invasive physiotherapy techniques such as TENS, low-level laser therapy [7, 8], and ultrasound [9]. Psychosocial interventions including biofeedback and cognitive-behavioral therapy also play a supportive role in reducing bruxism and stress-related muscle hyperactivity. Dietary modifications such as adopting a soft or pureed diet and avoiding excessive mandibular loading further support joint protection. When applied judiciously, these conservative approaches improve symptoms, enhance quality of life, and may delay or even reduce the need for surgical intervention.

3. Stem cell-based regenerative therapies

Mesenchymal stem cells (MSCs) exhibit self-renewal capacity and multipotent differentiation into chondrogenic, osteogenic, and adipogenic lineages, making them a central focus in regenerative medicine for TMJOA [10, 11]. Sources include bone marrow (BMSCs), adipose tissue (ADMSCs), dental pulp (DPSCs), synovium, and umbilical cord blood [10].

Preclinical and clinical studies indicate that intra-articular injection of MSCs alleviates TMJOA pathology, with outcomes such as reduced joint tenderness, improved mandibular function, and diminished local inflammation [12–14]. Proposed mechanisms include paracrine signaling, modulation of the inflammatory milieu, and differentiation into chondrocyte-like cells [11].

To enhance the MSC survival and functionality in the hostile joint microenvironment, scaffolds and hydrogels have been developed as delivery vehicles. Genipin-crosslinked 3D-printed gelatin scaffolds, for example, support MSC adhesion, viability, and chondrogenic differentiation, underscoring their utility in cartilage repair [15]. Injectable, ROS-responsive hydrogels such as RD-Gel replicate the extracellular matrix, provide bioactive cues, and shield cells from apoptosis. Studies delivering DPSCs *via* RD-Gel demonstrated enhanced stem cell viability, M2 macrophage polarization, and improved condylar cartilage regeneration in TMJOA models [13, 15].

These findings emphasize that scaffold-assisted MSC therapy maximizes regenerative potential. By anchoring cells, mimicking the native tissue microarchitecture, and modulating the joint microenvironment, scaffold integration significantly augments stem cell-based repair.

4. Exosome-based therapies

Exosome-based interventions are emerging as safer, cell-free alternatives to traditional MSC transplantation. Exosome lipid bilayer-bound extracellular vesicles released by MSCs and other cell types carry bioactive cargo including microRNAs, mRNAs, proteins, and lipids. These vesicles modulate inflammation, remodel the extracellular matrix, and stimulate chondrogenesis [13, 16].

Compared to whole-cell therapies, exosome have advantages of reduced tumorigenicity, lower immunogenicity, and greater clinical safety [17]. Preclinical evidence supports their regenerative efficacy: Exosome derived from urine stem cells enhanced chondrogenesis and inhibited pro-inflammatory signaling in TMJOA models, improving both cartilage architecture and synovial health [18]. Similarly, MSC-derived exosome demonstrated potent immunomodulatory activity, suppressing synovitis and promoting tissue repair [19].

Combination approaches using biomaterial scaffolds or nano-carriers can further improve exosome retention, targeting, and controlled release within the joint environment [20]. Collectively, exosome-based therapies replicate the beneficial paracrine effects of MSCs while avoiding the limitations of cell-based treatments, representing a significant step toward clinically translatable regenerative interventions for TMJOA.

5. Nano-carriers and targeted delivery

Nanotechnology offers precise, site-specific delivery of bioactive molecules to TMJOA lesions, enhancing therapeutic efficacy while minimizing systemic toxicity. Nano-carriers such as silica nanoparticles, lipid-based vesicles, and polymeric-nanospheres have been engineered to deliver growth factors, anti-inflammatory agents, and gene therapies in a sustained and localized manner [21].

Innovative self-assembling nanospheres function both as drug carriers and bioactive lubricants, reducing oxidative stress, preserving subchondral bone integrity, and slowing cartilage degradation in murine TMJOA models [22]. Similarly, mesoporous silica nanoparticles delivering hyaluronan-synthase-2 to synovicytes increased the production of high-molecular-weight hyaluronic acid, improving joint lubrication and prolonging anti-inflammatory effects [23].

Dual-targeted lipid nanoparticles (LNPs) encapsulating both anti-inflammatory microRNAs and chondrogenic agents such as kartogenin have shown synergistic effects, enhancing cartilage regeneration and reducing synovial inflammation in preclinical models [24].

These findings highlight the transformative potential of nanotechnology in TMJOA, offering controlled, multimodal, and site-specific therapeutic delivery systems that may redefine standard care.

6. Hydrogels and scaffolds

Hydrogels and scaffolds are indispensable in regenerative TMJOA therapy, as they mimic the native extracellular matrix (ECM) and create three-dimensional microenvironments conducive to cell survival and differentiation. Hydrogels possess physicochemical properties such as porosity, hydration, stiffness, and degradability that support the MSC viability and sustained release of bioactive agents [25, 26].

Emerging designs such as hydrogel-biosilica composites have demonstrated enhanced cartilage repair, promoting cell adhesion, matrix deposition, and tissue regeneration in animal models [27]. Stimuli-responsive hydrogels, particularly ROS-sensitive variants, dynamically interact with the inflammatory microenvironment, polarizing macrophages toward regenerative phenotypes and facilitating cartilage healing [28].

Scaffolds, fabricated from natural polymers (e.g., collagen, chitosan), synthetic polymers (e.g., PLGA, PEG), or hybrid composites, provide structural frameworks that guide tissue organization. Surface functionalization with growth factors such as IGF-1 and TGF-β1 enhances chondrogenic differentiation and ECM production [29]. Advances in 3D bio-printing enable patient-specific scaffold fabrication with tailored geometry, controlled cell distribution, and optimized integration with host tissue [30].

Together, hydrogels and scaffolds form synergistic platforms that support cellular and molecular regeneration, providing a versatile basis for clinical translation.

7. Combination and advanced strategies

Increasing evidence suggests that multimodal therapies outperform single-modality approaches in TMJOA regeneration. Combinations of MSCs with platelet-rich plasma (PRP), exosome, nanomaterial, or biophysical stimulation create synergistic environments that accelerate the cartilage repair and restore joint function [31–33]. PRP enhances MSC proliferation, immunomodulation, and trophic effects by supplying autologous growth factors [34]. Exosomes serve as paracrine mediators, further amplifying MSC-driven regeneration [35, 36].

Innovative nucleic acid-based systems such as tetrahedral framework nucleic acids (tFNAs) have been designed to deliver microRNAs with high efficiency. For instance, miR-124-loaded tFNAs promoted anti-inflammatory signaling and up-regulated chondrogenic gene expression in preclinical TMJOA models [37]. Concurrently, bio-functionalized scaffolds allow programmed release of bioactive molecules and mechanical stimuli, closely mimicking natural healing cascades [38].

These multimodal approaches underscore the need for individualized therapies that address the complex pathology of TMJOA. By integrating cellular, molecular, and material-based interventions, future therapies may achieve more durable and comprehensive joint regeneration.

8. Clinical translation and future directions

Preclinical studies consistently demonstrate that MSC-based therapy attenuates inflammation, promotes cartilage repair, and modifies the TMJOA microenvironment [14, 39]. However, translation into clinical practice remains challenging. Variability in MSC sourcing from bone marrow, adipose tissue, or synovium results in heterogeneity in differentiation potential, immunomodulatory capacity, and regenerative outcomes [40]. Delivery protocols also differ widely in terms of dosage, frequency, and use of adjuvants such as scaffolds or growth factors [41].

Clinical outcome measures the lack of standardization, with studies variously relying on subjective pain scales, imaging modalities, or biochemical markers, complicating cross-study comparisons [42]. Furthermore, long-term safety and efficacy data are limited. While short-term trials report the minimal adverse effects, the long-term fate of transplanted cells under chronic joint stress remains uncertain.

Progress will depend on harmonizing protocols, conducting well-designed randomized clinical trials and identifying reliable biomarkers predictive of therapeutic response. Establishing the standardized guidelines and interdisciplinary collaboration will be crucial for advancing MSC-based and adjunctive regenerative therapies are increasingly advancing from experimental concepts toward potential integration into established clinical practice [43].

9. Conclusion

Regenerative medicine is redefining the therapeutic landscape of TMJOA. By leveraging the reparative capacity of stem cells, the paracrine activity of exosome, the precision of nanotechnology, and the structural support of bioengineered scaffolds, these strategies aim not only to alleviate symptoms but also to restore joint architecture and long-term function. Multimodal approaches that integrate MSCs with PRP, exosome, or advanced scaffold systems demonstrate particular promise in preclinical models. Nevertheless, successful clinical translation will depend on the development of standardized protocols, rigorous randomized trials, and reliable biomarkers of treatment response. As evidence accumulates, regenerative therapies have the potential to progress from experimental interventions to mainstream clinical practice, offering durable and patient-specific solutions for TMJOA.

Acknowledgements

The author acknowledges the usage of Quilbot for language polishing of the manuscript.

Conflict of interest

The authors declare no conflict of interest.

Author details

Tharanikumar Sivakumar[1*], Chandrsekaran Krithika[1], U. Elaveyini[2], Chitathoor Sridhar[1], S. Nachiappan[3] and Ashok Prasanna[3]

1 Meenakshi Academy of Higher Education and Research, Chennai, India

2 Saveetha Medical College and Hospital, Chennai, India

3 Sathyabama Dental College and Hospital, Chennai, India

*Address all correspondence to: dr.tharanikumar1977@gmail.com

References

[1] Zakrzewska JM, Newton-John TRO, Durham J. Temporomandibular disorders. BMJ. 2015;**350**:h1154. DOI: 10.1136/bmj.h1154

[2] Scrivani SJ, Keith DA, Kaban LB. Temporomandibular disorders. The New England Journal of Medicine. 2008;**359**(25):2693-2705. DOI: 10.1056/NEJMra0802472

[3] de Leeuw R, Klasser GD. Orofacial Pain: Guidelines for Assessment, Diagnosis, and Management. 6th ed. Hanover Park, IL: Quintessence; 2018

[4] Manfredini D, Winocur E, Guarda-Nardini L, Lobbezoo F. Research diagnostic criteria for temporomandibular disorders: A systematic review of Axis I epidemiology findings. Oral Surgery, Oral Medicine, Oral Pathology, Oral Radiology, and Endodontics. 2011;**112**(4):453-462. DOI: 10.1016/j.tripleo.2011.04.021

[5] Al-Moraissi EA, Farea R, Qasem KA, Al-Wadeai MS, Al-Sabahi ME, Al-Iryani GM. Effectiveness of occlusal splint therapy in the management of temporomandibular disorders: Network meta-analysis of randomized controlled trials. International Journal of Oral and Maxillofacial Surgery. 2020;**49**(8):1042-1056. DOI: 10.1016/j.ijom.2020.01.004. Epub 2020 Jan 22

[6] Okeson JP. Management of Temporomandibular Disorders and Occlusion. 8th ed. St. Louis: Elsevier; 2019

[7] Matheus HRNS, Goncalves LM, Prado DH, et al. Stem cell-based therapies for temporomandibular joint osteoarthritis: Systematic review of preclinical studies. Osteoarthritis and Cartilage. 2022;**30**(9):S220-S221. DOI: 10.1016/S1063-4584(22)00747-6

[8] Fathy M, Hussien M, Hussien A. Effect of low-level laser application in conjunction with splint therapy for management of temporomandibular joint disorders. Al-Azhar Journal of Dental Science. 2021;**24**(1):49-54. DOI: 10.21608/ajdsm.2020.30503.1061

[9] Manfredini D, Favero L, Gregorini G, Cocilovo F, Guarda-Nardini L. Natural course of temporomandibular disorders with low pain-related impairment: A 2- to 3-year follow-up study. Journal of Oral Rehabilitation. 2013;**40**(6):436-442. DOI: 10.1111/joor.12047

[10] Barry F, Murphy M. Mesenchymal stem cells in joint disease and repair. Nature Reviews Rheumatology. 2013;**9**(10):584-594. DOI: 10.1038/nrrheum.2013.109

[11] Squillaro T, Peluso G, Galderisi U. Clinical trials with mesenchymal stem cells: An update. Cell Transplantation. 2016;**25**(5):829-848. DOI: 10.3727/096368915X689622

[12] Zhao Y, Xie L. An update on mesenchymal stem cell-centered therapies in temporomandibular joint osteoarthritis. Stem Cells International. 2021;**6619527**, 15pages. DOI: 10.1155/2021/6619527

[13] Ma J, Li J, Wei S, Ge Q, Wu J, Xue L, et al. Delivery of dental pulp stem cells by an injectable ROS-responsive hydrogel promotes temporomandibular joint cartilage repair via enhancing anti-apoptosis and regulating microenvironment. Journal of Tissue Engineering. 2024;**15**:20417314241260436. DOI: 10.1177/20417314241260436

[14] Collins NJ, Hart HF, Mills KAG. Osteoarthritis year in review 2018: Rehabilitation and outcomes. Osteoarthritis and Cartilage. 2019;**27**(3):378-391. DOI: 10.1016/j.joca.2018.11.010. Epub 2018 Dec 7

[15] Helgeland E, Mohamed-Ahmed S, Shanbhag S, Pedersen TO, Rosén A, Mustafa K, et al. 3D printed gelatin-genipin scaffolds for temporomandibular joint cartilage regeneration. Biomedical Physics & Engineering Express. 2021;7(5). DOI: 10.1088/2057-1976/ac1e68

[16] Raposo G, Stoorvogel W. Extracellular vesicles: Exosomes, microvesicles, and friends. The Journal of Cell Biology. 2013;**200**(4):373-383. DOI: 10.1083/jcb.201211138

[17] Zhou JP, Peng SS, Xu J, et al. Therapeutic potential of urine-derived stem cell exosomes in temporomandibular joint osteoarthritis. The FASEB Journal. 2024;**38**(15):e23852. DOI: 10.1096/fj.202400448RR

[18] Lee YH, Park HK, Auh QS, et al. Emerging potential of exosomes in regenerative medicine for temporomandibular joint osteoarthritis. International Journal of Molecular Sciences. 2020;**21**(4):1541. DOI: 10.3390/ijms21041541

[19] Yanez-Mo M, Siljander PR-M, Andreu Z, et al. Biological properties of extracellular vesicles and their physiological functions. Journal of Extracellular Vesicles. 2015;**4**:27066. DOI: 10.3402/jev.v4.27066

[20] Zhang S, Teo KYW, Chuah SJ, Lai RC, Lim SK, Toh WS. MSC exosomes alleviate temporomandibular joint osteoarthritis by attenuating inflammation and restoring matrix homeostasis. Biomaterials. 2019;**200**:35-47. DOI: 10.1016/j.biomaterials.2019.02.006

[21] Wang Y, Zhao M, Li W, et al. BMSC-derived extracellular vesicles induce cartilage reconstruction of TMJOA via autotaxin-YAP signaling. Frontiers in Cell and Development Biology. 2021;**9**:656153. DOI: 10.3389/fcell.2021.656153

[22] Wu J, Kuang L, Chen C, et al. miR-100-5p-abundant IPFP-MSC exosomes protect cartilage via mTOR inhibition. Biomaterials. 2019;**206**:87-100. DOI: 10.1016/j.biomaterials.2019.03.022

[23] Xu X, Liang Y, Li X, et al. Exosome-mediated delivery of kartogenin for chondrogenesis and cartilage regeneration. Biomaterials. 2021;**269**:120539. DOI: 10.1016/j.biomaterials.2020.120539

[24] Cosenza S, Ruiz M, Toupet K, Jorgensen C, Noël D. Mesenchymal stem cell–derived exosomes and microparticles protect cartilage and bone from degradation in osteoarthritis. Scientific Reports. 2017;**7**:16214. DOI: 10.1038/s41598-017-15376-8

[25] Mianehsaz E, Mirzaei HR, Mahjoubin-Tehran M, et al. Mesenchymal stem cell-derived exosomes: A new therapeutic approach to osteoarthritis? Stem Cell Research & Therapy. 2019;**10**:340. DOI: 10.1186/s13287-019-1445-0

[26] Chen X, Shi Y, Xue P, Ma X, Li J, Zhang J. Mesenchymal stem cell-derived exosomal microRNA-136-5p inhibits chondrocyte degeneration in traumatic osteoarthritis by targeting ELF3. Arthritis Research & Therapy. 2020;**22**(1):256. DOI: 10.1186/s13075-020-02325-6

[27] Zhang S, Chu WC, Lai RC, Lim SK, Hui JH, Toh WS. Exosomes from human embryonic MSCs enhance osteochondral

regeneration. Osteoarthritis and Cartilage. 2016;**24**(12):2135-2140. DOI: 10.1016/j.joca.2016.06.022

[28] Fan W, Li J, Yuan T, et al. Exosomes in osteoarthritis: Updated insights for diagnosis and therapy. Frontiers in Bioengineering and Biotechnology. 2022;**10**:908845. DOI: 10.3389/fbioe.2022.908845

[29] Yang B, Li X, Fu C, et al. Extracellular vesicles in osteoarthritis of peripheral joints and TMJ. Frontiers in Endocrinology. 2023;**14**:1158744. DOI: 10.3389/fendo.2023.1158744

[30] Boere J, Malda J, van de Lest CHA, van Weeren PR, Wauben MHM. Extracellular vesicles in joint disease and therapy. Frontiers in Immunology. 2018;**9**:2575. DOI: 10.3389/fimmu.2018.02575

[31] Mustonen AM, Nieminen P. Extracellular vesicles in osteoarthritis: Significance and therapeutic potential. Pharmaceuticals. 2021;**14**(4):315. DOI: 10.3390/ph14040315

[32] Withrow J, Murphy C, Liu Y, et al. Extracellular vesicles in the pathogenesis of rheumatoid arthritis and osteoarthritis. Arthritis Research & Therapy. 2016;**18**:286. DOI: 10.1186/s13075-016-1178-8

[33] Lee CH, Cook JL, Mendelson A, Moioli EK, Yao H, Mao JJ. Regeneration of the articular surface of the rabbit synovial joint by cell homing: A proof of concept study. Lancet. 2010;**376**(9739):440-448. DOI: 10.1016/S0140-6736(10)60668-X

[34] Wen J, He J, Meng J, et al. Intra-articular nanoparticle-based therapies for OA and RA management. Materials Today Bio. 2023;**19**:100597. DOI: 10.1016/j.mtbio.2023.100597

[35] Liao J, Yu C, Zhang S, et al. Advances in nanodrug therapies for osteoarthritis. Frontiers in Pharmacology. 2024;**15**:1402825. DOI: 10.3389/fphar.2024.1402825

[36] Yuan W, Wu Y, Huang M, Zhou X, Liu J, Yi Y, et al. A new frontier in temporomandibular joint osteoarthritis treatment: Exosome-based therapeutic strategy. Frontiers in Bioengineering and Biotechnology. 2022;**10**:1074536. DOI: 10.3389/fbioe.2022.1074536

[37] Zhao Z, Wang P, Li Z, et al. Targeted lipid nanoparticles distributed in hydrogel treat osteoarthritis by modulating cholesterol metabolism and promoting endogenous cartilage regeneration. Journal of Nanbiotechnology. 2024;**22**:786. DOI: 10.1186/s12951-024-02965-9

[38] Liu M, Zeng X, Ma C, et al. Injectable hydrogels for cartilage and bone tissue engineering. Bone Research. 2017;**5**:17014. DOI: 10.1038/boneres.2017.14

[39] Zhu S, Li J, Zhang Y, et al. Advanced injectable hydrogels for cartilage repair and regeneration. Frontiers in Bioengineering and Biotechnology. 2022;**10**:954501. DOI: 10.3389/fbioe.2022.954501

[40] Deng S, Cao H, Lu Y, et al. Injectable dECM-enhanced hyaluronic microgels with spatiotemporal release of cartilage-specific molecules to improve osteoarthritic chondrocyte's function. Collagen & Leather. 2024;**6**:14. DOI: 10.1186/s42825-024-00158-6

[41] Yang Z, Li H, Chen X, et al. Stem cell-laden hydrogel-based 3D bioprinting for bone and cartilage tissue engineering. Frontiers in Bioengineering and Biotechnology. 2022;**10**:865770. DOI: 10.3389/fbioe.2022.865770

[42] Daly AC, Pitacco P, Nulty J, Cunniffe GM, Kelly DJ. 3D printed microchannel networks to direct vascularisation during endochondral bone repair. Biomaterials. 2018;**162**:34-46. DOI: 10.1016/j.biomaterials.2018.01.057

[43] Levato R, Visser J, Planell JA, Engel E, Malda J, Mateos-Timoneda MA. Biofabrication of tissue constructs by 3D bioprinting of cell-laden microcarriers. Biofabrication. 2014;**6**(3):035020. DOI: 10.1088/1758-5082/6/3/035020

Chapter 9

Evaluating the Efficacy of Platelet-Rich Plasma, Hyaluronic Acid, and Botulinum Toxin in the Treatment of Temporomandibular Joint (TMJ) Disorders

Madiha Khan, Sufyan Ahmed and Aisha Faraz

Abstract

Temporomandibular joint (TMJ) disorders are a complex group of conditions that can cause significant pain, dysfunction, and impaired quality of life. As these disorders often involve both musculoskeletal and joint-related pathologies, treatment options must address the diverse factors contributing to the symptoms. Over the years, non-surgical interventions such as platelet-rich plasma (PRP), hyaluronic acid (HA), and botulinum toxin (BoNT) have emerged as effective therapeutic modalities. PRP harnesses the regenerative potential of platelets to promote tissue healing and reduce inflammation, particularly useful in managing cartilage degeneration and joint-related symptoms. HA, primarily known for its role in joint lubrication, alleviates pain and improves joint function, particularly in patients with osteoarthritis or early-stage TMJ dysfunction. BoNT, known for its muscle-relaxing properties, offers relief for muscle-induced pain, bruxism, and myofascial pain. This chapter explores the clinical applications, mechanisms, and efficacy of PRP, HA, and BoNT in the treatment of TMJ disorders. A comparative analysis of these therapies demonstrates their distinct roles in addressing the multifaceted nature of TMJ dysfunction. While each therapy offers specific benefits, emerging trends in combination therapies that integrate these modalities hold the potential for more comprehensive treatment plans. Additionally, the chapter discusses the role of personalized treatment approaches, incorporating biomarkers and advanced imaging, to better tailor interventions based on patient-specific characteristics. With an emphasis on clinical recommendations, this chapter provides a comprehensive guide to these innovative treatments, focusing on their application, limitations, and future directions in the management of TMJ disorders.

Keywords: TMJ, PRP, hyaluronic acid, interventions, botulinum toxin (BoNT), inflammation, dysfunction, degeneration

1. Introduction

Temporomandibular joint (TMJ) disorders (TMDs) represent a complex group of musculoskeletal conditions that affect the temporomandibular joint, the masticatory muscles, and associated craniofacial structures. Temporomandibular joint (TMJ) is one of the most complicated joints in the body [1]. Temporomandibular disorders (TMD) are known to be one of the most problematic disorders to patients since they are capable of instigating pain, altering oral functions and annoying dentists at the level of diagnosis and treatment. These disorders are the most frequent pathogenic reason of orofacial pain and functional limitation and are only surpassed by dental pain in frequency. Joint sounds, headache pain, mandibular movement limitation, and referred otologic symptoms, are common in patients with TMDs. Due to the complex form of the TMJ being a synovial joint having both hinge and gliding movements, there are numerous pathological conditions which are susceptible to the joint and most are multifactorial in origin [2]. The fact that it has become more prevalent in women, particularly in the reproductive age, has led to curiosity on the roles of hormones and psychological influences in pathogenesis. Even after decades of research, there are no standardized and universally successful treatment patterns toward TMDs. Although a majority of patients are responsive to conservative treatment, that is, non-steroidal anti-inflammatory drugs (NSAIDs), physical therapy, and occlusal splints, some are non-responsive (**Figure 1**) [3]. Such patients can have less invasive yet specific solutions like intra-articular interventions first hand before they think about going through surgical correction. The history of regenerative medicine has contributed to the availability of biologic therapy which includes platelet-rich plasma (PRP), hyaluronic acid (HA), and botulinum toxin A (BoNT-A) which exhibit specific mechanisms that can be used to rehab steward pain, cartilage erosion, and the presence of hyperactive muscles. This chapter intends to extensively analyze the reasoning, processes, and clinical-efficacy of these agents as a form of therapeutic modalities in treating TMJ illnesses (**Figure 2**) [4].

1.1 Overview of temporomandibular joint disorders

Temporomandibular joint disorders constitute a heterogeneous collection of conditions involving dysfunction or pathology of the temporomandibular joint and

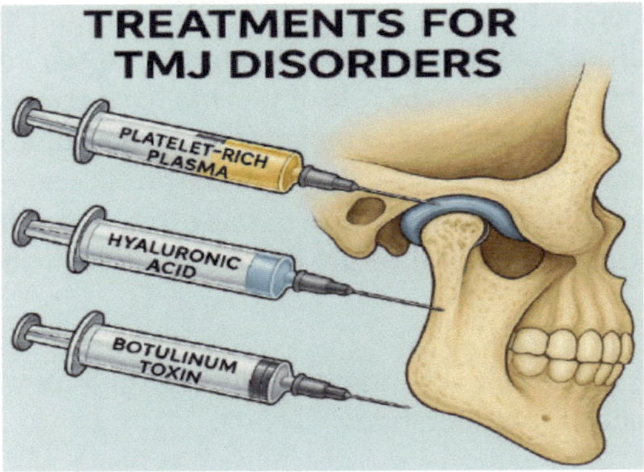

Figure 1.
Treatment for TMJ disorders.

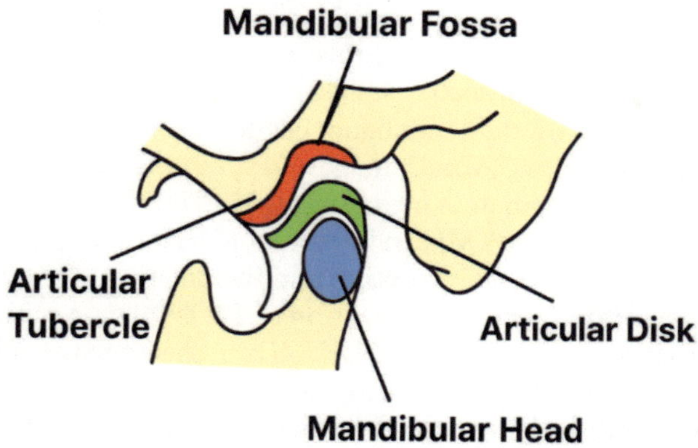

Figure 2.
Structure of TMJ.

its associated musculature. The TMJ is a special one in the sense that it is a bilateral articulation and a rotational and translational articulation [5]. Various disorders of such system may be caused by muscular hyperactivity, internal derangement of the disc-condyle complex, or degenerative changes of the joint. Based on the diagnosis of TMD as per the Research Diagnostic Criteria for TMD (RDC/TMD) and its revised form (DC/TMD), there are mainly three major categories of TMD that include muscle disorders, disc displacements, and arthralgia/arthritis/arthrosis. The prevalence of TMDs is widespread in the literature, but it is estimated to affect up to 25% of the entire population sometime during their lifetime. Other associated factors are: psychological stress, bruxism trauma, dental malocclusion, and postural imbalances [6]. Chronic pain, eating problems, sleep, and emotional distress are common factors among patients with TMD, which lead to a decrease in the quality of their lives. In young adults as well as teenagers, TMD may disrupt the process of normal development of the jaws and may cause chronic pain syndromes in old age [7]. The economic and social costs of health care systems are immense, both directly because of treatment expenses, as well as indirectly due to the lack of productivity and psychosocial effects. Usually, the diagnosis includes a multidisciplinary approach, such as dentists, oral surgeons, physical therapists, and pain specialists due to the variability of the condition in etiology and presentation. Modern imaging applications like MRI and CBCT are used critically in helping distinguish the subtypes and is critical in directing the choice of modalities of treatment. Biologics and injectables have led to alternative ways of management, particularly in the resistant cases of conventional therapy [8].

1.2 Pathophysiology and classification of TMJ disorders

The pathophysiology of TMJ disorders is complex and varies depending on the subtype of the disorder. On cellular levels, inflammation, oxidative stress, and biomechanical overloading are frequent topics of both myogenous and arthrogenous types of TMD. As an example, with internal derangement, the articular disc gets dislodged as a result of ligamentous laxity or injuries causing malfunctioning of joint mechanics, pain, and degeneration [9]. The secondary degenerative changes that can be seen in osteoarthritis, including thinning of the cartilage, inflammation of the synovium, and sclerosis of the subchondral bone can be obtained by chronic disc displacement. The most prevalent subtype of the TMD is the myofascial pain that is linked with the hyperactive masticatory muscles, trigger points, and referred pain patterns. Incentive sensitization and changes in nociceptive processing in the central nervous system may as well lead to chronicity in such cases [10]. Inflammatory arthropathies, such as synovitis and capsulitis, on the other hand, occur due either to immune-mediated or infection-induced processes. Joint Damage and symptomatology are given by the presence of inflammatory mediators including IL-10, TNF-α and prostaglandins. Osteoarthritic transitions in the TMJ can be similar to that in weight-bearing joints, but, due to the peculiar anatomical structure and functioning of the TMJ, its degeneration is more complicated. The categorization of TMDs plays a critical role in the proper choice of the treatment strategy [11]. TMDs in their turn are classified in a broad way into myogenous (muscle-related), arthrogenous (joint related), and mixed types. In arthrogenous disorders, we have further subtypes of disc displacements including with reduction and without reduction of the discs as well as inflammatory diseases and degenerative joint diseases. In determining such categories, imaging and functional assessments are very instrumental [12]. The realization of the pathophysiology is not only helpful in diagnosis but also in determination of responses to treatment. The goal of HA supplementation is to replace the viscosity and friction-reducing qualities of synovial fluid and the resulting benefit that PRP offers is the healing of the tissues, that is achieved through the release of growth factors. BoNT-A blocks the release of acetylcholine, a major symptom of the neuromuscular junction, which limits overactivity in muscles and pain transmission (**Figure 3**) [13].

Intra-articular injection of TMJ disorders is justified on the distribution principle of therapeutic agents directly to the per disease centre which increases its efficacy and at the same time reduces the systemic aspect of the side effect. This focal treatment has great advantage in a patient who does not respond to non-invasive management strategies or wants to prefer less invasive surgery. PRP, HA and BoNT-A have been increasingly being promoted as non-surgical tools due to their efficacy to create change on the joint milieu and overall clinical results [14]. Platelet-rich plasma (PRP) is a platelet suspension in plasma, comprising autologous concentration of platelet-derived growth factor (PDGF), transforming growth factor-beta (TGF-beta), and vascular-endothelial growth factor (VEGF) growth factors. This activates cell multiplication, angiogenesis, and matrix production in the extracellular space, which repair the damaged tissue. Cumulative clinical research has proved the potential of PRP to alleviate pain, increase or improve the movement of the joints, and

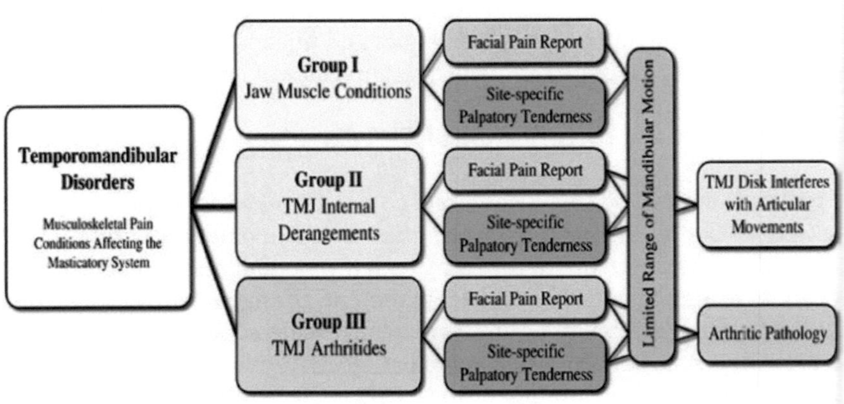

Figure 3.
TMJ disorders and their classification.

tissue regeneration in both TMJ internal derangement and osteoarthritis [15]. Shock absorption. The glycosaminoglycan, hyaluronic acid, is a natural part of synovial fluid that lubricates joints and acts as a shock absorber. In TMDs, the goal of intra-articular HA injections is the recovery of joint viscoelastic qualities, suppression of an inflammatory process, and enhancement of joint performance [16]. Several clinical studies have demonstrated that HA can be helpful when it comes to relieving TMJ pain, and also help increase the mandibular range of motion especially in patients with degenerative joint diseases. Although botulinum toxin A is traditionally applied to the myofascial pain syndrome, these emerging functions have been seen to have resulted in the intra-articular and pericapsular injections of TMJ pain [17]. Blocking in the release of acetylcholine, BoNT-A results in relaxation of muscles, the reduction of excess loading on joints, and the disruption of the signaling pathways of pain. It has the particular usefulness in muscular hyperactive patients; patients with bruxism; mixed TMD patients. In this chapter, there is an endeavor to review the existing literature and give a review of the role of PRP, HA, and BoNT-A in contemporary care delivered to patients with TMJ disorders [18].

2. Platelet-rich plasma (PRP) in TMJ disorders

Platelet-rich plasma (PRP) therapy has gained significant attention as a potential treatment for temporomandibular joint (TMJ) disorders. These disorders, which affect the joint responsible for jaw movement, are often associated with chronic pain, limited mouth opening, and a decreased quality of life. The traditional approach to managing TMJ disorders typically includes conservative methods such as physical therapy, splints, and non-steroidal anti-inflammatory drugs (NSAIDs). However, these treatments often fail to provide long-term relief, especially in cases of more severe dysfunction. Consequently, the regenerative potential of PRP has made it a subject of interest in treating these disorders, offering a minimally invasive, effective solution to patients suffering from chronic pain and joint degeneration [19].

2.1 Biological mechanism of PRP

The basic biological procedure of PRP in TMJ disease is founded on PRP capability of speeding up tissue recovery, diminishing irritation, and improving the recuperating cycle. PRP comes out of the blood of the patient which is rich with growth factors which are in the form of platelets which it concentrates. Platelets are very instrumental in the repair of tissues and this occurs through the release of proteins by the platelets that activate healing mechanisms within the body. Such growth factors are platelet-derived growth factor (PDGF), transforming growth factor-beta (TGF-beta), vascular endothelial growth factor (VEGF), and fibroblast growth factor (FGF) which also act to stimulate cell proliferation, collagen formation, and angiogenesis [20]. Such aspects promote the regeneration of injured tissues, such as cartilage, ligaments, as well as muscles, which are all essential elements of TMJ. As it has growth factors and cytokine stimulation, the PRP stimulates the healing of the soft tissues and cartilage once it is injected to the affected region of the TMJ, where it causes regeneration of the surrounding tissues. The outcome is increased tissue performance and anti-inflammation. The capacity of PRP to speed up tissue healing is especially notable when TMJ disorder is considered, in which case damage of the cartilage and ligaments of the joint can compose a critical factor in its

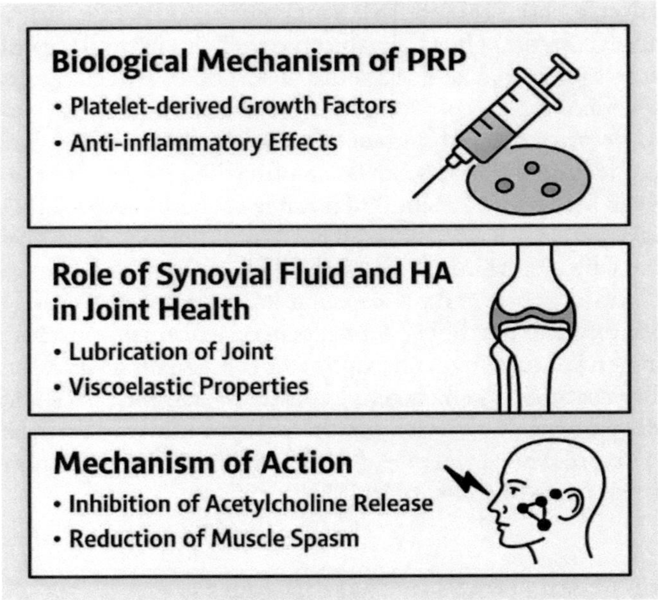

Figure 4.
Biological mechanism of PRP.

dysfunction. Inflammatory response that accompanies such damage is also reduced as the result of the work of PRP that helps reduce pain and swelling and promote cellular healing (**Figure 4**) [21].

2.2 Preparation techniques

The preparation of PRP involves a simple yet critical process that ensures the final product is concentrated with platelets and growth factors essential for tissue regeneration. The initial stage in the PRP process is taking at least 10 milliliters to 60 milliliters of the patient's blood sample, and this relies on the amount of blood needed based on the injection process. The blood collected will then be put in a centrifuge, which is a machine that causes the blood to spin at high velocities, separating the components of the blood on the basis of their density [20]. In centrifugation, the cells are placed in a centrifuge; this separates the red blood cells, the white blood cells, and the plasma, as well as concentrating the platelets in the plasma. The centrifugation process usually separates three layers of blood, that is, red blood cells, a buffy coat, which contains the white blood cells and platelets, and at the top will be the platelet-rich plasma [21]. The platelet-rich plasma is withdrawn, after which it is injected into the area of the TMJ that requires treatment. In other, but rare, cases, leukocytes (white blood cells) can be removed or kept in PRP preparation to prevent the excessive inflammatory response or to take advantage of the possible anti-inflammatory effects of white blood cells [22]. The number of platelets can vary between twofold to fivefold that represented in whole blood, depending on the PRP system. Platelets concentration in PRP is an important aspect that may affect its therapeutic efficacy. An improved outcome is found when the platelet concentration is higher as this results in a higher release of growth factors that are required to regenerate tissue. Moreover, various systems used to prepare PRP might differ in the concentration of platelets, and protocol

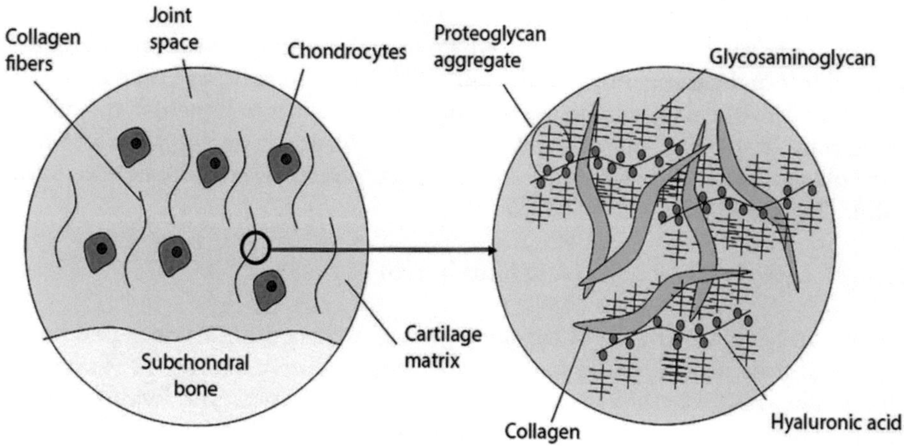

Figure 5.
Effects of HRA and PRP on TMJ mobility.

standardization on the preparation of various systems is deem vital in providing the standardization in clinical effect (**Figure 5**) [23].

2.3 Clinical evidence and outcomes

The merits have been demonstrated clinically that the PRP can be used to treat TMJ disorder with promising results with variable outcomes attributed to variable selection of patients, severity of the disease, and PRP preparation method. Various studies have proved that PRP may lead to a considerable reduction of pain, the increase of the mobility of joints, and the overall improvement of the TMJ functionality [24]. As an example, a randomized controlled trial by Lee et al. [25] revealed that patients receiving PRP injections experienced a considerable decrease in pain and an augmentation in mouth opening in contrast to individuals who had inspired a placebo injection. In such a way, the study by Schmitter et al. [26] pointed out the results of treating TMJ dysfunction by means of PRP injections that resulted in the improvements of TMJ function and the reduction of the number of clicking and popping sounds that are frequently observed in TMJ dysfunction patients. These data indicate that the regenerative effect can be used within the context of PRP to treat both structural and functional defects of TMJ disorders [27]. There have however not been equally strong results in all studies, and some have suggested the variability in response among the patients. The use of PRP as a therapy could be affected by various factors that include the way the PRP is prepared, timing of injections as well as the pathology of the TMJ. Although there are cases of great improvement in some patients, others will just demonstrate small improvements, and research is still required to determine the best regimen [28].

3. Hyaluronic acid (HA) in TMJ disorders

Hyaluronic acid (HA) is a natural substance found in the body, particularly in the synovial fluid of joints, where it plays a vital role in maintaining joint health. In the context of Temporomandibular Joint (TMJ) disorders, HA is gaining recognition as a promising treatment for its ability to restore joint lubrication, reduce pain, and improve joint function. TMJ disorders, which include conditions such as osteoarthritis and internal derangement of the joint, often lead to pain, inflammation, and impaired mobility of the jaw. The use of HA injections aims to replenish the natural synovial fluid in the TMJ, providing better lubrication and reducing friction between the articular surfaces, thus helping to alleviate symptoms and restore normal joint function (**Figure 6**) [29].

3.1 Role of synovial fluid and HA in joint health

Health and the well-being of synovial joints, such as the TMJ, is dependent on the synovial fluid whose role is to lubricate, absorb shock, and feed the articular cartilage. The fluid mostly has water, electrolytic substances and hyaluronic acid, with HA considered one of the most significant ones. HA helps in providing viscosity and elasticity of the synovial fluid so that it can serve as a lubricant thereby minimizing any friction along the joint surfaces during locomotion. Moreover, HA has a protective property on the cartilage since it assists in restraining its degradation and aids in the regeneration of the joint tissues. In TMJ disorders, there is a possible reduction in concentration of HA in the synovial fluid causing undue friction, thereby causing increased irritation within the joint that may compound the pain and restrict motion. The viscosity of the synovial fluid is regained when HA is injected into TMJ, and it can help in alleviating the pain, inflammation, and further breakdown of the joint in addition to enhancing movement and functioning of the jaw [30].

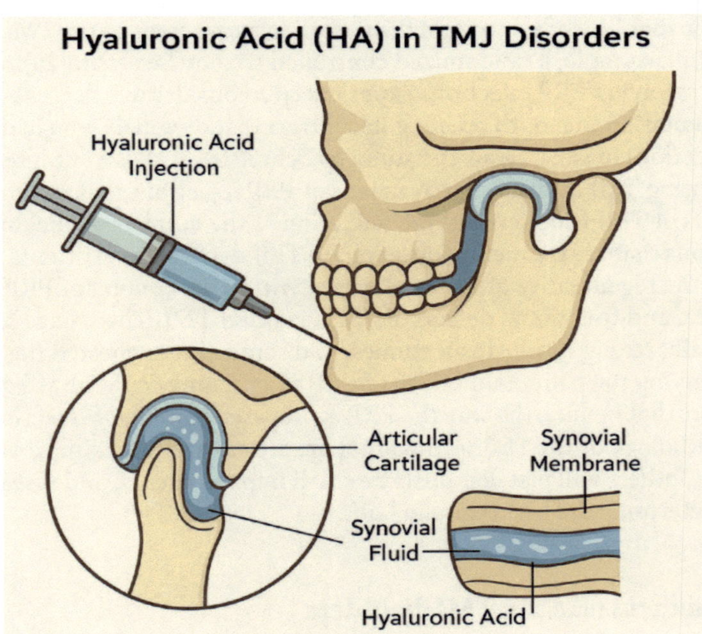

Figure 6.
HA in TMJ disorder.

3.2 Types and properties of HA preparations

The preparations of hyaluronic acid applied in clinical practice differ in molecular weight that influences their characteristics and clinical effect. Molecules of low-molecular-weight (LMW) HA are smaller, making them more fluid in nature, and they are absorbed faster in the body. This form of HA is usually preferred due to its tissue-penetrating capabilities, thus rendering it appropriate to be applied in the treatment of joint inflammation and involvement of deep tissues. On the contrary, the high-molar weight HA (HMW HA) is thicker, containing larger molecules that offer long-term lubrication and anti-destructive effect on the joint. HMW HA is more likely to stay longer in the joint and hence effective in offering long-lasting relief to symptoms of TMJ disorders. Besides the molecular weight, HA preparations can be grafted to improve their duration and stability [31].

3.3 Clinical studies and comparative efficacy

Various clinical trials have anticipated the efficacy and efficacy of HA injections in the treatment of TMJ disorders in TMJ disorders patients with osteoarthritis or degenerative illnesses of the joint. Clinical data indicate that HA may make substantial changes in the manifestations of pain, limited range of motion, and joint pain. Results obtained in a randomized controlled trial by Bouloux et al. [32] show that patients treated by HA injection demonstrated a notable decrease of pain and improved mouth opening that was not shown in patients in whom a placebo was used. A different research conducted by Schmitter et al. [26] revealed that HA is more effective than conservative interventions, such as splints or physical therapy, to handle TMJ symptoms. However, a study conducted by Conti et al. [33] revealed that HA injections were as efficient as corticosteroid injections or even more in pain improvement and improvement of joint functioning. Nonetheless, research shows that the effectiveness of HA is already well-established in most patients, yet in some cases, it may vary due to a variety of factors, including the severity of the disorder, patient response, and a possibly used form of HA (**Figure** 7) [34].

3.4 Therapeutic benefits and constraints

Hyaluronic acid injections offer several therapeutic benefits for patients suffering from TMJ disorders. Among the major benefits of HA treatment, it is important to mention the possibility of pain relief. HA helps ease the pain that is evident when the jaw is moving because it lubricates the joint, a feature that lowers the friction. Further on, HA injection may enhance the joint activity which ensures the range of movements and relieves such symptoms as clicking or locking that typically accompanies TMJ disorders. The effects are usually long-term, and in some cases, the patients are relieved several months on getting a single injection. The other advantage of the HA therapy is that it is less invasive. The injection procedure can be done on outpatient basis, and the patient does not need much downtime or recovery other than making it convenient to many patients [35]. There are, nevertheless, certain limitations to HA therapy. Although it may give temporary relief, they do not give long-lasting relief, and more injections may be required in order to keep symptoms at bay. Also, HA injections may be of high amount, and they may not be reimbursed by insurance scheme, which may be a liability to access by some group of people. Moreover, in

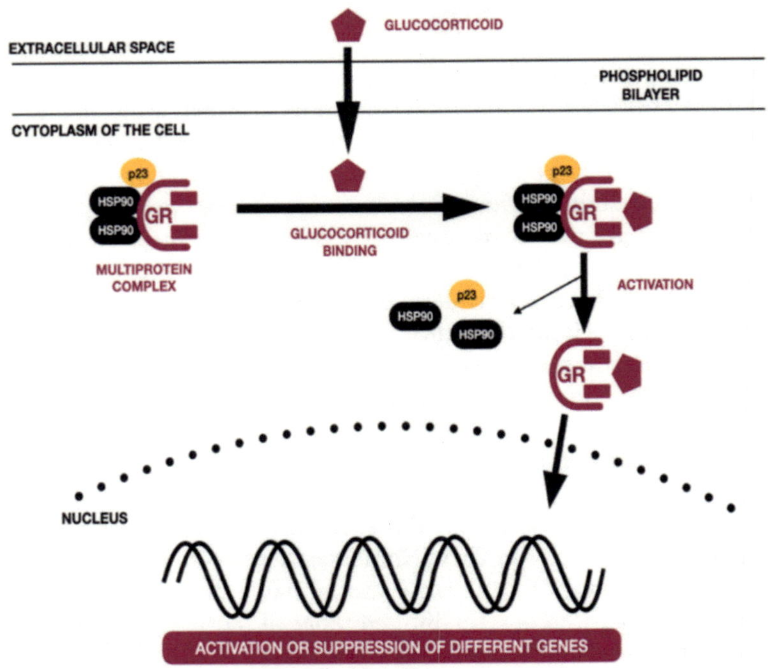

Figure 7.
Mechanism of action of HA and PRP.

exceptional cases, there is a chance of an allergic reaction or local inflammation after the injection. When considering HA as possible treatment option for TMJ disorders, the variability in the responses of the patients and the fact that periodic injections are a necessity, is one of the main aspects. Nevertheless, given these drawbacks, HA is a fruitful form of treatment of TMJ disorders presenting a surgical-free, efficient method in the management of numerous patients [36].

4. Botulinum toxin (BoNT) in TMJ disorders

Botulinum toxin (BoNT), commonly known for its cosmetic applications, has proven to be a valuable treatment option for temporomandibular joint (TMJ) disorders, particularly in managing muscular pain, spasms, and dysfunction. TMJ disorders often involve pain, stiffness, and difficulty in jaw movement, primarily resulting from muscular overactivity, bruxism, or myofascial pain. Botulinum toxin helps alleviate these symptoms by reducing muscle activity. Initially used in cosmetic procedures, BoNT has found its place in medical applications for its ability to block neurotransmission and relax the muscles, thus offering significant relief to individuals suffering from TMJ disorders. This section delves into the mechanisms, indications, clinical evidence, and potential risks associated with using BoNT in the treatment of TMJ dysfunction (**Figure 8**) [37].

4.1 Mechanism of action

Botulinum toxin works by inhibiting the release of acetylcholine, a neurotransmitter responsible for transmitting nerve signals to muscles, at the neuromuscular

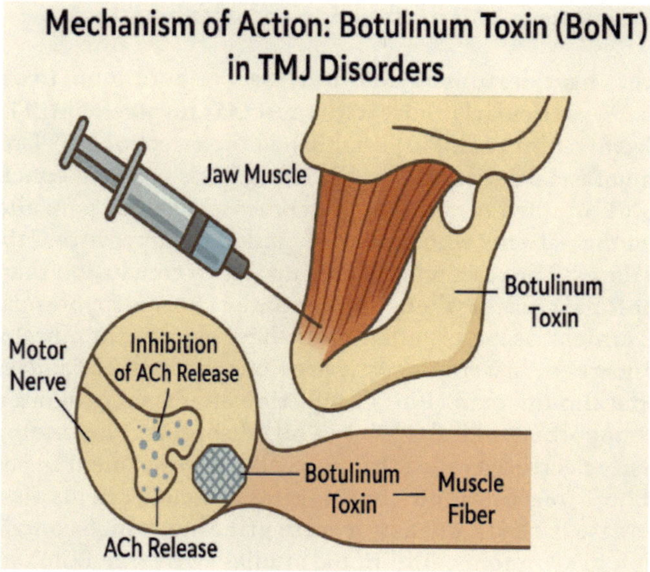

Figure 8.
Mechanism of action of BoNT in TMJ disorder.

junction. This prevents the muscle from contracting and reduces muscle hyperactivity, which is a common cause of pain and dysfunction in TMJ disorders. Specifically, in TMJ disorders, the toxin is injected into muscles such as the masseter and temporalis, which are often involved in clenching, grinding, and other abnormal jaw movements. By reducing excessive muscle activity, BoNT alleviates pain, decreases muscle spasms, and improves jaw mobility. The effects of BoNT are temporary, typically lasting between 3 and 6 months, depending on the patient and the dosage. During this period, patients often experience significant improvements in pain relief and jaw function [38].

4.2 Indications and injection protocols

Botulinum toxin is indicated for patients with TMJ disorders primarily involving muscle dysfunction, including myofascial pain syndrome, bruxism, and temporomandibular joint hyperactivity. It is especially beneficial for patients who do not respond to more conventional treatments like splints, anti-inflammatory medications, or physical therapy. In terms of injection protocols, BoNT is administered into the affected muscles, with the masseter muscle being the most commonly targeted. The typical injection involves 20–30 units per side, though this can vary depending on the severity of symptoms and individual patient needs. If necessary, additional muscles like the temporalis and pterygoid muscles may be targeted. Although there may be some discomfort during the procedure, it is relatively quick and does not require general anesthesia. Most injections are given outpatient. Injections are done with precision, and proper training is essential to ensure the correct muscles are injected, as incorrect administration can lead to side effects such as difficulty swallowing or facial asymmetry. The procedure generally requires minimal recovery time, and patients can resume normal activities immediately after the injection [39].

4.3 Evidence-based use in TMJ dysfunction and myofascial pain

Several studies have demonstrated the efficacy of botulinum toxin for treating TMJ disorders, particularly those with muscular involvement. The study conducted by Manfredini et al. [40] established the effect of BoNT injection in patients with myofascial pain and TMJ disorders. This research concluded that injection of BoNT attained meaningful outcomes measuring pain alleviation and jaw mobility among patients who previously failed to improve on other normal remedial procedures. The researchers came up with a conclusion that BoNT might be one of the optimal choices when it comes to the chronic myofascial pain treatment in TMJ disorders, as far as patients who have significant muscle-related findings are concerned. In a similar way, previous research has addressed the interaction of botulinum toxin (BoNT) injection effects on pain intensity caused by bruxism in temporomandibular joint (TMJ) disorders. The findings indicated that pain intensity decreased, with the noticeable improvement in jaw functioning following BoNT injections into the masseter muscle. Patients also reported a substantial decrease in the frequency of teeth grinding, which contributed to an overall reduction in symptoms. Additional studies analyzing BoNT use in patients with TMJ osteoarthritis demonstrated reductions in pain levels alongside the positive functional outcomes. Comparative analyses have further shown that BoNT therapy is more effective than corticosteroid injections or occlusal splints, particularly due to its superior pain-relieving effect and ability to induce mild muscle relaxation. Furthermore, BoNT administration has been associated with decreased frequency of bruxism episodes and improved mouth opening, making it a valuable treatment option for many patients.

4.4 Risks, side effects, and limitations

While botulinum toxin is generally safe when administered by a trained professional, it is not without risks. The mild effects happen in most cases and are local and involve swelling, bruising around the injection area, or mild discomfort and are often resolved after a few days. Mild headache or nausea can also be experienced by patients but these are not common and are very short-lived. The lesser but more severe risk of BoNT injections is the unintended movement of the toxin to other places outside the intended muscle, resulting in the unintended outcome like the inability to swallow, talk, or drool. Such complications tend to arise when the toxin is not injected properly or given in large doses, and it is therefore vital that the practitioners observe the proper etiquettes and dose. Another limitation is transience of the effects of BoNT. Although symptom reduction is mainly effective on many people, its effects diminish after a few months necessitating the infusion treatment to continue which poses a challenge to patients. Having several treatments might act against the patient, when one thinks about the cost of the procedure, as not all cases are covered by insurance. Moreover, although BoNT is useful in treating muscle-related TMJ conditions, it will not be of greater help to patients with joint problems and structural problems and those with large cartilage degradation. Given that treatment should be comprehensive and BoNT can be added to the treatment regimen, it is often accompanied by physical therapy along with splinting and other interventions to treat all aspects of TMJ dysfunction.

5. Comparative analysis of PRP, HA, and BoNT

The use of platelet-rich plasma (PRP), hyaluronic acid (HA), and botulinum toxin (BoNT) has gained considerable attention in the management of temporomandibular joint (TMJ) disorders. These three treatment modalities offer minimally invasive, non-surgical options for patients suffering from TMJ dysfunction, particularly those with muscle-related pain, cartilage degeneration, and inflammation. While each therapy has shown promising results, understanding the comparative efficacy, patient outcomes, and methodological differences between them is essential for optimizing clinical decision-making. This section provides a comparative analysis of PRP, HA, and BoNT, focusing on clinical trial methodologies, key outcome measures, and head-to-head efficacy.

5.1 Methodological review of clinical trials

Clinical trials comparing PRP, HA, and BoNT in TMJ disorders generally involve randomized controlled trials (RCTs), cohort studies, and case series. These studies vary in design, patient selection criteria, treatment protocols, and outcome measurements. PRP studies typically focus on its regenerative properties, aiming to evaluate the healing of cartilage and the reduction of inflammation. HA trials usually emphasize its role in improving joint lubrication and reducing pain, particularly in cases of TMJ osteoarthritis. On the other hand, BoNT studies are often centered around its muscle-relaxing effects, targeting myofascial pain and bruxism-induced dysfunction. One key methodological challenge is the inconsistency in dosage and injection protocols. For instance, while PRP preparation protocols vary widely in terms of platelet concentration and the inclusion of leukocytes, HA preparations differ in molecular weight, cross-linking, and concentration. Similarly, BoNT dosing and injection sites may differ across studies, making direct comparisons difficult. Some trials use standardized dosages (e.g., 20–30 units for masseter injections), while others adjust the dose based on patient-specific factors such as muscle mass or the severity of TMJ dysfunction. Another issue in the methodological review is the lack of long-term follow-up in many studies. While short-term results are promising, long-term efficacy and safety data for these treatments are still limited. Furthermore, patient characteristics, such as the presence of osteoarthritis, muscle hyperactivity, or structural joint issues, can influence treatment outcomes, complicating the interpretation of comparative results.

5.2 Outcome measures: Pain, function, and quality of life

The primary outcome measures in clinical trials evaluating PRP, HA, and BoNT in TMJ disorders include pain reduction, functional improvement, and quality of life. Pain is typically assessed using visual analog scales (VAS) or numerical rating scales (NRS), with a focus on jaw pain intensity, discomfort during chewing, and nocturnal bruxism. Functional improvement is often measured by the range of motion (ROM) of the jaw, including the maximum mouth opening and the reduction in symptoms like clicking or locking. In addition to pain and function, many studies also assess improvements in the overall quality of life (QoL) using validated questionnaires. The most commonly used QoL instruments include the Oral Health Impact Profile (OHIP) and the Short Form-36 (SF-36), which measure aspects like emotional well-being, physical function, and social limitations due to TMJ symptoms. These tools help capture the broader impact of TMJ disorders on daily living, not just in terms of pain but also in terms of how patients perceive their ability to perform routine activities such as eating, speaking, and socializing. A systematic review of studies on PRP in TMJ disorders found significant improvements in pain scores and jaw mobility after treatment, with many patients reporting reduced use of pain medications and enhanced functional capacity [25]. Similarly, HA injections have been shown to improve pain relief and joint function, particularly in TMJ osteoarthritis cases, with patients experiencing enhanced lubrication and reduced joint stiffness [26]. BoNT, on the other hand, is highly effective in reducing muscle-induced pain and improving jaw function, especially in patients with bruxism or myofascial pain syndrome [40].

5.3 Head-to-head comparative efficacy

Head-to-head comparisons of PRP, HA, and BoNT in TMJ disorders are relatively scarce, but several studies have attempted to evaluate the relative effectiveness of these treatments. There is a comparative trial of Conti et al. [33], which proposed PRP in relation to HA and corticosteroid injections in patients with TMJ osteoarthritis. It was revealed in the study that PRP and HA gave similar results in pain relief and range of multifunction of the joints, however PRP was more effective in long-term results with its efficacy lasting till 12 months. On the contrary, corticosteroids injected proved efficient only in the short run, giving the patients only short time relief of their symptoms which resurfaced a few months later. Bordoni et al. [41] undertook a study based on comparison between the use of BoNT and HA among patients with TMJ disorders with both muscular and joint involvement. These findings showed that BoNT injections were better in relief of muscle-related pain and bruxism and HA injections had better effects on lubrication of joints and pain alleviation in a patient with osteoarthritis. These data indicate that, in the context of management of musculoskeletal dysfunction, the two methods used can be additive, as the lack of muscular function is treated with BoNT, and the joint one can be treated with HA. On the whole, the relative effectiveness of PRP, HA, and BoNT in treating the TMJ disorders is predetermined, most likely, by the character of the disease being treated. PRP only seems to work best in cartilage repair and long-lasting pain reduction especially when dealing with osteoarthritis and degenerative joint disease. The strongest point of HA is joint lubrication and pain relief in patients with minor and moderate joint degradation. In the meantime, BoNT has been used most effectively in terms of dealing with muscle problems, such as bruxism or myofascial pain, eliminating hyperactivity in muscles [42].

6. Emerging trends and future directions

The management of temporomandibular joint (TMJ) disorders is evolving as new treatment modalities, such as platelet-rich plasma (PRP), hyaluronic acid (HA), and botulinum toxin (BoNT), gain prominence for their effectiveness in treating muscle-related pain, joint degeneration, and inflammation. However, despite these advancements, there remains a need for more personalized and comprehensive approaches to improve patient outcomes. Emerging trends in TMJ disorder treatment involve combination therapies and the integration of biomarkers to guide personalized treatment approaches. These innovations have the potential to further optimize care and expand therapeutic options, improving the long-term management of TMJ disorders.

DOI: http://dx.doi.org/10.5772/intechopen.1011988

6.1 Combination therapies

One of the most promising emerging trends in TMJ disorder treatment is the use of combination therapies, where different treatment modalities are used synergistically to address multiple aspects of the disorder. For example, combining PRP or HA injections with BoNT therapy could help address both muscle-related pain and cartilage degeneration simultaneously, offering a more comprehensive solution than single treatments alone. In patients with significant muscular dysfunction and joint inflammation, the synergistic effects of BoNT and HA could reduce muscle spasms, improve joint lubrication, and decrease pain, leading to more effective long-term relief. Combining conservative therapies such as physical therapy with injectables like PRP or HA is also an emerging strategy. While PRP or HA injections can target the underlying tissue degeneration and joint inflammation, physical therapy can assist in enhancing muscle strength and mobility in the jaw. This combination can optimize treatment outcomes by addressing both the structural and functional components of TMJ disorders. Furthermore, incorporating non-invasive modalities such as occlusal splints alongside injectable therapies can help provide relief for patients with bruxism and nocturnal teeth grinding, which often exacerbate TMJ symptoms. Splints can prevent further damage to the TMJ while BoNT injections alleviate muscle-related pain, creating a multi-faceted approach to treatment. Although some studies have shown promising results, more clinical research is required to identify the most effective treatment combinations, dosages, and frequency of interventions. Combination therapies are still in their infancy. The development of protocols that guide the use of multiple therapies in a coordinated manner could pave the way for more personalized and effective treatments for TMJ disorders (**Figure 9**) [43].

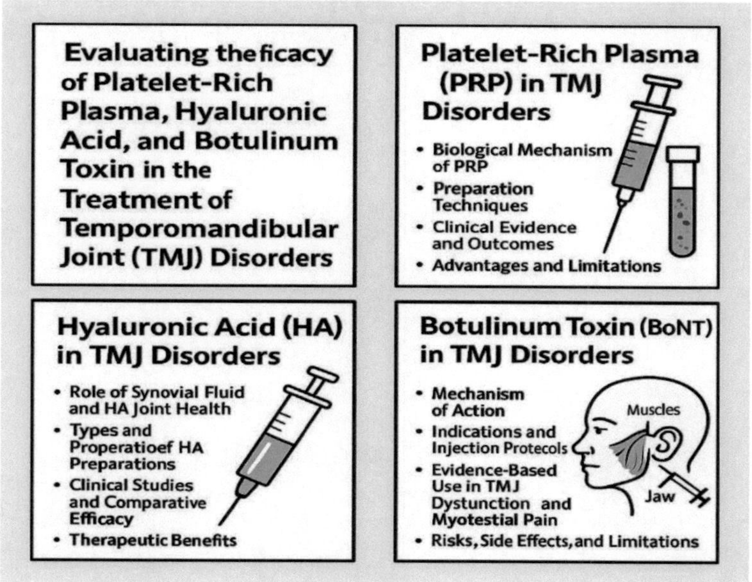

Figure 9.
Efficacy of PRP, HA, and BoNT in TMJ disorder.

6.2 Biomarkers and personalized treatment approaches

As our understanding of the pathophysiology of TMJ disorders continues to expand, biomarkers are emerging as key tools in personalized treatment approaches. Biomarkers are measurable signs of a disease's presence or severity that can help understand the underlying mechanisms that cause TMJ dysfunction. By identifying specific biomarkers associated with joint inflammation, cartilage degradation, or muscle dysfunction, clinicians may be able to tailor treatment plans to individual patients, improving outcomes and minimizing unnecessary treatments. To determine the degree of inflammation in the TMJ, for instance, inflammatory markers like C-reactive protein (CRP) and interleukins could be utilized. Elevated levels of these biomarkers might indicate that a patient would benefit more from treatments like PRP or HA, which target inflammation and tissue repair. Similarly, markers of cartilage degradation, such as matrix metalloproteinases (MMPs), could help identify patients who are more likely to respond to HA therapy, which aims to restore joint lubrication and protect cartilage from further damage. The role of genetic and molecular profiling in TMJ disorders is being investigated, in addition to markers of inflammation and cartilage degradation. Studies are beginning to investigate genetic predispositions to conditions such as osteoarthritis, which is a common cause of TMJ degeneration [44]. Identifying genetic markers that predispose individuals to TMJ disorders could allow for earlier diagnosis and intervention, as well as more precise treatment options tailored to the individual's genetic profile. Another area of personalized treatment involves the use of functional imaging techniques, such as magnetic resonance imaging (MRI) and ultrasound, to better understand the structural and functional aspects of the TMJ. These imaging tools can be used to assess joint health, identify areas of degeneration or inflammation, and guide the selection of the most appropriate treatment. For example, patients with significant cartilage degeneration may benefit more from PRP injections, while those

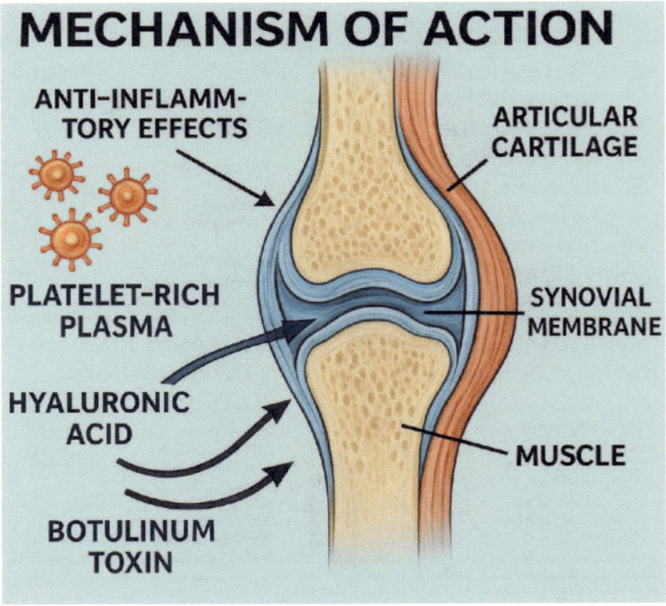

Figure 10.
How PRP, HA, and BoNT affect muscles.

with muscle-related pain may see greater relief from BoNT injections. As personalized medicine continues to evolve, the integration of biomarkers, genetic profiling, and advanced imaging into clinical practice holds great promise for improving the precision and effectiveness of TMJ disorder treatments. These advances will allow clinicians to move beyond a one-size-fits-all approach and provide more individualized, evidence-based care that is better suited to the unique needs of each patient (**Figure 10**).

7. Conclusion

Temporomandibular joint (TMJ) disorders represent a significant clinical challenge, affecting a large portion of the population with symptoms ranging from chronic pain and jaw dysfunction to impaired quality of life. Advances in the treatment of TMJ disorders have led to the development of several minimally invasive therapies, such as platelet-rich plasma (PRP), hyaluronic acid (HA), and botulinum toxin (BoNT), each offering unique benefits depending on the nature and severity of the disorder. While individual therapies have shown promise, emerging trends suggest that combination treatments and personalized approaches hold great potential for optimizing patient outcomes [45].

7.1 Clinical recommendations

Based on the current body of evidence, several clinical recommendations can be made for the management of TMJ disorders using PRP, HA, and BoNT:

1. *PRP injections*: PRP is particularly beneficial for patients with degenerative TMJ disorders, such as osteoarthritis or cartilage degeneration. It is recommended for patients who have failed conservative treatments and are seeking regenerative therapy to restore joint function and promote tissue healing. PRP's regenerative properties make it an ideal treatment option for patients with long-term joint damage, especially when combined with physical therapy for improved rehabilitation.

2. *HA injections*: HA is most effective in patients who have mild to moderate TMJ osteoarthritis or joint inflammation. It is particularly beneficial for improving joint lubrication, reducing inflammation, and alleviating pain associated with joint degeneration. HA injections should be considered as a first-line treatment for patients with early to moderate-stage TMJ osteoarthritis or those experiencing limited pain relief from conservative measures. Repeated injections may be necessary for sustained symptom control.

3. *Botulinum toxin (BoNT) Injections*: BoNT is recommended for patients with myofascial pain, bruxism, and muscle-related TMJ dysfunction. It is most effective in reducing muscle spasms, pain from clenching, and teeth grinding. BoNT should be considered for patients with significant muscular involvement, especially when there is a history of nocturnal bruxism or muscle hyperactivity. It may be used in conjunction with HA or PRP to address both muscular and joint components of TMJ disorders.

4. *Combination therapies*: For patients who present with both muscle-related pain and joint degeneration, combination therapies should be explored. PRP or HA

injections can target joint lubrication and tissue repair, while BoNT can be used to alleviate muscular tension and bruxism. The combination of these treatments may provide more comprehensive and long-lasting relief, improving overall joint function and reducing pain.

5. *Personalized treatment approaches*: As research continues to evolve, personalized treatment plans based on biomarkers, genetic profiling, and advanced imaging techniques should be integrated into clinical practice. These approaches allow for more tailored therapies that address the specific pathophysiology of the patient's TMJ disorder, improving both short- and long-term outcomes.

7.2 Final reflections

The treatment of TMJ disorders is continuously advancing, with newer therapies like PRP, HA, and BoNT providing promising non-surgical alternatives to traditional methods. While each treatment has its strengths and limitations, the key to improving patient outcomes lies in a holistic, individualized approach. Clinicians must carefully assess the nature of the disorder, whether it is primarily musculoskeletal, degenerative, or inflammatory, before deciding on the appropriate treatment or combination of therapies. Emerging trends, such as the integration of combination therapies and the use of biomarkers to guide personalized care, represent exciting future directions in TMJ disorder management. These innovations hold the potential to refine treatment protocols, ensuring that patients receive the most effective and tailored therapies available. Furthermore, the use of advanced imaging and functional assessments to monitor treatment progress and adjust interventions will become integral in providing comprehensive care. Despite the progress made in the field, challenges remain, particularly in determining the optimal dosing and frequency of injections, as well as understanding the long-term effects of these therapies. More robust, long-term clinical trials and research into the underlying mechanisms of TMJ disorders will be crucial in shaping the future of treatment. Ultimately, the goal is to offer patients not only relief from pain and dysfunction but also a sustainable approach to managing their TMJ disorders, improving their quality of life, and restoring normal jaw function.

Conflict of interest

There are no conflicts of interest.

Author details

Madiha Khan*, Sufyan Ahmed and Aisha Faraz
Oral and Maxillofacial Surgery, Abbasi Shaheed Hospital, Karachi, Pakistan

*Address all correspondence to: dr.khanmadiha@gmail.com

References

[1] Manafikhi M, Ataya J, Heshmeh O. Evaluation of the efficacy of platelet rich fibrin (I-PRF) intra-articular injections in the management of internal derangements of temporomandibular joints – A controlled preliminary prospective clinical study. BMC Musculoskeletal Disorders. 2022;**23**:454. DOI: 10.1186/s12891-022-05421-7

[2] Madani A, Ahrari F, Fallahrastegar A, Daghestani N. A randomized clinical trial comparing the efficacy of low-level laser therapy (LLLT) and laser acupuncture therapy (LAT) in patients with temporomandibular disorders. Lasers in Medical Science. 2020;**35**(1):181-192

[3] Florjanski W, Malysa A, Orzeszek S, Smardz J, Olchowy A, Paradowska-Stolarz A, et al. Evaluation of biofeedback usefulness in masticatory muscle activity management—A systematic review. Journal of Clinical Medicine. 2019;**8**(6):766

[4] Nitecka-Buchta A, Nowak-Wachol A, Wachol K, Walczyńska-Dragon K, Olczyk P, Batoryna O, et al. Myorelaxant effect of transdermal cannabidiol application in patients with TMD: A randomized, double-blind trial. Journal of Clinical Medicine. 2019;**8**(11):1886

[5] Nitecka-Buchta A, Buchta P, Tabeńska-Bosakowska E, Walczyńska-Dragoń K, Baron S. Myorelaxant effect of bee venom topical skin application in patients with RDC/TMD Ia and RDC/TMD Ib: A randomized, double-blinded study. BioMed Research International. 2014;**2014**:296053. DOI: 10.1155/2014/296053

[6] Sung S, Kim D, Park M, Hwang S, Yoon Y, Park J. Electroacupuncture for temporomandibular disorders: A systematic review of randomized controlled trials. Healthcare (Basel). 2 Nov 2021;**9**(11):1497. DOI: 10.3390/healthcare9111497

[7] Park H-B, Yang J-H, Chung K-H. Characterization of the cytokine profile of platelet rich plasma (PRP) and PRP-induced cell proliferation and migration: Upregulation of matrix metalloproteinase-1 and -9 in HaCaT cells. The Korean Journal of Hematology. 2011;**46**(4):265-273

[8] Alkerdi K, Alsabek L, Alkhouli M, Al-Nerabieah Z, Jaafo H. Evaluation of the effect of injectable platelet-rich fibrin (I-PRF) in reducing the resorption of fat graft during facial lipostructure: A randomized clinical trial. Dental and Medical Problems. 2022;**59**(1):131-136

[9] Bhattacharya HS, Gummaluri SS, Astekar M, Gummaluri RK. Novel method of determining the periodontal regenerative capacity of T-PRF and L-PRF: An immunohistochemical study. Dental and Medical Problems. 2020;**57**(2):137-144

[10] Pietruszka P, Chruścicka I, Duś-Ilnicka I, Paradowska-Stolarz A. PRP and PRF—Subgroups and divisions when used in dentistry. Journal of Personalized Medicine. 2021;**11**(10):944

[11] Kavadar G, Demircioglu DT, Celik MY, Emre TY. Effectiveness of platelet-rich plasma in the treatment of moderate knee osteoarthritis: A randomized prospective study. Journal of Physical Therapy Science. 2015;**27**(12):3863-3867

[12] Graziani F, Ivanovski S, Cei S, Ducci F, Tonetti M, Gabriele M. The

in vitro effect of different PRP concentrations on osteoblasts and fibroblasts. Clinical Oral Implants Research. 2006;**17**(2):212-219

[13] Albanese A, Licata ME, Polizzi B, Campisi G. Platelet-rich plasma (PRP) in dental and oral surgery: From the wound healing to bone regeneration. Immunity & Ageing. 2013;**10**(1):1-10

[14] Miron RJ, Fujioka-Kobayashi M, Hernandez M, Kandalam U, Zhang Y, Ghanaati S, et al. Injectable platelet rich fibrin (i-PRF): Opportunities in regenerative dentistry? Clinical Oral Investigations. 2017;**21**(8):2619-2627

[15] Fujioka-Kobayashi M, Katagiri H, Kono M, Schaller B, Zhang Y, Sculean A, et al. Improved growth factor delivery and cellular activity using concentrated platelet-rich fibrin (C-PRF) when compared with traditional injectable (i-PRF) protocols. Clinical Oral Investigations. 2020;**24**(12):4373-4383

[16] McCain JP, Hossameldin RH. Advanced arthroscopy of the temporomandibular joint. Atlas of the Oral and Maxillofacial Surgery Clinics of North America. 2011;**19**(2):145-167

[17] Helkimo M. Studies on function and dysfunction of the masticatory system. IV. Age and sex distribution of symptoms of dysfunction of the masticatory system in Lapps in the north of Finland. Acta Odontologica Scandinavica. 1974;**32**(4):255-267

[18] Gupta S, Sharma A, Purohit J, Goyal R, Malviya Y, Jain S. Comparison between intra-articular platelet-rich plasma injection versus hydrocortisone with local anesthetic injections in temporomandibular disorders: A double-blind study. National Journal of Maxillofacial Surgery. 2018;**9**(2):205-208

[19] Hancı M, Karamese M, Tosun Z, Aktan TM, Duman S, Savaci N. Intra-articular platelet-rich plasma injection for the treatment of temporomandibular disorders and a comparison with arthrocentesis. Journal of Cranio-Maxillofacial Surgery. 2015;**43**(1):162-166

[20] Harba AN, Harfoush M. Evaluation of the participation of hyaluronic acid with platelet-rich plasma in the treatment of temporomandibular joint disorders. Dental and Medical Problems. 2021;**58**(1):81-88

[21] Al-Delayme MA, Alnuamy SH, Hamid FT, Azzamily TJ, Ismaeel SA, Sammir R, et al. The efficacy of platelets rich plasma injection in the superior joint space of the tempromandibular joint guided by ultra sound in patients with non-reducing disk displacement. Journal of Maxillofacial and Oral Surgery. 2016;**16**(1):43. DOI: 10.1007/s12663-016-0911-9 [Accessed: July 6, 2025]

[22] Jacob SM, Bandyopadhyay TK, Chattopadhyay PK, Parihar VS. Efficacy of platelet-rich plasma versus hyaluronic acid following arthrocentesis for temporomandibular joint disc disorders: A randomized controlled trial. Journal of Maxillofacial and Oral Surgery. 2022;**21**(4):1199-1204. DOI: 10.1007/s12663-021-01519-y. Epub 2021 Feb 8. PMID: 36896087; PMCID: PMC9989114

[23] Mishra A, Tummala P, King A, et al. Buffered platelet-rich plasma enhances mesenchymal stem cell proliferation and chondrogenic differentiation. Tissue Engineering. Part C, Methods. 2009;**15**(3):431-435. DOI: 10.1089/ten.tec.2008.0534

[24] Ahn S-J, Kim T-W, Lee D-Y, et al. Evaluation of internal derangement of the temporomandibular joint by panoramic radiographs compared with

magnetic resonance imaging. American Journal of Orthodontics and Dentofacial Orthopedics. 2006;**129**:479-485. DOI: 10.1016/j.ajodo.2005.12.009

[25] Lee JY, Kim DJ, Lee SG, Chung JW. A longitudinal study on the osteoarthritic change of the temporomandibular joint based on 1-year follow-up computed tomography. Journal of Cranio-Maxillofacial Surgery. 2012;**40**(8):e223-e228

[26] Schmitter M, Wacker K, Pritsch M, Giannakopoulos NN, Klose C, Faggion C, et al. Preliminary longitudinal report on symptom outcomes in symptomatic and asymptomatic women with imaging evidence of temporomandibular joint arthritic changes. The International Journal of Prosthodontics. 2010;**23**(6):544-551

[27] Shan YZ, Chi Y, Min JC, et al. Magnetic resonance imaging in the diagnosis of intra-articular adhesions of the temporomandibular joint. The British Journal of Oral & Maxillofacial Surgery. 2009;**47**:389-392. DOI: 10.1016/j.bjoms.2008.09.007

[28] Charles NB, Thomas G, Glenn TC, et al. Use of sodium hyaluronate in treating temporomandibular joint disorders: A randomized, double-blind placebo-controlled clinical trial. Journal of Oral and Maxillofacial Surgery. 1993;**51**:232-242. DOI: 10.1016/S0278-2391(10)80163-6

[29] Marx RE. Platelet-rich plasma: Evidence to support its use. Journal of Oral and Maxillofacial Surgery. 2004;**62**:489-496. DOI: 10.1016/j.joms.2003.12.003

[30] Comert Kilic S, Gungormus M. Is arthrocentesis plus platelet-rich plasma superior to arthrocentesis plus hyaluronic acid for the treatment of temporomandibular joint osteoarthritis: A randomized clinical trial. International Journal of Oral and Maxillofacial Surgery. 2016;**45**(12):1538-1544. DOI: 10.1016/j.ijom.2016.06.009

[31] Hancı M, Karamese M, Tosun Z, et al. Intra-articular platelet-rich plasma injection for the treatment of temporomandibular disorders and a comparison with arthrocentesis. Journal of Cranio-Maxillo-Facial Surgery. 2015;**43**:162-166. DOI: 10.1016/j.jcms.2014.11.002

[32] Bouloux GF, Chou J, Krishnan D, Aghaloo T, Kahenasa N, Smith JA, et al. Is hyaluronic acid or corticosteroid superior to lactated ringer solution in the short-term reduction of temporomandibular joint pain after arthrocentesis? Journal of Oral and Maxillofacial Surgery. 2017;**75**(1):52-62, 63-72

[33] Conti PCR, dos Santos CN, Kogawa EM, de Castro Ferreira Conti AC, de Araujo Cdos R. The treatment of painful temporomandibular joint clicking with oral splints: A randomized clinical trial. Journal of the American Dental Association. 2006;**137**(8):1108-1114

[34] Alpaslan GH, Alpaslan C. Efficacy of temporomandibular joint arthrocentesis with or without injection of sodium hyaluronate in treatment of internal derangements. Journal of Oral and Maxillofacial Surgery. 2001;**59**:613-618. DOI: 10.1053/joms.2001.23368

[35] Pihut M, Szuta M, Ferendiuk E, et al. Evaluation of pain regression in patients with temporomandibular dysfunction treated by intra-articular platelet-rich plasma injections: A preliminary report. BioMed Research International. 2014;**2014**:132369. DOI: 10.1155/2014/132369

[36] Manfredini D, Bonnini S, Arboretti R, et al. Temporomandibular

joint osteoarthritis: An open label trial of 76 patients treated with arthrocentesis plus hyaluronic acid injections. International Journal of Oral and Maxillofacial Surgery. 2009;**38**:827-834. DOI: 10.1016/j.ijom.2009.03.715

[37] Smith MM, Ghosh P. The synthesis of hyaluronic acid by human synovial fibroblasts is influenced by the nature of the hyaluronate in the extracellular environment. Rheumatology International. 1987;**7**(3):113-122. DOI: 10.1007/BF00270463

[38] Asari A, Miyauchi S, Matsuzaka S, et al. Molecular weight-dependent effects of hyaluronate on the arthritic synovium. Archives of Histology and Cytology. 1998;**61**(2):125-135

[39] Darwish G. A comprehensive analysis of the efficacy of injectable medications in relieving temporomandibular joint discomfort: A systematic review. Journal of Clinical Practice and Research. 2024;**46**(1):1-10

[40] Manfredini D, Guarda-Nardini L, Winocur E, Piccotti F, Ahlberg J, Lobbezoo F. Research diagnostic criteria for temporomandibular disorders: A systematic review of axis I epidemiologic findings. Oral Surgery, Oral Medicine, Oral Pathology, Oral Radiology, and Endodontology. 2011;**112**:453-462

[41] Bordoni B, Varacallo M. Anatomy, Head and Neck, Temporomandibular Joint. StatPearls Publishing; 2018–present

[42] Sikora M, Sielski M, Chęciński M, Nowak Z, Chlubek D. Repeated intra-articular administration of platelet-rich plasma (PRP) in temporomandibular disorders: A clinical case series. Journal of Clinical Medicine. 2021;**11**(15):4281. DOI: 10.3390/jcm11154281 [Accessed: July 6, 2025]

[43] Chęciński M, Chęcińska K, Turosz N, Brzozowska A, Chlubek D, Sikora M. Current clinical research directions on temporomandibular joint intra-articular injections: A mapping review. Journal of Clinical Medicine. 2022;**12**(14):4655. DOI: 10.3390/jcm12144655 [Accessed: July 6, 2025]

[44] Xu J, Ren H, Zhao S, et al. Comparative effectiveness of hyaluronic acid, platelet-rich plasma, and platelet-rich fibrin in treating temporomandibular disorders: A systematic review and network meta-analysis. Head & Face Medicine. 2023;**19**:39. DOI: 10.1186/s13005-023-00369-y

[45] Choukroun J, Ghanaati S. Reduction of relative centrifugation force within injectable platelet-rich-fibrin (PRF) concentrates advances patients' own inflammatory cells, platelets and growth factors: The first introduction to the low speed centrifugation concept. European Journal of Trauma and Emergency Surgery. 2018;**44**(1):87-95. DOI: 10.1007/s00068-017-0767-9

Chapter 10

Physiotherapeutic Approaches in the Management of Temporomandibular Disorders

Sarah Allal

Abstract

Temporomandibular disorders (TMD) comprise a multifactorial group of musculoskeletal and neuromuscular dysfunctions affecting the masticatory system. This chapter provides a comprehensive overview of physiotherapeutic strategies used in TMD management, covering both manual and instrumental techniques. Clinical applications, mechanisms of action, and evidence-based insights are presented for therapies such as manual manipulation, shock wave therapy, vibration, radiofrequency, Transcutaneous electrical nerve stimulation (TENS), proprioceptive rehabilitation, and topical phytotherapy. The importance of individualized treatment plans, interdisciplinary care, and patient empowerment through therapeutic education is emphasized. Drawing from clinical experience and a review of recent literature, the chapter offers a structured, integrative model for optimizing functional recovery and long-term quality of life in TMD patients.

Keywords: temporomandibular disorders, physiotherapy, manual therapy, non-invasive treatment, self-care, orofacial pain, rehabilitation, photobiomodulation

1. Introduction

Physiotherapy, which encompasses all non-pharmacological and non-surgical external treatments, includes a wide range of tools and protocols: physical therapy, electrotherapy, thermotherapy, radiofrequency, shock waves, vibration therapy, phytotherapy, and even light or aroma therapy. It involves cross-disciplinary competencies shared among physiotherapists, dentists, pain specialists, and physical medicine practitioners.

Over the past 30 years, physiotherapy has seen a significant rise in fields such as orthopedics, neurology, pulmonology, and neurosurgery. It has become a reference treatment for certain conditions—such as lateral epicondylitis or community-acquired low back pain [1, 2]. However, its use remains limited in maxillofacial surgery, dentistry, or pain medicine. Its role in the treatment of temporomandibular disorders (TMD) is still being defined.

Despite an increasing number of referrals for maxillofacial physical therapy, its application is often misunderstood or poorly documented by practitioners.

IntechOpen

Frequently relegated behind pharmacological approaches (anti-inflammatories, analgesics, and muscle relaxants), intraoral devices, or injections (e.g., botulinum toxin), physiotherapy struggles to find its place in care protocols due to a lack of visibility and structural support. This is mainly due to the scarcity of robust scientific data, uneven access to trained therapists, and the complexity of initial clinical assessment.

However, these so-called "next-generation" techniques—far from being secondary—deserve a central place in the care of TMD patients. Non-invasive and adaptable, they offer a diverse range of actions (muscle relaxation, neuromodulation of pain, functional improvement) and encourage the development of self-care strategies by patients. They target underlying pathophysiological mechanisms—such as inflammation, hypernociception, stiffness, discal alterations, edema, or fibrous retractions—by aiming to restore disrupted physiological functions.

The physiotherapeutic approach thus requires a nuanced understanding of mechanical and neurofunctional imbalances and necessitates careful adaptation to the patient's profile. It involves thinking in terms of physiology, pathophysiology, and treatment individualization. Far from a standardized model, this approach seeks to reconcile clinical precision with therapeutic alliance in a care dynamic rooted in practical realities and the concrete—yet often limited—capacities of the patient. Nevertheless, the vast diversity of applications, while beneficial, can also disorient or intimidate both practitioners and patients. Hence, it is essential to provide a structured, accessible, and comprehensive framework to better navigate this therapeutic domain and integrate it into a coherent treatment plan.

2. External manipulations

2.1 Description

Manual therapies are the most frequently used physiotherapeutic approach in the management of TMD. Performed by specialized physiotherapists, osteopaths, chiropractors, or trained physicians, these techniques aim to restore joint mobility, reduce muscle hypertonicity, and relieve pain.

Among the most commonly used techniques are passive or oscillatory mobilizations of the temporomandibular joint. These help restore fluid joint movement, enhance synovial fluid diffusion, and stimulate deep joint receptors to promote reflex neuromuscular regulation. When applied as prolonged capsular stretching, they can soften pericapsular structures and stimulate synovial fluid production *via* capsular mechanoreceptors.

Anteroposterior glides, applied through gentle traction or controlled translation, are indicated to address range-of-motion limitations, particularly in cases of disc displacements, mechanical blockages, or recurrent subluxations. They contribute to realigning joint surfaces and restoring functional congruency.

Deep massage of masticatory muscles is used to release tension, reduce trigger points, and improve local microcirculation. These massages are often combined with targeted pressure on myofascial trigger points, especially in the masseter, temporalis, and cervical muscles. Their deactivation leads to rapid pain relief and improved muscle function. However, attention must be paid to pressure intensity—too light is ineffective, while too strong may provoke muscular resistance or aggravate the pain.

Passive stretching of the masticatory, neck, and infrahyoid muscles helps restore optimal muscle length, improve tissue flexibility, and release myofascial restrictions. Complementary myolymphatic drainage techniques may also be used to reduce post-traumatic or inflammatory edema and promote local detoxification. Mouth opening stretches should always be performed alongside progressive cervical hyperextension to maintain proper disc positioning. Patients must be taught to coordinate these two movements and remain attuned to their pain threshold, ensuring the stretch does not exceed tolerable limits in amplitude or duration. Patients should accept some discomfort associated with these exercises while the therapeutic support emphasizes relaxation and trust.

These techniques address a broad spectrum of clinical presentations: muscular or articular pain, functional lockjaw, mandibular trajectory deviations, limited mouth opening, and associated postural alterations. They may be combined or integrated into broader protocols, depending on the disease stage and specific patient needs.

2.2 Literature data

Several clinical trials, although limited in sample size, have demonstrated the significant effectiveness of manual therapy in managing TMD, with excellent tolerability. Recent studies support these techniques not only for symptomatic relief but also for promoting neuroplastic reorganization of mandibular motor control. Kalamir et al. [3] reported that approximately 70% of patients treated with manual mobilizations experienced significant pain reduction and lasting functional improvement [4]. These findings are reinforced by multiple randomized controlled trials. For example, Tuncer et al. showed the superior efficacy of a manual therapy program combined with home exercises over conventional care, with significant improvements in pain scores and mouth opening [5]. In their meta-analysis, Calixtre et al. [6] emphasized that manual therapy techniques not only reduce pain immediately but also improve mandibular range of motion and quality of life for several weeks after treatment.

More recent studies have evaluated the specific effects of deep massage and passive stretching applied to masticatory muscles, confirming their muscle-relaxing effects and reduction of abnormal electromyographic activity, particularly in the masseter muscle.

2.3 Perspectives and challenges

Manual therapy offers a personalized, reversible, non-invasive, and low-cost approach. Its excellent tolerance makes it particularly suitable even in cases of refractory chronic pain. However, inter-practitioner variability and the lack of consensus on technical parameters (intensity, duration, frequency) limit its standardization.

A better categorization of responsive patient profiles, clearer evaluation of dose-response effects, and delineation of the specific roles of each technique (mobilization, stretching, massage, etc.) remain necessary. Combining manual therapy with other approaches—such as therapeutic education, muscle strengthening, and postural control—seems promising for effective multimodal care. Ultimately, integrating manual techniques into official therapeutic guidelines for TMD will require large-scale, multicenter comparative studies with standardized assessments of mandibular function, pain, and disability.

3. Extracorporeal shock wave therapy (ESWT)

3.1 Description

Extracorporeal shock wave therapy (ESWT) is based on the emission of high-intensity acoustic waves delivered either in a focused or radial pattern to deep tissues. Initially developed for lithotripsy, it has since gained popularity in the treatment of chronic tendinopathies and musculoskeletal pain and is now finding its place in temporomandibular disorders (TMD).

For facial indications, the ESWT device is typically a pneumatic radial shockwave system, such as the Storz Medical Masterpuls MP100® or an equivalent. It allows controlled delivery of mechanical impulses *via* an ergonomic handpiece equipped with a 15–20 mm diameter applicator, with adjustable frequency (1–20 Hz) and intensity (1–4 bars). Parameters are individualized based on patient tolerance and the characteristics of the targeted tissues.

The mechanical stimulation induced by the impulses creates controlled micro-trauma that triggers a cascade of biological responses favorable to tissue repair. The most commonly targeted zones are the masseter muscles, lateral pterygoid muscles (*via* extraoral access), and painful ligamentous or tendinous insertions associated with functional restrictions.

Shock waves induce peripheral desensitization by decreasing substance P release and reducing nociceptor sensitivity. They also enhance microcirculation through angiogenesis and facilitate collagen fiber reorganization. Additionally, central modulation of pain transmission may occur, likely *via* activation of Aβ fibers and inhibition of ascending pain pathways.

ESWT is particularly indicated in chronic myofascial TMD, especially in cases of trigger points resistant to manual therapy, diffuse masseteric pain, or muscular-related limited mouth opening. It may also be useful as an adjunct to proprioceptive or postural rehabilitation.

Treatment is typically administered in one session per week for 3–5 weeks. Impulse intensity is adjusted to patient tolerance to avoid post-treatment pain exacerbation. Cryotherapy can be applied afterward to support healing.

3.2 Literature data

The efficacy of ESWT in managing myofascial pain has been investigated in several clinical studies, primarily in locomotor regions (shoulder, plantar fascia, and low back), with findings applicable to the maxillofacial field. In a prospective study of 28 patients with myogenous TMD, a 60–80% improvement in pain was observed, along with functional gains in mouth opening [7], without significant adverse effects and following a reproducible protocol.

Similar results have been found in a randomized controlled trial using radial shockwave protocols for pelvic floor disorders [8], showing significant reductions in chronic muscle pain after three to five sessions. In tendinopathies, plantar fasciitis, and low back pain, several trials [7, 9–11] demonstrate long-lasting pain reduction, improved tissue flexibility, activation of reparative mechanisms (*via* induction of microlesions), and stimulation of local vascularization.

The most frequently cited mechanisms of action include nociceptive terminal desensitization, fibroblast activation, TRPV1 receptor modulation, and stimulation of pro-regenerative substances like VEGF.

The most common protocols use 1500–3000 impulses per session at frequencies ranging from 8 to 15 Hz. Most devices are pneumatic radial systems, although some studies utilize deeper-acting electromagnetic focused devices. These allow for tailored intensity adjustment, and newer-generation portable devices increase accessibility in private practice settings.

3.3 Perspectives and challenges

Shockwave therapy presents a promising option for chronic muscle pain, including in the orofacial region, due to its anti-inflammatory, anti-fibrotic, and regenerative effects. However, data specific to TMD remain scarce, and technical parameters vary widely between studies. The diversity of devices, frequencies, and energy densities makes direct comparison of results challenging.

Robust multicenter trials including active control groups, objective outcome measures (e.g., kinematics, MRI, and functional scales), and medium- to long-term follow-up are needed to refine the specific indications for orofacial use. Concurrently, practitioner training and the validation of standardized protocols will be critical for safely integrating this technique into TMD treatment pathways.

4. Vibratory therapies

4.1 Description

As with extracorporeal shock waves (ESWT), vibratory therapies may raise concerns—especially when applied to the face—but these fears are often based on misconceptions rather than scientific evidence. In sports medicine, localized vibration—*via* massage guns or oscillating platforms—is widely used to relieve muscle soreness, improve recovery, and prepare tissues for exertion. Multiple studies demonstrate significant reductions in delayed-onset muscle soreness (DOMS) and increased neuromuscular flexibility, even among elite athletes [12].

These therapies involve the application of mechanical oscillations at variable frequencies, typically between 20 and 150 Hz. Once confined to post-exercise recovery, vibratory techniques are increasingly used for chronic musculoskeletal pain, including in the maxillofacial region.

Devices used include handheld massage guns, manual vibratory therapy instruments (e.g., Novafon), or oscillating platforms. These tools stimulate soft tissues, activate deep mechanoreceptors, and provide analgesic, muscle-relaxing, and proprioceptive effects.

Muscle relaxation is thought to result from inhibition of myotatic reflexes and reduced neuromuscular excitability. Fibrous and periarticular tissues benefit from a defibrosing effect due to vibratory shear, improving suppleness and gliding. Deep mechanoreceptors, such as Piezo1 and Piezo2 channels, are activated and may trigger repair responses, inflammatory modulation, or even osteogenesis.

Vibration also contributes to peripheral desensitization and central modulation of pain through the Gate Control mechanism, as well as enhancing capillary flow and lymphatic drainage.

In practice, these techniques are indicated for myofascial pain in the masseter and temporalis muscles, postoperative stiffness, residual post-inflammatory tension, and proprioceptive dysfunctions in the orofacial region. Frequency, duration, and application mode should be tailored to patient tolerance.

Contraindications include local infection, unhealed fractures, open wounds, unstable atheromatous plaques, dislodged or unstable calculi, atlantoaxial instability, and known malignancies. In situations like pregnancy, pacemaker use, or known arteriovenous malformations or aneurysms, a precautionary principle should be applied despite a lack of confirmed harm.

Local vibration is typically applied at 50–100 Hz using a soft-tipped device over less padded bony areas (canine pillars, zygomatic arch, parasymphyseal region). Sessions last from 5 to 20 minutes, several times a week. A self-administered version is possible after a brief instructional phase.

4.2 Literature data

Numerous studies in sports medicine have confirmed the efficacy of vibration in reducing DOMS, improving neuromuscular flexibility, and accelerating post-exercise recovery [12–14].

In orthopedics, vibration has been shown to enhance vascularization, reduce inflammation, and improve proprioception and postural stability, as highlighted by systematic reviews on whole-body vibration in chronic low back pain and other painful musculoskeletal conditions [15–18].

In the facial region, controlled clinical trials have shown that high-frequency vibration (100 Hz) significantly reduces pain in TMD patients (vibratory analgesia), with stronger effects than those seen at 20 Hz—suggesting central modulation of pain perception. A pilot study using a local device (Novafon Pro SK2 at 50–100 Hz) in 28 patients also reported significant reductions in muscle, joint, and headache pain after 1 week of treatment [19].

4.3 Perspectives and challenges

Vibratory therapies appear to be safe, cost-effective, and easily reproducible, particularly for patient self-management. Their potential for home use, along with excellent tolerance, makes them ideal for therapeutic education and functional maintenance. However, more numerous and better-controlled studies are needed to determine optimal parameters (frequency, duration, application site) and clarify potential contraindications. The mechanical defibrosing effect, in particular, deserves further exploration to assess its contribution to tissue restoration in chronic TMD.

5. Radiofrequency therapy

5.1 Description

Radiofrequency (RF) therapy is a physical modality that uses high-frequency electromagnetic waves—typically between 0.3 and 1 MHz—to produce controlled endogenous heating of soft tissues. Unlike conventional thermotherapy, which transfers heat externally by conduction, RF generates heat within deep tissues *via* capacitive or resistive mechanisms, targeting specific areas such as the masticatory muscles, fascia, joint capsules, or periarticular ligaments.

The RF devices used in rehabilitation are usually equipped with mobile electrodes—capacitive for water-rich tissues and resistive for fibrous structures—and allow precise adjustments of power, frequency, and treatment duration. Sessions last between 20 and 30 minutes, applied one to three times per week, depending on the chosen protocol and patient tolerance. The objective is to raise local tissue temperature to 42–45°C, a threshold at which significant biological effects occur without causing burns or cellular damage.

RF acts at multiple physiological levels. In chronically contracted muscles, it promotes effective relaxation by breaking residual actin-myosin bridges, increasing fiber extensibility, and enhancing muscular compliance. It is particularly beneficial in hypertonic masseter or temporalis muscles, common in myogenous TMD. In connective tissues—such as fascia, capsular ligaments, or cervico-mandibular fascia—generated heat leads to collagen reorganization, softening of fibrous zones, and improved local viscoelasticity.

RF also exerts anti-inflammatory effects by downregulating pro-inflammatory cytokines (IL-6 and TNF-α) and modulating peripheral nociceptor activity. Additionally, it enhances microcirculation through reflex vasodilation, aiding in lymphatic and venous drainage, especially in chronic post-inflammatory edema. The local chemical environment becomes less favorable to pain, which explains the significant clinical improvement often reported in patients with persistent facial pain.

5.2 Literature data

Numerous studies confirm the effectiveness of RF therapy in treating chronic musculoskeletal pain, with significant outcomes reported in various anatomical regions: moderate to marked pain reduction in shoulder, sacroiliac joint, and spinal disorders; over 50% pain relief in knee osteoarthritis, with effects lasting up to 2 years; substantial improvements in cervical pain (especially facet-related), with response rates between 70 and 88%. In TMD, several controlled trials have demonstrated clear pain reduction and improved mouth opening, both in the masticatory muscles and the temporomandibular joint itself, particularly using pulsed RF techniques [10, 20–22].

5.3 Perspectives and challenges

Radiofrequency therapy offers a promising modality in managing chronic musculoskeletal pain, especially in complex myofascial syndromes and post-surgical sequelae. Its combined action on pain, inflammation, fibrosis, and circulation makes it a versatile and potentially central tool in TMD treatment. However, despite its proven efficacy in numerous studies, its use remains limited in orofacial care due to several barriers.

Firstly, the technology is not widely available in standard rehabilitation clinics, as it requires dedicated RF equipment that can cost several thousand euros. The most advanced devices offer stable, safe, and adjustable energy delivery, along with precise settings (frequency, intensity, duration) and interchangeable electrodes for different anatomical areas. This type of investment is usually found in multidisciplinary or specialized rehabilitation centers.

Secondly, the lack of standardized, large-scale validated protocols limits its integration into official guidelines. Treatment parameters vary widely between studies (duration, frequency, electrode type, number of sessions), making it difficult to compare results and optimize clinical indications.

Moreover, although its analgesic and muscle-relaxing effects are well documented, the precise cellular mechanisms—especially regarding neuro-immunological interactions—remain poorly understood in maxillofacial tissues.

Large-scale, multicenter clinical trials with active comparators, standardized functional assessments, and long-term follow-up are needed to better define its indications by patient profiles, pain types, and anatomical targets. Clear technical guidelines and dedicated practitioner training would also be key to scaling up its use in TMD care.

6. Transcutaneous electrical nerve stimulation (TENS)

6.1 Description

Transcutaneous electrical nerve stimulation (TENS) is a widely used electrotherapy technique for treating musculoskeletal and neuropathic pain. It involves applying low-intensity electrical currents through the skin using surface electrodes placed over strategic areas—such as dermatomes, muscular trigger points, or nerve pathways.

The analgesic effects of TENS are explained by several complementary neurophysiological mechanisms, depending on the type of stimulation applied.

In its conventional high-frequency form (80–120 Hz), TENS selectively activates large-diameter sensory nerve fibers (Aβ fibers). Their stimulation inhibits nociceptive transmission at the spinal dorsal horn level, a process known as the "gate control" theory [23], wherein non-nociceptive signals "close the gate" to painful stimuli.

Low-frequency forms (1–10 Hz), with more intense stimulation, act through the activation of endogenous opioid pathways. They induce the release of beta-endorphins, met-enkephalins, and other analgesic neuromodulators at the spinal and supraspinal levels, producing a longer-lasting, though sometimes delayed, analgesic effect.

Other modalities, such as burst TENS (pulsed frequencies), or modulated amplitude/frequency modes, aim to optimize physiological adaptation and delay the onset of nerve accommodation in prolonged treatments.

TENS is thus primarily indicated for peripheral neurogenic pain, myofascial syndromes, postoperative pain, and chronic musculoskeletal pain—especially when pharmacological treatments are ineffective or poorly tolerated.

TENS is valued for its simplicity, safety, and excellent tolerance. It is commonly used for cervical, lumbar, or trigeminal pain; tension-type headaches and certain migraines; postoperative pain (including maxillofacial and dental surgeries); facial pain, masseteric discomfort, and post-traumatic TMJ pain; peripheral neuralgias (sciatica, cruralgia, cervicobrachial neuralgia); and pain associated with scar fibrosis or myofascial retractions.

Its use is also common in immediate postoperative settings, as part of multimodal analgesia strategies, helping to limit opioid consumption.

While generally safe, TENS has some relative or absolute contraindications, including the presence of a pacemaker or implanted neurostimulator (risk of electromagnetic interference); pregnancy, especially early stages (as a precaution); uncontrolled epilepsy (for cranial applications); and dermatological lesions or infections at the electrode sites. It should also be used cautiously in sensitive areas without supervision (e.g., anterior neck, carotid region, and precordium).

DOI: http://dx.doi.org/10.5772/intechopen.1011989

6.2 Literature data

Several meta-analyses [20] indicate pain relief in 50–60% of TMD patients, especially in myofascial forms. TENS is also recognized for its excellent safety profile, making it a suitable option for self-treatment, particularly in therapeutic education programs.

6.3 Perspectives and challenges

Its low cost, ease of use, and portability make TENS an ideal choice for home care programs. However, the wide variability of protocols (frequencies, durations, electrode placements) still limits standardization. Further research targeting optimal parameters according to TMD subtypes would be beneficial in formalizing TENS use in multimodal care protocols.

7. Proprioceptive rehabilitation

7.1 Description

Proprioceptive rehabilitation aims to restore or improve the fine perception of joint position, movement, and internal tissue tension within the musculoskeletal system. It relies on targeted stimulation of mechanoreceptors (muscle spindles, Golgi tendon organs, cutaneous, and articular receptors) to optimize neuromotor coordination, postural stability, and movement fluidity.

Once considered a secondary component of functional rehabilitation, proprioception is now central in the management of chronic muscular imbalances, recurrent pain, and postural disorders. In the context of temporomandibular disorders (TMD), it helps re-establish fine motor control of the masticatory apparatus, often impaired by pain, muscle compensation, or joint dysfunctions.

Proprioceptive work is based on sensorimotor feedback loops. It engages the central nervous system's ability to integrate afferent signals from peripheral receptors and adapt motor responses in real-time.

In chronic pain patients, these loops are often disrupted: reflex muscle inhibition, loss of segmental differentiation, and maladaptive motor responses. Proprioceptive rehabilitation thus "re-educates the brain for movement" by restoring bodily mapping and neuromuscular synergies specific to each task.

Progression generally follows increasing instability (asymmetric postures, inclined planes, and dynamic supports) and motor complexity (adding voluntary movement, dual-tasking, altered visual or auditory cues), with or without technological aids (balance platforms, pressure sensors, and virtual reality systems).

In maxillofacial care, proprioceptive rehabilitation is indicated in multiple situations: pre- and postoperative phases of orthognathic surgery or TMJ interventions (e.g., prostheses and TMJ anchors), orofacial dyspraxia or tongue malposition, and in general TMD.

Exercises may include mandibular work on unstable surfaces (balls and proprioceptive cushions), with or without visual feedback; maintaining neutral jaw position (MIH or CR) with eyes closed; coordinating mandibular-cervical movements; dissociating jaw motion from head motion; and retraining bilateral mastication and swallowing.

7.2 Literature data

A double-blind, randomized controlled study published in 2024 [24] assessed the effects of proprioceptive neuromuscular facilitation (PNF) stretching in patients with TMD and forward head posture. The protocol targeted both cervical and mandibular muscles to restore coherent sensorimotor synergy. Results showed significant improvement in mouth opening, marked pain reduction, and measurable correction of cervical posture after 6 weeks of intervention. This provides strong support for integrating PNF-based exercises in proprioceptive rehabilitation strategies for TMD, especially when part of a broader craniocervical dysfunction context.

7.3 Perspectives and challenges

Proprioceptive rehabilitation is a key approach for TMD, particularly in patients with subtle but disabling motor control disorders. It has the notable advantage of excellent tolerance, but requires good patient cooperation and cognitive engagement. It promotes fine and durable neuromotor reprogramming when individualized and integrated into comprehensive care. Further randomized controlled trials are needed to standardize protocols and validate the effectiveness of each modality, individually or in combination.

8. Muscle strengthening

8.1 Description

Long confined to the domains of sports and orthopedics, muscle strengthening is now recognized as an essential component in the rehabilitation of chronic musculoskeletal disorders, including maxillofacial conditions. Far from simply "toning" muscles, this approach aims to restore functional symmetry, rebalance muscle chains, and re-establish the body's capacity for precise, efficient, and sustained movement. In the context of temporomandibular disorders (TMD), muscle strengthening helps correct imbalances caused by pain or parafunctional habits, stabilize the temporomandibular joint, and restore coordinated motor control of the orofacial region.

The goal is to achieve both morphological and functional recovery: reintegrating the masticatory muscles into more efficient neuromotor patterns, strengthening deep neck and floor-of-mouth stabilizers, and improving muscle endurance for daily functions such as chewing, swallowing, and speaking. This requires work on strength, coordination, endurance, and precision, in a progressive and comprehensive rehabilitation program.

Target muscles often include the masseters, pterygoids, and temporalis, as well as deep cervical flexors, suprahyoid and infrahyoid muscles, and broader muscle groups involved in cervicocephalic posture. These areas are often imbalanced due to chronic pain and compensatory patterns—some overactive and tight, others inhibited or weakened. Muscle strengthening seeks to re-harmonize these imbalances.

Exercise modalities vary depending on therapeutic goals: gentle isometric contractions to restore conscious muscle activation, controlled dynamic movements to increase range and precision, or functional exercises mimicking everyday activities. Emphasis is placed on movement quality rather than intensity. Strengthening may also involve unstable postures or combined tasks to foster better sensorimotor integration in real-life conditions.

In TMD, exercises may include guided mouth opening, lateral excursions against resistance (manual or elastic), or bilateral mastication using resistant materials. When cervical pain is present, retraining deep cervical stabilizers is often beneficial, as hypotonia in these muscles is commonly associated with mandibular and postural dysfunctions.

8.2 Literature data

Clinical studies show that targeted muscle strengthening improves joint stability by 60–75% in patients with recurrent dislocations or mandibular instability. For example, Seyhan and Atalay demonstrated in a randomized controlled trial that a program combining cervicothoracic strengthening and mandibular exercises significantly reduced pain and improved posture and masticatory function [25]. Similarly, Crăciun et al. reported marked functional improvements in TMD after a cervical-jaw stabilization program [23]. The combined effect with proprioceptive rehabilitation appears particularly beneficial, reducing painful episodes and promoting smoother mastication.

8.3 Perspectives and challenges

Often overlooked in traditional TMD management, the strengthening phase is crucial for achieving lasting functional recovery. It should not involve hypertrophying or fibrosing the masticatory muscles. Protocol standardization remains limited, and further studies are needed to define optimal loads, frequencies, and modalities tailored to specific clinical profiles.

9. Topical phytotherapy

9.1 Description

Although historically marginalized in modern functional rehabilitation practices, phytotherapy is regaining relevance in an integrative and individualized approach to chronic pain management. It offers valuable support in complement to mechanical or neurophysiological treatments, particularly when targeting low-grade inflammatory states, persistent pain modulation, or restoration of altered psycho-neuro-immunological balance.

In the context of temporomandibular disorders (TMD), the rational use of specific plant extracts can help alleviate muscular and articular pain, reduce emotional tension, and support tissue recovery processes. The aim is not to replace conventional pharmacology with herbal medicine, but rather to propose targeted support based on well-known properties of certain plants, in synergy with other therapeutic modalities.

Commonly used plants include those with direct anti-inflammatory effects such as devil's claw (harpagophytum), rich in harpagosides, and turmeric, whose curcumin acts on pro-inflammatory cytokine cascades. These extracts, well-tolerated in oral use, may be proposed in standardized capsule form, especially for chronic articular or myofascial pain.

Other plants are sought for their muscle-relaxing properties, such as passionflower, valerian, or California poppy, which act centrally to promote global neuromuscular relaxation. These are suitable for patients with persistent hypertonia, nocturnal parafunctions, or anxiety-related sleep disturbances.

Essential oils provide an interesting topical or olfactory route. Wintergreen (rich in methyl salicylate) has notable analgesic and anti-inflammatory effects, especially when massaged locally over the masseters or neck. True lavender and ylang-ylang, used in diffusion or diluted topical application, may enhance the calming effect of relaxation or gentle mobilization sessions [26].

Additionally, plants that support microcirculation and lymphatic drainage—such as blackcurrant, red vine, or ginkgo—may be used in cases of facial edema following trauma or surgery.

Caution is warranted, as interactions with conventional medications are possible, and phytotherapy should always be individualized based on patient history and the coherence of the overall treatment plan.

9.2 Literature data

One study [27] demonstrated that regular application of a herbal-based balm on masticatory muscles could reduce pain by up to 30%, when used alongside conventional physiotherapy. Preliminary research also suggests that topical CBD may offer additional benefits in inflammatory muscle pain [28], although evidence remains limited.

Regarding individual active compounds, several systematic reviews have highlighted the relevance of topical capsaicin (derived from chili peppers) [27–31] in managing chronic musculoskeletal pain, with a number needed to treat (NNT) of about 8 and a significant pain reduction without systemic effects.

Similarly, formulations combining camphor, menthol, eucalyptol, eugenol, and vanillin have shown over 80% pain reduction in some inflammatory musculoskeletal disorders, with a favorable safety profile [32, 33].

Recent studies on eucalyptus globulus essential oil indicate analgesic and anti-inflammatory activity *via* μ-opioid receptor modulation, supporting its use in facial myofascial pain [34].

9.3 Perspectives and challenges

Topical phytotherapy offers a gentle, well-tolerated, and accessible approach—ideal for enhancing treatment adherence and empowering patients in their daily self-management. Its local action without major systemic side effects makes it a valuable adjunct in the long-term care of chronic TMD.

Nevertheless, the wide heterogeneity of available products, lack of standardization in active compound concentrations, and interindividual variability in response continue to limit its integration into clinical recommendations. Well-controlled randomized clinical trials comparing natural formulations and standard treatments are needed to validate the efficacy of each plant extract or combination in precise indications.

Better pharmacological characterization and composition standardization would help make phytotherapy a more reliable and clinically integrated therapeutic option in multimodal facial pain management.

It also represents a highly relevant axis for therapeutic education and self-care programs. Educating patients on safe and consistent use of natural topicals could enhance long-term care strategies for TMD.

10. Postural re-education

10.1 Description

Posture is far more than the mechanical alignment of body segments—it reflects a complex balance between muscular, skeletal, neurological, and sensory systems. When posture becomes dysregulated, often subtly and progressively, it leads to redistributed mechanical loads, overuse of certain stabilizing muscles, and, in some cases, chronic pain. In the context of temporomandibular disorders (TMD), postural issues are both a consequence and a perpetuating factor of dysfunction.

It is now well established that cervical spine alignment directly influences mandibular kinematics, masticatory muscle tone, and even resting tongue position. Head protraction, cervical kyphosis, or upper spine instability can disturb TMJ function, alter chewing force vectors, and induce secondary muscle hypertonicity—particularly in the masseters, pterygoids, and infrahyoid muscles.

Postural re-education in this context goes beyond correcting a "bad" position. It aims to retrain body awareness, restore efficient muscular synergies, and support dynamic stability compatible with daily life demands. It fosters a new, energetically efficient tone organization that respects deep musculoskeletal balance.

Treatment usually begins with physical and proprioceptive recentration. This involves bringing the cranial axis back over the pelvis, releasing restrictions in overactive muscular chains, and encouraging patients to rediscover neglected support zones—such as the sternum, pelvic floor, or cranial base. Through simple yet precise exercises, the therapist guides patients to develop spatial awareness, regulate postural tone, and reactivate stabilizing reflex loops.

In TMD patients with postural involvement, multiple compensations are common: shoulder elevation on one side, occlusal plane tilting, asymmetric foot support, or oculomotor disturbances. Postural re-education therefore integrates TMJ within a global body system—linked to vision, breathing, and plantar support. Work can be done sitting, standing, or lying down, using gentle techniques: muscle chain approaches (GDS, Mézières), Busquet method, postural stretching, therapeutic yoga, or sensory-based methods such as Feldenkrais or Alexander Technique.

When implemented rigorously and progressively, this process reduces symptoms and prevents relapse by restoring the body's adaptive capabilities. Many studies have confirmed the value of postural re-education in managing low back pain, cervical pain, and chronic musculoskeletal disorders. Emerging data suggest similar benefits in TMD—particularly when accompanied by global postural instability.

What makes this approach powerful is its individualization. Every patient has a unique postural organization shaped by bodily history, past trauma, professional habits, and emotional patterns. Posture is never neutral—it compensates, protects, and expresses. The therapist's role is to decode this language and offer, through attentive support, a more functional, liberated, and balanced organization.

10.2 Literature data

Several studies have demonstrated the link between forward head posture and TMD symptom severity. A systematic review concluded that combined postural and TMD interventions improved pain and function more effectively than isolated approaches. Oleksy et al. [35] showed that cervical rehabilitation alone significantly improved TMJ function in patients with idiopathic neck pain [36]. Furthermore, a clinical trial demonstrated that adding global postural training to physiotherapy improved mouth opening and reduced pain thresholds in TMD patients. Finally, Yu et al. [37] showed that combining cervicoscapular and mandibular exercises led to better muscular and joint outcomes than segmental approaches alone [35, 38].

10.3 Perspectives and challenges

Postural re-education is a foundational, yet often overlooked, element in chronic TMD—particularly in patients with altered posture or generalized motor control issues. It promotes sustainable recovery by addressing distant contributors to dysfunction. However, standardization remains difficult due to the wide variability in postural profiles [39].

It is crucial to strengthen protocol development based on clinical data, integrating objective measures (e.g., kinematic analysis and cervical proprioception tests).

Educational work with patients about the links between posture, jaw function, and pain could also improve treatment adherence. In this regard, postural re-education would benefit from inclusion in therapeutic education programs, with a dedicated self-care component aimed at maintaining clinical gains between sessions.

11. Conclusion

Physiotherapy offers a multifaceted, human-centered approach to the management of temporomandibular disorders (TMD). More than a collection of techniques, it represents a care philosophy rooted in observation, patient collaboration, and therapeutic adaptability.

Through manual therapies, instrumental technologies, proprioceptive re-education, and complementary modalities, the physiotherapist does not merely treat symptoms, but accompanies the patient in reclaiming function, dignity, and confidence.

This approach is most powerful when embedded in an interdisciplinary framework involving surgeons, dentists, physiotherapists, psychologists, pain specialists, and educators. TMD often go beyond mechanical dysfunctions—they reflect postural, emotional, and behavioral patterns that demand a holistic and coordinated response.

In this context, physiotherapy becomes a new way of understanding the suffering body—an invitation to reconnect with oneself not as a collection of dysfunctions, but as a reservoir of healing potential.

Despite promising clinical outcomes, physiotherapy still lacks high-level scientific evidence to secure its place in official TMD guidelines. Rigorous, large-scale studies with long-term follow-up and precise evaluation tools are essential. The diversity of interventions makes it difficult to isolate specific effects.

Moreover, patient variability makes rigid standardization both unrealistic and counterproductive. A given technique may be transformative for one person and ineffective—or even detrimental—for another. This calls for clinical finesse and flexible, guided protocols. In addition, access to qualified practitioners varies greatly across regions.

Thus, physiotherapy choices must consider not only the benefit-risk balance, but also beliefs and habits, local availability of treatments, patient preferences, and financial constraints. Future efforts should focus on clearer guidelines and better recognition and reimbursement of physiotherapy. Ideally, this would include the creation of dedicated therapeutic education programs for TMD, similar to diabetes education models.

Today's patients no longer wish to remain passive recipients—they want to understand, anticipate, and participate. They seek to learn the anatomy of their jaw, recognize warning signs, safely use self-care tools (massage devices and topical balms), and break the cycle of chronic pain.

Empowering the patient improves adherence and outcomes—but more importantly, it transforms the therapeutic relationship itself.

Among emerging physiotherapeutic approaches, mechanical vibration therapy stands out for its potential to support self-care through therapeutic education. It is timely to define and evaluate a dedicated protocol for TMD management.

As traditional siloed models reach their limits, we must build bridges—between surgery and rehabilitation, science and intuition, clinic and home. Physiotherapy for TMD is not just a treatment—it is a care philosophy, a partnership with the body, and a commitment to holistic healing.

Acknowledgements

The author wishes to express her gratitude to the patients who have inspired this clinical work and colleagues who have shared their insights in interdisciplinary care. Particular thanks go to the Department of Maxillofacial Surgery at the Dijon University Hospital (CHU de Dijon), and to the collaborators at the CHU de Saint-Étienne, the Centre Hospitalier d'Auxerre, and the Centre Hospitalier de Bourg-en-Bresse. Special appreciation is also extended to the members of the Committee for the Fight Against Pain (CLUD) and to the dedicated maxillofacial physiotherapist partners who have enriched this work with their clinical expertise. No specific funding was received for this work.

Conflict of interest

The author declares no conflict of interest.

Notes

This chapter reflects 6 years of dedicated engagement in the study and advancement of therapeutic strategies for treating and healing painful and functional craniofacial disorders. It is the result of continuous theoretical and practical exploration, fueled by a clinical commitment to improving care and deepening understanding of these complex conditions.

Author details

Sarah Allal
Maxillofacial Surgery Practice, Maxillofacial Turquoise, Bourg-en-Bresse, France

*Address all correspondence to: sarah.allal.cmf@google.com

References

[1] Landesa-Piñeiro L, Leirós-Rodríguez R. Physiotherapy treatment of lateral epicondylitis: A systematic review. Journal of Back and Musculoskeletal Rehabilitation. 2022;**35**(3):463-477

[2] Stoll T, Germann D, Hagmann H. Physiotherapy in lumbar disc herniation. Therapeutische Umschau. 2001;**58**(8):487-492

[3] Kalamir A, Pollard H, Vitiello AL, Bonello R. Manual therapy for temporomandibular disorders: A review of the literature. Journal of Bodywork and Movement Therapies. 2007;**11**(1):84-90

[4] Paço M, Peleteiro B, Duarte J, Pinho T. The effectiveness of physiotherapy in the management of temporomandibular disorders: A systematic review and meta-analysis. Journal of Oral & Facial Pain and Headache. 2016;**30**(2):93-102

[5] Tuncer AB, Ergun N, Tuncer AH, Karahan S. Effectiveness of manual therapy and home physical therapy in patients with temporomandibular disorders: A randomized controlled trial. Journal of Bodywork and Movement Therapies. 2013;**17**(3):302-308

[6] Calixtre LB, Moreira RFC, Franchini GH, Alburquerque-Sendín F, Oliveira AB. Manual therapy for the management of pain and limited range of motion in subjects with signs and symptoms of temporomandibular disorder: A systematic review of randomized controlled trials. Journal of Oral Rehabilitation. 2015;**42**(11):847-861

[7] Rajfur K, Rajfur J, Matusz T, Walewicz K, Dymarek R, Ptaszkowski K, et al. Efficacy of focused extracorporeal shock wave therapy in chronic low back pain: A prospective randomized 3-month follow-up study. Medical Science Monitor. 2022;**28**:e936614

[8] Liu K, Zhang Q, Chen L, Zhang H, Xu X, Yuan Z, et al. Efficacy and safety of extracorporeal shockwave therapy in chronic low back pain: A systematic review and meta-analysis. Journal of Orthopaedic Surgery and Research. 2023;**18**(1):455

[9] An S, Li J, Xie W, Yin N, Li Y, Hu Y. Extracorporeal shockwave treatment in knee osteoarthritis: Therapeutic effects and possible mechanism. Bioscience Reports. 2020;**40**(11):BSR20200926

[10] Melese H, Alamer A, Getie K, Nigussie F, Ayhualem S. Extracorporeal shock wave therapy on pain and foot functions in subjects with chronic plantar fasciitis: Systematic review of randomized controlled trials. Disability and Rehabilitation. 2022;**44**(18):5007-5014

[11] Akehurst H, Grice JE, Angioi M, Morrissey D, Migliorini F, Maffulli N. Whole-body vibration decreases delayed onset muscle soreness following eccentric exercise in elite hockey players: A randomized controlled trial. Journal of Orthopaedic Surgery and Research. 2021;**16**(1):589

[12] Lu X, Wang Y, Lu J, You Y, Zhang L, Zhu D, et al. Does vibration benefit delayed-onset muscle soreness? A meta-analysis and systematic review. The Journal of International Medical Research. 2019;**47**(1):3-18

[13] Cheng L, Wang K, He B, Yan Y. Effect of vertical vibration stimulation at different frequencies on delayed muscle soreness in athletes: A randomized trial. Frontiers in Public Health. 2022;**10**:980454

[14] Zafar T, Zaki S, Alam MF, Sharma S, Babkair RA, Nuhmani S, et al. Effect of whole-body vibration exercise on pain, disability, balance, proprioception, functional performance and quality of life in people with non-specific chronic low back pain: A systematic review and meta-analysis. Journal of Clinical Medicine. 2024;**13**(6):1639

[15] Remer F, Keilani M, Kull P, Crevenna R. Effects of whole-body vibration therapy on pain, functionality, postural stability, and proprioception in patients with subacute and chronic non-specific low back pain: A systematic review. Wiener Medizinische Wochenschrift (1946). 2025;**175**(1-2):20-40

[16] Dong Y, Wang H, Zhu Y, Chen B, Zheng Y, Liu X, et al. Effects of whole body vibration exercise on lumbar-abdominal muscles activation for patients with chronic low back pain. BMC Sports Science, Medicine and Rehabilitation. 2020;**12**(1):78

[17] Li Q, Liu P, Wang Z, Li X. Vibration therapy to improve pain and function in patients with chronic low back pain: A systematic review and meta-analysis. Journal of Orthopaedic Surgery and Research. 2023;**18**(1):727

[18] Scialanca G, Serritella E, Di Giacomo P, Vompi C, Di Paolo C. Local vibration therapy for the treatment of facial pain. In: Proceedings of the Italian National Research Council. 2019

[19] ResearchGate. The Mechanism of Beneficial Effect of Radiofrequency Therapy on Masticatory Muscles in Temporomandibular Disorders - A Literature Review [Internet]. Available from: https://www.researchgate.net/publication/342924725 [Accessed: July 3, 2025]

[20] Farì G, de Sire A, Fallea C, Albano M, Grossi G, Bettoni E, et al. Efficacy of radiofrequency as therapy and diagnostic support in the management of musculoskeletal pain: A systematic review and meta-analysis. Diagnostics. 2022;**12**(3):600

[21] Manchikanti L, Knezevic NN, Knezevic E, Abdi S, Sanapati MR, Soin A, et al. A systematic review and meta-analysis of the effectiveness of radiofrequency neurotomy in managing chronic neck pain. Pain and Therapy. 2023;**12**(1):19-66

[22] ResearchGate. Long-Term Efficacy and Patient Satisfaction of Pulsed Radiofrequency Therapy in Temporomandibular Disorders: A Randomized Controlled Trial [Internet]. 2025. Available from: https://www.researchgate.net/publication/357444580 [Accessed: July 3, 2025]

[23] Melzack R, Wall PD. Pain mechanisms: A new theory. Science. 1965;**150**(3699):971-979

[24] Serrano-Muñoz D, Beltran-Alacreu H, Martín-Caro Álvarez D, Fernández-Pérez JJ, Aceituno-Gómez J, Arroyo-Fernández R, et al. Effectiveness of different electrical stimulation modalities for pain and masticatory function in temporomandibular disorders: A systematic review and meta-analysis. The Journal of Pain. 2023;**24**(6):946-956

[25] Saleh MS, Mohamed WM, Elsayed WH, Abdelatief EEM. Proprioceptive neuromuscular facilitation stretching exercises for treatment of temporomandibular dysfunction in patients with forward head posture: A double-blinded, randomized, controlled trial. Journal of Back and Musculoskeletal Rehabilitation. 2024;**37**(5):1259-1268

[26] Mahboubi M, Mokari Z. The efficacy of eucalyptus globulus essential oil in the management of pain. International Journal of Pain. 2024;**15**(2):70-79

[27] Crăciun MD, Geman O, Leuciuc FV, Holubiac IŞ, Gheorghiță D, Filip F. Effectiveness of physiotherapy in the treatment of temporomandibular joint dysfunction and the relationship with cervical spine. Biomedicine. 2022;**10**(11):2962

[28] Li LCF, Wong RWK, Rabie ABM. Clinical effect of a topical herbal ointment on pain in temporomandibular disorders: A randomized placebo-controlled trial. Journal of Alternative and Complementary Medicine. 2009;**15**(12):1311-1317

[29] Seyhan M, Atalay ES. Is core stability training effective in temporomandibular disorder? A randomized controlled trial. Clinical Oral Investigations. 2023;**27**(12):7237-7246

[30] ResearchGate. Topical Cannabinoids for the Management of Musculoskeletal Pain: Understanding and Review. [Internet]. Available from: https://www.researchgate.net/publication/366324080 [Accessed: July 4, 2025]

[31] Romero V, Lara JR, Otero-Espinar F, Salgado MH, Modolo NSP, de Barros GAM. Capsaicin topical cream (8%) for the treatment of myofascial pain syndrome. Brazilian Journal of Anesthesiology. 2019;**69**(5):432-438

[32] Tshering G, Posadzki P, Kongkaew C. Efficacy and safety of topical capsaicin in the treatment of osteoarthritis pain: A systematic review and meta-analysis. Phytotherapy Research. 2024;**38**(7):3695-3705

[33] Burke BE, Baillie JE. Randomized placebo controlled trial of phytoterpenes in DMSO for the treatment of plantar fasciitis. Scientific Reports. 2024;**14**(1):17621

[34] Mason L, Moore RA, Derry S, Edwards JE, McQuay HJ. Systematic review of topical capsaicin for the treatment of chronic pain. BMJ. 2004;**328**(7446):991

[35] Oleksy Ł, Kielnar R, Mika A, Jankowicz-Szymańska A, Bylina D, Sołtan J, et al. Impact of cervical spine rehabilitation on temporomandibular joint functioning in patients with idiopathic neck pain. BioMed Research International. 2021;**2021**:6886373

[36] Miçooğulları M, Yüksel İ, Angın S. Effect of pain on cranio-cervico-mandibular function and postural stability in people with temporomandibular joint disorders. The Korean Journal of Pain. 2024;**37**(2):164-177

[37] Yu LJ, Yan X, Kim TH. Effects of combined jaw and cervicoscapular exercises on mouth opening and muscle properties in cervical extension type. Scientific Reports. 2025;**15**(1):19049

[38] Bakó E, Fehérvári P, Garami A, Dembrovszky F, Gunther EE, Hegyi P, et al. Efficacy of topical essential oils in musculoskeletal disorders: Systematic review and meta-analysis of randomized controlled trials. Pharmaceuticals. 2023;**16**(2):144

[39] Usefulness of Posture Training for Patients: With Temporomandibular Disorders. ResearchGate [Internet]. 2025. Available from: https://www.researchgate.net/publication/12635853_Usefulness_of_posture_training_for_patients_With_temporomandibular_disorders [Accessed: July 5, 2025]

Section 3

Future Perspectives in Temporomandibular Joint Disorders

Chapter 11

Perspective Chapter: Temporomandibular Joint Disorders – New Perspectives in Diagnosis and Treatment

Mohamed M. Ghoneim, Mohamed Arafa and Taha Fayad

Abstract

Temporomandibular joint (TMJ) disorder diagnosis involves evaluating jaw pain, clicking or grinding sounds, and limited mouth opening. Disk displacement, where the joint disk slips out of place, is a common issue. A thorough examination, including imaging tests such as MRI or CT scans, helps diagnose the condition. Your doctor will assess your symptoms, medical history, and jaw function to determine the best course of treatment. Early diagnosis is a key to relieving pain, improving jaw function, and preventing further damage. If you're experiencing persistent jaw pain or discomfort, consult a healthcare professional for a proper evaluation and personalized treatment plan.

Keywords: TMJ, TMD, orofacial pain, arthrocentesis, TMJ clicking

1. Introduction

Temporomandibular disorders (TMD) represent a complex group of musculoskeletal conditions affecting the temporomandibular joint (TMJ), masticatory muscles, and associated structures. As the most common cause of non-dental orofacial pain, TMD significantly impacts the quality of life through pain, functional limitations, and frequent comorbidities such as headaches and psychological distress [1, 2]. Despite their prevalence—affecting 5–15% of adults, with rising incidence—diagnosis and management remain challenging due to the disorders' multifactorial etiology and heterogeneous presentations [1, 3].

Recent advances have shifted understanding toward a biopsychosocial model, where physical factors (e.g., disc displacement, trauma) intersect with psychosocial stressors (e.g., anxiety, depression) and systemic conditions (e.g., fibromyalgia) [1, 2]. The evolution of evidence-based tools like the *Diagnostic Criteria for TMD (DC/TMD)* has standardized classification, emphasizing both physical diagnoses (Axis I) and psychosocial contributors (Axis II) [2, 3]. This

IntechOpen

chapter explores contemporary perspectives on TMD etiology, classification, and emerging diagnostic paradigms, challenging outdated theories while highlighting integrative approaches to patient care.

2. Etiology and classification of temporomandibular joint disorders

2.1 Etiology

TMD arise from a multifactorial interplay of physical and psychosocial factors. As noted by Li and Leung, structural anomalies (e.g., disc displacement) do not always correlate with symptoms, highlighting the role of biopsychosocial mechanisms:

"While structural anomalies of the TMJ may predispose patients to symptoms of TMD, it should be noted that not all those with structural abnormalities suffer from the same level of clinical symptoms. Apart from physical causes, the association between biopsychosocial factors and TMD has been described by many" [1].

Kapos et al. (2020) emphasize that TMD pain is not localized to the jaw alone but linked to systemic and psychological comorbidities:

"Similar to other chronic pain conditions, recent research reinforces the biopsychosocial nature of common painful TMD (myalgia and/or arthralgia) and their interconnections with general health" [2].

Key etiological factors include:

1. Physical triggers: Trauma, joint overloading, or degenerative changes (e.g., osteoarthritis) [1].

2. Psychosocial stressors: Stress, depression, and anxiety amplify pain perception. The COVID-19 pandemic exacerbated TMD symptoms due to lockdown-related stress [1].

3. Systemic associations: Comorbid conditions such as fibromyalgia and sleep disturbances are common [2].

2.2 Classification

The DC/TMD system (cited in both papers) categorizes TMD into:

- Axis I (Physical Diagnoses):

- Painful conditions: Myalgia (local, myofascial, or with referral), arthralgia, and headache attributed to TMD.

- Non-painful conditions: Disc displacement (with/without reduction), degenerative joint disease (DJD), and subluxation [1, 2].

- Axis II (Psychosocial Impact):

- Assesses pain-related disability (e.g., Graded Chronic Pain Scale) and psychological distress (e.g., PHQ-4) [2].

Kapos et al. (2020) note:

"The DC/TMD offers a standardized and operationalized method to examine the masticatory structures physically (Axis I) and to screen for psychosocial and comorbid factors (Axis II)" [2].

Key controversy.

Both papers reject occlusal theories as outdated. Li and Leung (2021) state:

"In the past, a causative relationship between occlusion and TMD had been suggested, but it is now considered an outdated theory not supported by robust evidence" [1].

3. Innovations in diagnosis of temporomandibular joint (TMJ) disorders

Recent advancements in diagnosing temporomandibular dysfunction (TMD) emphasize the integration of imaging technologies and novel analytical methods to improve accuracy. Below are key innovations highlighted in the recent literature:

3.1 Advanced imaging modalities

3.1.1 Magnetic resonance imaging (MRI)

Considered the gold standard for soft tissue evaluation, MRI excels in assessing disc position, joint effusion, and bone marrow edema. It is particularly valuable for diagnosing disc displacement with/without reduction and inflammatory conditions like synovitis [3, 4].

- Clinical utility: High sensitivity for detecting degenerative changes (e.g., osteophytes, subchondral cysts) and dynamic joint dysfunction [4].

3.1.2 Cone-beam computed tomography (CBCT)

CBCT provides high-resolution 3D imaging of bony structures with lower radiation doses than conventional CT. It is ideal for detecting fractures, osteoarthritic changes, and condylar hyperplasia/hypoplasia [4].

- Advantage: Superior for preoperative planning and evaluating subtle osseous abnormalities (e.g., erosions, ankylosis) [4].

3.1.3 Ultrasonography (US)

Emerging as a non-invasive alternative for disc displacement diagnosis, US is useful for real-time guidance during arthrocentesis and viscosupplementation. While less accurate than MRI, it is cost-effective and avoids ionizing radiation [3, 4].

3.2 Artificial intelligence (AI) and signal analysis

3.2.1 AI neural networks

Moxley et al. (2023) demonstrated that an AI-based diagnostic tool achieved 96.9% sensitivity and 95.5% specificity in differentiating TMD from other orofacial pain conditions (e.g., migraines, referred cardiac pain) [4].

- Advantage: Reduces diagnostic errors by analyzing complex symptom patterns and imaging data [3].
- Electronic signal analysis:

A novel method using electronic stethoscopes and wavelet transforms distinguished TMJ hypermobility from TMD with 98.8% sensitivity, addressing a common misdiagnosis pitfall [4].

3.3 Functional and biochemical markers

3.3.1 Salivary endocannabinoid profiling

Preliminary studies suggest unique endocannabinoid (eCB) patterns in TMD patients, though further validation is needed to establish diagnostic biomarkers [4].

3.3.2 Electromyography (EMG)-based indices

EMG analysis of masticatory muscle activity (e.g., temporalis, masseter) revealed significant differences in TMD patients during clenching and rest, offering potential adjunctive diagnostic criteria [4].

3.4 Standardized MRI scoring systems

A validated MRI scoring system (Wurm et al.) assesses disc position, osseous changes, and joint morphology with high inter-rater reliability (ICC: 0.85–0.99), enhancing diagnostic consistency [4].

3.5 Nuclear medicine techniques

3.5.1 SPECT/CT and bone scintigraphy

This is useful for detecting metabolic bone activity (e.g., osteomyelitis, neoplasms) but limited in differentiating inflammatory from degenerative changes [3].

3.5.2 Imaging selection criteria

Clinical Implications: The selection of imaging modality should always be guided by clinical presentation, patient needs, and cost-benefit considerations to ensure accurate diagnosis and optimal management of TMD.

Ferreira et al. (2016) emphasize tailoring imaging choices to clinical needs:

- MRI for soft tissue and disc pathology.
- CBCT for trauma or bony degeneration.
- US for dynamic assessments or contraindications to MRI [3].
- Cost vs. benefit: Low-cost radiographs (e.g., panoramic, transcranial) remain valuable for initial screening of gross bony abnormalities [3].

4. Emerging treatment paradigms of TMJ disorders

The CADTH report highlights several emerging treatment approaches for temporomandibular joint disorders (TMD), focusing on psychological, physiotherapeutic, pharmacological, and surgical interventions. Key findings include:

4.1 Psychological interventions

- Long-term cognitive behavioral therapy (CBT), alone or combined with biofeedback, showed statistically significant improvements in pain compared to usual care. However, short-term CBT with biofeedback was associated with unfavorable results [5, 6].

4.2 Physiotherapy

- Low-level laser therapy (LLLT): LLLT demonstrated favorable results for pain reduction and improved mouth opening compared to placebo [7].

- Acupuncture: Needle acupuncture was more effective than sham acupuncture for pain relief, though evidence for mouth opening and TMJ clicking was inconclusive [8, 9].

- Manual therapy: Targeted manual therapy for the orofacial region and jaw exercises showed significant pain reduction and improved mouth opening [10].

4.3 Pharmacological interventions

- Injections: Cyclobenzaprine hydrochloride, botulinum toxin, and inferior/double space injections of hyaluronate or prednisolone were effective for pain relief [11, 12].

- Oral/topical agents: Melatonin and topical NSAIDs had favorable but inconclusive results [13, 14].

4.4 Surgical interventions

- Open surgery was more effective than arthroscopic surgery for pain relief and mouth opening [15, 16].

4.5 Splint therapy

- Stabilization splints were more effective than non-occluding appliances for pain relief [17, 18].

5. Current controversies in TMJ diagnosis and treatment

The diagnosis and treatment of temporomandibular dysfunction (TMD) remain areas of significant debate. One major controversy lies in the reliability of current diagnostic tools. While magnetic resonance imaging (MRI) is considered the "gold standard," its effectiveness is limited in cases where patients exhibit symptoms without obvious pathological or mechanical disruptions. This has led to challenges in accurately classifying TMD into its subgroups (muscle disorders, disc displacement, and arthralgia/arthritis/arthrosis), which complicates treatment planning [3].

Another contentious issue is the application of artificial intelligence (AI) in TMD diagnosis. Although the artificial neural network (ANN) developed by Kreiner et al. demonstrated high sensitivity (96.9%) and specificity (95.5%) in diagnosing TMD, its widespread adoption is hindered by the need for further validation and concerns about replacing clinical judgment. Similarly, the use of salivary endocannabinoid profiles as diagnostic markers shows promise, but the lack of distinct patterns in TMD patients compared to other orofacial pain disorders limits its current applicability [3].

In therapeutics, conservative management (e.g., occlusal splints, physiotherapy) is often prioritized over surgical interventions, but the efficacy of novel therapies such as aromatherapy massage and manual muscle relaxation techniques remains debated due to limited sample sizes and short-term follow-ups in studies. For instance, while radial extracorporeal shock wave therapy (rESWT) and light/LASER therapies showed pain reduction in TMD patients, conflicting evidence in other musculoskeletal applications raises questions about their reliability [3].

6. Future research directions

Future research should focus on refining diagnostic tools to improve accuracy and accessibility. The novel MRI scoring system by Wurm et al., validated for inter- and intra-rater reliability, offers a standardized approach but requires broader clinical adoption and training. Similarly, signal analysis for TMJ hypermobility diagnosis, with its high sensitivity (98.8%) and specificity (100%), could reduce misdiagnoses if further validated [3].

Advancements in AI, such as expanding ANN algorithms to incorporate more diverse patient data, could enhance diagnostic precision and differentiate TMD from overlapping conditions such as migraines or referred cardiac pain. Additionally, investigating salivary endocannabinoid profiles in larger cohorts may identify specific biomarkers for TMD, enabling non-invasive screening [3].

Therapeutic innovations should prioritize rigorous clinical trials to establish long-term efficacy. For example, radial extracorporeal shock wave therapy and light/LASER therapies warrant further study to confirm their benefits in TMD management. Manual techniques such as post-isometric relaxation and myofascial release, though promising, need standardized protocols and comparative studies against conventional treatments.

In conclusion, addressing these controversies and advancing research in AI, biomarkers, and minimally invasive therapies will be pivotal in improving TMD care. As Moxley et al. noted, "Further research is recommended to advance the care of patients suffering from TMD" [3].

7. Conclusion

Temporomandibular disorders represent a complex interplay of biomechanical, psychological, and systemic factors that challenge both diagnosis and management. As highlighted throughout this chapter, contemporary understanding has moved beyond simplistic mechanical explanations to embrace a biopsychosocial model that acknowledges the multifactorial nature of TMD. The DC/TMD framework provides clinicians with valuable tools for comprehensive assessment, integrating both physical diagnoses and psychosocial contributors. While significant progress has been made in standardizing classification and treatment approaches, TMD management remains an evolving field. Future research directions should focus on personalized treatment strategies, biomarker identification, and further elucidation of the complex mechanisms underlying these disorders. Ultimately, successful management of TMD requires a patient-centered approach that addresses not just the physical symptoms but also the psychological and social dimensions of this challenging condition.

Author details

Mohamed M. Ghoneim[1]*, Mohamed Arafa[2] and Taha Fayad[3]

1 Faculty of Dentistry, Department of Oral and Maxillofacial Surgery, Sinai University, North Sinai, Egypt

2 Faculty of Dentistry, Department of Oral Histopathology, Sinai University, North Sinai, Egypt

3 Faculty of Dentistry, Sinai University, North Sinai, Egypt

*Address all correspondence to: ghoneimm194@gmail.com

References

[1] Li DTS, Leung YY. Temporomandibular disorders: Current concepts and controversies in diagnosis and management. Diagnostics. 2021;**11**(3):459. DOI: 10.3390/diagnostics11030459

[2] Kapos FP et al. Temporomandibular disorders: A review of current concepts in aetiology, diagnosis, and management. Oral Surgery. 2020;**13**(4):321-334. DOI: 10.1111/ors.12473

[3] Moxley B, Stevens W, Sneed J, Pearl C. Novel diagnostic and therapeutic approaches to temporomandibular dysfunction: A narrative review. Life (Basel). 2023;**13**(9):1808

[4] Ferreira LA, Grossmann E, Januzzi E, de Paula MVQ, Carvalho ACP. Diagnosis of temporomandibular joint disorders: Indication of imaging exams. Brazilian Journal of Otorhinolaryngology. 2016;**82**(3):341-352

[5] Zhang Y, Montoya L, Ebrahim S, Rashiq S, Dick BD, Moulin DE, et al. Hypnosis/relaxation therapy for temporomandibular disorders: A systematic review and meta-analysis of randomized controlled trials. Journal of Oral Rehabilitation. 2015;**42**(11):847-861

[6] Aggarwal VR, Lovell K, Peters S, Javidi H, Joughin A, Goldthorpe J. Psychosocial interventions for the management of chronic orofacial pain. Cochrane Database of Systematic Reviews. 2011;**11**:CD008456

[7] Xu GZ, Jia J, Jin L, Li JH, Wang ZY, Cao DY. Low-level laser therapy for temporomandibular disorders: A systematic review with meta-analysis. Pain Research and Management. 2018;**2018**:4230583

[8] Jung A, Shin BC, Lee MS, Sim H, Ernst E. Acupuncture for treating temporomandibular joint disorders: A systematic review and meta-analysis of randomized, sham-controlled trials. Journal of Dentistry. 2011;**39**(5):341-350

[9] Cho SH, Whang WW. Acupuncture for temporomandibular disorders: A systematic review. Journal of Orofacial Pain. 2010;**24**(2):152-162

[10] Armijo-Olivo S, Pitance L, Singh V, Neto F, Thie N, Michelotti A. Effectiveness of manual therapy and therapeutic exercise for temporomandibular disorders: Systematic review and meta-analysis. Physical Therapy. 2016;**96**(1):9-25

[11] Häggman-Henrikson B, Alstergren P, Davidson T, Högestätt ED, Östlund P, Tranaeus S, et al. Pharmacological treatment of orofacial pain - health technology assessment including a systematic review with network meta-analysis. Journal of Oral Rehabilitation. 2017;**44**(10):800-826

[12] Liu Y, Wu JS, Tang YL, Tang YJ, Fei W, Liang XH. Multiple treatment meta-analysis of intra-articular injection for temporomandibular osteoarthritis. Journal of Oral and Maxillofacial Surgery. 2018;**76**(6):1165-1175

[13] Mujakperuo HR, Watson M, Morrison R, Macfarlane TV. Pharmacological interventions for pain in patients with temporomandibular disorders. Cochrane Database of Systematic Reviews. 2010;**10**:CD004715

[14] Melo RA, de Resende CMBM, Rocha LFC, de Almeida EO, Barbosa GAS, de Souza RF. Short-term effectiveness of conservative therapies

in pain, quality of life, and sleep in patients with temporomandibular disorders: A systematic review and meta-analysis. Journal of Oral Rehabilitation. 2018;**45**(12):884-894

[15] Al-Moraissi EA, Wolford LM, Ellis E 3rd, Neff A. The hierarchy of different treatments for arthrogenous temporomandibular disorders: A network meta-analysis of randomized clinical trials. Journal of Cranio-Maxillofacial Surgery. 2015;**43**(8):1381-1389

[16] Nagori SA, Jose A, Gopalakrishnan V, Roy ID, Chattopadhyay PK, Roychoudhury A. The efficacy of dextrose prolotherapy over placebo for temporomandibular joint hypermobility: A systematic review and meta-analysis. Journal of Oral Rehabilitation. 2018;**45**(12):998-1006

[17] Pficer JK, Dodic S, Lazic V, Trajkovic G, Milic N, Milicic B. Occlusal stabilization splint for patients with temporomandibular disorders: Meta-analysis of randomized controlled trials. Journal of Oral Rehabilitation. 2017;**44**(11):947-955

[18] Fricton J, Look JO, Wright E, Alencar FG Jr, Chen H, Lang M, et al. Systematic review and meta-analysis of randomized controlled trials evaluating intraoral orthopedic appliances for temporomandibular disorders. Journal of Orofacial Pain. 2010;**24**(3):237-254

Chapter 12

Integration of Artificial Intelligence and Regenerative Medicine in Surgical Management of TMJ Disorders

Ajit Sinha and Noopur Srivastava

Abstract

Temporomandibular-joint (TMJ) disorders are complex conditions typically characterised by pain, joint dysfunction and progressive tissue degeneration. This chapter explores how two cutting-edge domains—artificial intelligence (AI) and regenerative medicine—can converge to improve the surgical management of TMJ disorders. Recent AI advances, including deep-learning systems that classify condylar osteoarthritis (OA) on panoramic views, detect anterior-disc displacement on magnetic resonance imaging (MRI), and collate multi-centre evidence in an umbrella review, now deliver pooled sensitivity and specificity ≥0.80 for key TMJ diagnosis. These tools promise faster more objective assessments than conventional reading of radiographs or magnetic resonance (MR) images. In parallel, regenerative strategies, such as injectable stem-cell-laden hydrogels that repair condylar cartilage, platelet-rich-plasma (PRP) protocols that outperform, or equal, hyaluronic-acid controls in network meta-analysis, and bi-layer hydrogel/ β-TCP (β-tricalcium-phosphate scaffold scaffolds able to regenerate osteochondral defects in vivo, are moving from bench to early phase clinics. Tissue-engineered TMJ discs fabricated from aligned collagen-gylcosaminoglycan matrices show native-like anisotropy and biomechanics. The chapter discusses how AI can refine patient selection, surgical planning and intra-operative guidance for these biologic interventions, citing evidence that convolutional neural network (CNN) models already equal or surpass expert clinicians in key diagnostic tasks. We also review engineered scaffolds that replicate native joint structures and withstand physiological loading. Finally, we outline present limitation-large annotated datasets, regulatory approval for AI diagnostics, variability in cell-based therapies and future directions, such as explainable federated-learning, exosome-based "cell-free" treatments and three-dimensional (3-D) bioprinting of osteochondral constructs. Together, the fusion of AI and regenerative medicine signals a forthcoming era of precision, minimally invasive, restorative TMJ surgeries.

Keywords: temporomandibular-joint disorders, artificial intelligence, regenerative medicine, stem-cell therapy, platelet-rich plasma, tissue engineering, surgical management, TMJ osteoarthritis, AI diagnostics precision surgery

1. Introduction

Temporomandibular disorders (TMDs) are common; large population studies report clinical or sub-clinical symptoms in ≈ 60–70% of adults [1–10]. They may involve inflammatory degeneration of the articular disc, condylar cartilage, sub-chondral bone and peri-auricular musculature, leading to chronic pain and impaired jaw function [11, 12].

Management options range from splints, physiotherapy and pharmacotherapy to minimally invasive arthrocentesis/arthroscopy, disc repair or removal and, in end-stage disease, totally alloplastic joint replacement [13].

Yet, outcomes remain sub-optimal: most current treatments are palliative and rarely achieve durable restoration of native structures or biomechanics [12, 13]. In regenerative TMJ osteoarthritis, therapies tend to relieve symptoms without reversing cartilage loss, and even total-joint prostheses—a last resort—leave open questions about long-term mandibular biomechanics and implant longevity [14].

These limitations underscore the need for innovative, biology-guided and data-driven approaches. Two rapidly advancing fields offer that promise:

1. Artificial intelligence (AI): A recent umbrella review summarised 27 primary studies and found pooled sensitivity = 0.83 and specificity = 0.85 for an AI system that diagnoses TMDs across imaging modalities [4]. Deep-learning classifiers already outperform residents in detecting condylar osteoarthritis on panoramic radiographs (area under the curve (AUC) ≈ 0.89) [2] and achieve >90% accuracy for anterior-disc displacement on MRI [3]. A meta-analysis of diagnostic-test accuracy confirmed that such models match or exceed those formulated by expert clinicians across datasets [5]. These capabilities enable faster, more objective assessment and personalised surgical planning.

2. Regenerative medicine: Injectables, reactive-oxygen-species (ROS)-responsive hydrogel delivering dental-pulp stem cells have regenerated condylar cartilage and improved sub-chondral bone in vivo [6]. A bi-layer hydrogel/β-TCP scaffold restored osteochondral defects in rapid condyles, illustrating scaffold-guided repair [15]. Meta-analysis of randomised trials shows that platelet-rich plasma (PRP) injections, especially when combined with arthrocentesis, produce clinically important pain relief and mouth-opening gains up to 6 months [16]. Meanwhile, tissue-engineered TMJ discs fabricated from aligned collagen-gylcosaminoglycan matrices now replicate native and anisotropy and compressive properties, marking real progress towards biologic disc replacement [8].

Integrating AI-driven diagnosis/planning with these regenerative modalities could transform TMJ surgery: AI triage may identify early, focal degeneration, amenable to stem-cell or PRP therapy, while patient-specific 3-D-printed scaffolds, optimised by AI design algorithms, may be implanted arthroscopically to restore joint anatomy. The following chapter explores this synergy, the evidence supporting it and the hurdles that must be overcome to bring genuinely restorative, precision surgery to routine TMJ care.

2. Scope of the chapter

This chapter provides a state-of-the-art synthesis of how artificial intelligence (AI) and regenerative medicine are converging to transform surgical care for temporomandibular-joint (TMJ) disorders. It is aimed at oral-maxillofacial surgeons, radiologist, biomedical engineers and postgraduate investigators who need (i) a critical appraisal of the newest AI algorithms capable of reading TMJ imaging with expert-level accuracy, (ii) a clear picture of the fast-maturing biologic tool-kit-mesenchymal-stem-cell (MSC) therapy, platelet-rich plasma (PRP), smart hydrogel 3-D-printed scaffolds and extracellular-vesicle (EV) products, and (iii) a road map for integrating these technologies in real-world surgical work flows. Particular emphasis is placed on evidence published since 2020, because both AI and regenerative signs had accelerated sharply in that time. Seminal umbrella reviews on AI for TMJ diagnosis and foundational papers on tissue-engineered discs and vesicle-based therapeutic frame the discussion [4, 8, 17].

Chapter structure

1. Artificial intelligence in TMJ diagnosis and surgical planning—the chapter opens with today's best—performing deep-learning systems. Convolutional neural networks (CNNs) now achieve area-under-the-curve (AUC) values close to 0.90 for condylar osteoarthritis on panoramic or cone-beam computed tomography (CBCT) images, often surpassing junior clinicians in both sensitivity and reading time [2]. Transforming-enhanced pipelines for multi-sequence MRI reach >90% accuracy in classifying anterior-disc displacement and provide heat-map explanations that build surgeon trust [3]. The section then shows how automated 3-D segmentation and finite-element modelling are already being used to pre-shape custom alloplastic joint or bioprinted scaffolds, and previews early computer-vision prototypes that label cartilage and synovial in situ during arthroscopy.

2. Regenerative-medicine approaches for TMD disorders—Attention turns to biologic repair. Readers track the bench-to-bedside voyage of MSC injections (bone marrow, adipose, dental pulp) and evaluate a network meta-analysis demonstrating that PRP combined with arthrocentesis yields significantly greater pain relief and mouth-opening gains than lavage alone [18]. Breakthrough biomaterial follows: a reactive-oxygen-species (ROS)-responsive hydrogel delivers dental-pulp MSCs only in inflamed joints and doubles cartilage-repair scores in pre-clinical models [6], while a bi-layer hydrogel/β-tricalcium-phosphate scaffold simultaneously regenerates fibro-cartilage and sub-chondral bone in rabbit condyles [19]. The section closes with anisotropic collagen-glycosaminoglycan discs that mimic native visco-elasticity and survive 1-million loading cycles in vitro [8].

3. Integrating AI and regenerative strategies in surgical practice—Having detailed both tool-kits, we show how they converge in the operating theatre. A prototypical work flow starts when an AI triage model flags subtle erosive changes in routine orthodontics CBCT; the same system exports a 3-D printable scaffold file, which is bioprinted from poly-ε-caprolactone/ β-TCP, seeded with autologous MSCs and implanted under augmented-reality guidance that overlays AI-segmented cartilage margins. Post-operative data—jaw-tracking wearables, pain scores and follow-up imaging—feed a patient-specific "digital twin", allowing the algorithm to predict graft maturation and recommend booster biologic injections.

4. Current limitations and challenges—a balanced appraisal follows. For AI, we discuss the demand for large, multi-ethnic datasets, risks of algorithmic bias, "black-box" opacity and the stringent U.S. Food and Drug Administration/Eu-

ropean Union (FDA/EU) regulatory pathways that Software as a Medical Device (SaMD) must clear [4]. On the regenerative side, variability in cell potency, sterility control, cost-of-goods and unknown decades-long durability under para-functional loading are examined [6, 8, 19]. Cross-cutting issues—surgeon learning curves, reimbursement gaps and the ethics of AI decision support—round out the critique.

5. Future directions and conclusion—The finale projects a near future of cell-free extracellular-vesicle therapeutics with lower tumour risk yet robust paracrine signalling [17], gene-edited MSC lines for sustained chondrogenesis and privacy-preserving federated-learning frameworks that train robust diagnostic models across institutions without sharing raw images [20]. Hybrid robotic-endoscope systems with AI feedback loops and adaptive-design clinical trials are mapped out, and the chapter closes by arguing that the AI-regenerative convergence will shift TMJ surgery from palliative mechanics to genuine biological precision repair.

2.1 Narrative expansion

Over the last half-decade, *AI diagnostics have vaulted from proof-of-concept to near-clinical-grade accuracy*. CNNs trained on as few as 2000 panoramic projections now flag condylar flattening and sub-chondral sclerosis with an AUC of 0.89, halving resident reading times while maintaining expert-level sensitivity [2]. Likewise, a deep-learning pipeline integrating proton-density and T2-weighted MRI sequences recently achieved 93% accuracy for disc-position classification and produced pixel-level saliency maps that localised displacement, providing surgeons with intuitive visual feedback [3].

2.2 Regenerative medicine is keeping pace

A ROS-triggered hydrogel loaded with dental-pulp MSCs regenerated condylar cartilage and improved sub-chondral bone in vivo, outperforming both cell-free gel and free MSC injections [6]. Clinical meta-analysis suggests that PRP plus arthrocentesis confers an additional *8–10 mm* in maximal interincisal opening at 6 months compared with lavage alone—although heterogeneity still tempers certainty [18]. Meanwhile, a cell-mediated hydrogel/β-TCP scaffold restored both cartilage and bone layers in rabbit TMJ defects, signalling the dawn of osteochondral unit engineering [19]. Tissue-engineered discs fabricated from aligned collagen-glycosaminoglycan matrices now replicate native anisotropy and compressive resilience, reinvigorating the quest for biologic disc replacement [8].

2.3 The most exciting frontier is their integration

Imagine a federated-learning model, trained on privacy-protected data from multiple centres, which alerts dentists to early erosive changes on a teen's orthodontic CBCT; the platform simultaneously generates a scaffold blueprint optimised for biomechanical load distribution, which is printed, seeded with the patient's MSCs and implanted under AR guidance. Post-operative monitoring streams back into the patient's digital twin, allowing real-time predictions of graft ossification and suggesting booster PRP or EV therapy, if healing stalls. Each step leverages AI to sharpen decision-making and regenerative tools to rebuild tissue, moving TMJ care from palliation to *biologic precision surgery*.

3. Artificial intelligence in TMJ disorders: Enhancing diagnosis and planning

Artificial-intelligence (AI) research in the cranio-maxillofacial field has accelerated within the past five years, and temporomandibular-joint (TMJ) disease has become a fertile test-bed for new models. TMJ disorders range from internal derangements such as disc displacement to degenerative joint disease and inflammatory arthritides; their diagnosis is traditionally an image-intensive, highly subjective exercise that relies on panoramic radiographs, cone-beam CT (CBCT) or multi-sequence MRI interpreted alongside clinical findings [12].

A 2025 umbrella review synthesising 27 primary studies reported pooled sensitivity and specificity of about 0.83–0.85 for machine-learning pipelines that automate at least one step of that workflow [4].

3.1 Deep-learning detection of structural pathology

On two-dimensional (2-D) imaging, Iwase et al. trained a CNN on 2146 panoramic TMJ projections and obtained an AUC 0.89 for condylar osteoarthritis while cutting average reading time from 42 s (residents) to 0.03 s [2].

A companion CBCT study by Eşer et al. preserved external-validation AUC 0.86, indicating reasonable generalisability across modalities [21].

In the 3-D domain, Yu et al. fed proton-density and T2-weighted MRI volumes into a transformer-augmented network that reached 93% accuracy (sensitivity 0.91, specificity 0.95) for anterior-disc-displacement classification and produced Grad-CAM (Gradient-weighted Class Activation Mapping) saliency maps that localised the pathological posterior band—an early step towards explainable AI [3].

3.2 Multimodal fusion is extending capability further

Choi et al. combined panoramic radiography with stethoscope-captured joint-sound waveforms and boosted the F1-score for early degenerative change to 0.72, outperforming senior clinicians on a prospective test set [22].

These gains are echoed in a 2023 meta-analysis confirming deep-learning superiority over conventional radiomics for TMJ osteoarthritis in both accuracy and labour cost [8].

3.3 Prognostication and treatment selection

Diagnosis is only the first decision point. A 2024 Proceeding of the National Academy of Sciences of the United States of America (PNAS) study by Al Turkestani et al. built a patient-specific gradient-boosting model on 1047 longitudinal MRI scans; it predicted 12-month cartilage-thickness trajectories and symptomatic improvement with an AUC 0.78, providing individual risk curves to aid shared decision-making [23].

3.4 Anatomical segmentation and 3-D surgical planning

Pixelwise segmentation remains a bottleneck in computer-aided design (CAD) of prostheses and scaffolds. Jha et al. reported a 3-D U-Net that delineates mandibular condyles on CBCT with a Dice score 0.94 ± 0.02 and exports stereolithography (STL) files in under 2 minutes—fast enough for point-of-care printing of patient-specific titanium or bioprinted osteochondral implants [24].

Parallel pipelines now segment articular discs on MRI with Dice >0.90; the model by Nozawa et al. (Dentomaxillofac Radiol 2022) feeds virtual-surgery workstations used for disc-plication planning [25]. Finite-element solvers linked to these segmentations can simulate bite-force distribution and predict prosthetic wear, adding biomechanical insight to pre-operative consults [24].

3.5 Functional monitoring and follow-up

AI does not clock out after wound closure. Mouchoux et al. demonstrated a least-mean-squares tracking algorithm that quantifies condylar trajectories on real-time MRI 76% faster than manual tracking while halving spatial error (<0.03 mm), opening the door to objective, image-based rehabilitation metrics [26]. Ongoing multi-centre projects are using federated-learning frameworks to train such motion-analysis models without sharing raw data, preserving privacy while expanding dataset diversity [20].

3.6 Implementation hurdles and future research

Three gaps must narrow before AI becomes a routine "co-pilot": (i) Data diversity—most models remain single-centre and scanner-specific; (ii) Explainability and medico-legal trust, partially addressed by saliency mapping (e.g., Grad-CAM) but still under regulatory scrutiny [27]; (iii) Workflow integration into PACS (Picture Archiving and Communication System), planning software and theatre stacks. FDA guidance on AI/ML-based Software as a Medical Device and hybrid "glass-box" model architectures are active research avenues aimed at closing these gaps [28].

If successful, AI will link the diagnostic desktop, the design studio and the follow-up scanner into a continuously learning ecosystem that shepherds TMJ care from early triage to long-term outcome tracking.

4. Regenerative-medicine approaches for TMJ disorders

Regenerative medicine pursues biological repair rather than mechanical replacement, aiming to restore condylar cartilage, rebuild a diseased disc and modulate the joint's inflammatory milieu. Three therapeutic pillars dominate current research: mesenchymal-stem-cell (MSC) therapy, platelet-rich plasma (PRP) and tissue engineering with smart biomaterials.

4.1 Mesenchymal-stem-cell (MSC) therapy

Pre-clinical work shows that intra-articular MSCs can repopulate fibro-cartilage and dampen synovitis in osteoarthritic TMJs. In *rat* and *rabbit* models, bone-marrow or umbilical-cord MSC injections lowered modified Mankin scores by ≈ 40% and restored type-II-collagen staining within 6 weeks [29, 30].

Adipose-derived MSCs delivered on a hyaluronic-acid micro-scaffold achieved comparable cartilage thickness and suppressed tumour necrosis factor alpha (TNF-α) compared with untreated controls [31].

Paracrine signalling—not merely cell engraftment—appears central; in vitro and in vivo studies show MSC exosomes enriched in miR-140-5p, together with secreted transforming growth factor beta (TGF-β) and interleukin 10 (IL-10), drive chondrogenesis and dampen catabolic pathways [32].

Early human evidence. A first-in-human, randomised, controlled tissue-stromal-vascular-fraction (tSVF) trial is now recruiting TMJ-OA (osteoarthritis) patients to receive autologous adipose tSVF after arthrocentesis (primary outcomes: pain and mouth opening at 6 months) [33].

In parallel, a phase-I study of a ROS-responsive hydrogel loaded with dental-pulp stem cells (15 patients) reported significant gains in maximal mouth opening (+ 7 mm) and condylar cartilage thickness at 12 months, with no serious adverse events [6].

Remaining questions on cell source, dose, carrier and long-term safety (e.g., ectopic calcification) mean MSC-based interventions are still considered experimental.

4.2 Platelet-rich plasma (PRP) and growth-factor injectables

PRP delivers a concentrated autologous pool of TGF-β, insulin-like growth factor (IGF-1), platelet-derived growth factor (PDGF) and vascular endothelial growth factor (VEGF) released from platelet α-granules, which together orchestrate angiogenesis, anti-inflammation and chondrogenesis [34].

A 2023 network meta-analysis of 12 randomised controlled trials ($n = 421$) ranked PRP as the top intervention for maximal-mouth-opening (MMO) gain at one month and among the two best for pain relief at three- to six-month follow-up, outperforming hyaluronic-acid and saline comparators [7]. Subgroup data indicated even greater benefit when PRP is injected after arthrocentesis, likely because lavage removes pro-inflammatory mediators and enhances platelet adherence.

Durability is less certain: A 2025 systematic review focused on PRP after arthrocentesis observed that analgesic and MMO gains wane beyond 12 months, signalling the need for booster injections or adjunct biologics [16]. Researchers are therefore evaluating platelet-rich fibrin (PRF), autologous conditioned serum and PRP fortified with concentrated-growth-factor (CGF) gels. In a goat model, CGF membranes placed arthroscopically over surgically created condylar cartilage defects regenerated smooth fibro-cartilage and reduced histological damage compared with suture repair alone, underscoring the synergy between platelet-derived matrices and minimally invasive surgery [35].

4.3 Tissue engineering and smart biomaterials

Over the past decade, tissue engineering for the TMJ has moved from proof-of-concept hydrogels to sophisticated multi-layer, patient-specific constructs that approximate native biomechanics and cellular micro-architecture. Two anatomical targets dominate research: (A) the articular disc and (B) the osteochondral condylar unit.

4.3.1 TMJ disc engineering: From hydrogels to hierarchical, load-bearing laminates

4.3.1.1 Structural requirements

The native disc is a biconcave fibro-cartilage only 1–2 mm thick, yet capable of handling shear stresses >2 MPa and cyclic loads of ≈ 500 N at 1 Hz [36]. Replicating that visco-elastic window demands anisotropic fibre alignment, controlled porosity (~70%) and collagen/elastin ratios that balance toughness with flexibility.

4.3.1.2 Scaffold families

- *Hybrid decellularised/PCL laminates*: Seo et al. combined decellularised porcine discs (type-II-collagen framework) with electro-spun poly-ε-caprolactone (PCL) nanofibres, boosting tensile strength 2.5-fold and Young's modulus to 4.1 ± 0.6 MPa while preserving cell-adhesion cues. Rabbits implanted with the hybrid regained 92% of baseline joint space by week 24 and showed no foreign-body reaction histologically [37].

- *Silk-fibroin/SIS composites*: Duan et al. 3-D-printed an interpenetrating silk-fibroin mesh inside small-intestinal-submucosa (SIS). Dynamic compression tests (10^5 cycles, 1 Hz) revealed <6% height loss, outperforming pure collagen discs [38].

- *Gradient micro-fluidic hydrogels*: Murphy's group created a methacrylated-gelatin (GelMA) hydrogel with a radial stiffness gradient (150 kPa → 45 kPa) using micro-fluidics; bone-marrow stromal cell (BMSC)-laden discs cultured for 4 weeks generated region-specific extracellular matrix (ECM) and resisted delamination, underscoring the value of biomimetic mechanical gradients [39].

4.3.1.3 Cell and bio-cue incorporation

Strategies range from seeding autologous disc cells or MSCs to embedding slow-release transforming growth factor beta 3 (TGF-β3) nanoparticles that amplify proteoglycan synthesis [40]. Exosome-laden hydrogels further accelerate matrix deposition—MSC exosomes rich in miR-29a reduced matrix metalloproteinase 13 (MMP-13) expression by ≈ 60% in inflamed disc cultures [41].

4.3.1.4 Clinical translation outlook

No human-grade disc implant has yet cleared regulatory hurdles, but a first-in-human pilot using a collagen-PCL laminate (n = 5) is scheduled in Spain for 2026. Key endpoints will include MRI-measured joint space, pain scores and device migration.

4.3.2 Condylar reconstruction and osteochondral scaffolds

4.3.2.1 Biomechanical challenge

The mandibular condyle carries a 0.5-mm fibro-cartilage cap over trabecular bone that endures masticatory loads exceeding ≈1000 N; any graft therefore needs a dual-layer architecture and immediate load-bearing strength (**Table 1**) [8].

4.3.2.2 Smart release and remodelling

Zoledronate-functionalised bio-glass limits early osteoclastic activity, while magnesium (Mg)-doped β-TCP enhances angiogenesis, together accelerating osseointegration [42]. Coupling such drug-releasing scaffolds with AI-derived finite-element stress maps will let surgeons tune composition to a patient's bite-force profile.

Strategy	Key features	Pre-clinical outcome
Patient-specific PCL/β-TCP scaffold (CBCT-derived) [8]	400-μm pores, 65% porosity; BMSC seeding; β-TCP-driven osteogenesis	Rabbit critical-size defect: cartilage 0.42 mm (vs 0.48 mm native) and 80% elastic-modulus restoration at 12 weeks ✓
PLA/PCL + bio-glass gradient [42]	3-D lattice, 58S bio-glass surface; zoledronate loading to curb resorption	Goat hemi-mandibulectomy: BV/TV ↑ 30% over scaffold-only control ✓
In-body bioreactor grown condyle [43]	PCL scaffold seeded with periosteal cells, matured 8 weeks in latissimus dorsi then transplanted	Porcine model: vascularised graft, no necrosis; peak bite-force 88% baseline at 6 months ✓
Injectable hydrogel/β-TCP paste (ROS-responsive) [6]	Gel releases dental-pulp MSCs + β-TCP granules	Rat TMJ-OA: OARSI ↓ 60%, sub-chondral bone ↑ 35% ✓

Table 1.
Representative osteochondral reconstruction strategies for the TMJ condyle and Key pre-clinical outcomes (materials, design features, and summarised results).

4.3.2.3 From bench to bedside

Current clinical repairs still rely on costochondral grafts or Co-Cr-Mo prostheses. The first compassionate-use, patient-specific PCL/β-TCP condyle (Australia 2024) has reached 24-month follow-up; CT already shows ≈90% bone in-growth and preserved fossa congruence. Long-term MRI cartilage signal and wear testing will decide its viability relative to metal prostheses.

5. Integrating AI and regenerative medicine in surgical practice

The convergence of artificial-intelligence (AI) analytics with regenerative biomaterials is transforming how surgeons select, plan, execute and follow up biologic interventions for temporomandibular-joint (TMJ) disorders. What once depended on a surgeon's qualitative eye and a fixed surgical kit is now evolving into a data-driven, patient-specific workflow that continuously refines itself with every case.

5.1 Pre-operative triage and prognostication

Deep-learning MRI classifiers can detect sub-millimetre disc thinning or early osteochondral cysts with >90% sensitivity [3]. By stratifying joints into "mild, modifiable" versus "advanced, reconstructive" phenotypes, these models steer candidates towards minimally invasive biologic injections or scaffold-based reconstruction months earlier than manual reads. Risk-prediction dashboards that fuse image scores, pain trajectories and wearable jaw-kinematics have already forecast six-month success after arthrocentesis ± platelet-rich plasma (PRP) with an AUC ≈ 0.78 [44]. This lets teams reserve stem-cell-laden hydrogels for the highest-yield cases.

5.2 Virtual design of patient-specific grafts

Once a biologic strategy is chosen, automatic CBCT/MRI segmentation produces a watertight 3-D mesh of a patient's condyle or disc in <2 min (Dice ≈ 0.94) [45].

A built-in finite-element engine applies individual bite-force vectors—extracted from AI-interpreted occlusal scans—to locate stress peaks. A multi-material printer then thickens poly-ε-caprolactone (PCL) struts or increases β-tricalcium-phosphate (β-TCP) infill exactly where stiffness is needed, yielding an osteochondral scaffold tuned to that joint. For disc repair, GelMA hydrogels are cast with radial stiffness gradients (150 → 45 kPa) taken from the same stress map, re-creating the posterior-band compliance that cushions retrusive loading [46].

5.3 Augmented-reality placement and feedback

In theatre, a lightweight computer-vision network classifies cartilage, disc and synovium pixels in arthroscopic video at 30 fps, colouring degenerated cartilage red and perforated disc yellow. A recent pilot study in porcine knee arthroscopy (general-joint surrogate) showed the overlay cut debridement time by 35% and improved localisation accuracy of PRP/MSC injectate versus freehand [47].* The same engine can warn when the injection needle drifts outside AI-defined safe zones, lowering iatrogenic-perforation risk.

5.4 Post-operative digital-twin monitoring

After wound closure, smartphone face-mesh algorithms track mandibular range-of-motion arcs with <2 mm error and stream daily metrics to a federated-learning server [20]. The evolving model benchmarks each patient against thousands of prior recoveries; if mouth-opening lags its predicted curve, the surgeon is pinged to consider a booster PRP session or early physiotherapy escalation.

5.5 Continuous learning and governance

Every new case updates the federated backbone without exporting raw data, preserving privacy while enlarging the analytic base. Saliency maps and counterfactual heat lines satisfy transparency requirements under European Union Medical Device Regulation (EU-MDR) and forthcoming FDA SaMD guidance, mitigating "black-box" concerns. Scanner-specific bias, good manufacturing practice (GMP)-grade scaffold manufacture and reimbursement codes for AI-planned biologics remain active policy frontiers.

By linking AI perception with biomaterial performance, TMJ surgery is shifting from "best-guess" timing and off-the-shelf hardware to truly adaptive, biologic precision repair—a closed loop in which diagnosis, design, delivery and rehabilitation are all data-enriched and patient-specific.

6. AI-driven scaffold design and virtual rehearsal

6.1 Generative design on demand

After CBCT/MRI upload, a cloud engine now auto-segments the condyle or glenoid fossa and overlays a voxel-level stress field derived from bite-force vector analysis. Within ≈ 15 min, it proposes a lattice whose *strut diameter, β-TCP ratio and pore size vary continuously* along the lines of maximum principal stress. Jeong *et al.* printed such patient-specific PCL/β-TCP scaffolds (Ø 400-μm pores, 65% porosity) and showed a 38% higher compressive modulus and 50% faster bone-volume restoration than hand-drawn CAD parts—all without extra design time [48].

Materials tuned for biology, not just mechanics Optimisation modules sift through a library of β-TCP weight fractions and unit-cell topologies to hit *dual* targets: an ~12-month degradation half-life and chondrogenic pore cues. In β-TCP scaffolds, Diao *et al.* found 250–400-μm pores triggered the highest ALP activity *and* produced 80% defect bridging in a rat calvarial model [49].

6.2 Virtual rehearsal inside a "digital-twin" theatre

A one-click export spins up a physics-based replica of the joint. Surgeons can trial drilling paths, plication angles or graft insertion, while the twin forecasts contact stresses and cartilage strain for each what-if scenario. A systematic review across cranio-maxillofacial cases showed that digital-twin rehearsal altered the operative plan in 28% of cases and trimmed theatre time by ≈ 18% [50].

6.3 Augmented-reality guidance and AI-assisted delivery

Pre-op segmentations stream to a head-mounted display (HoloLens-class). Cartilage slated for debridement glows red; safe margins green. In a phantom study using the VOSTARS (Video and Optical See-Through Augmented Reality Surgical System) headset, mean edge-localisation error fell by 2 mm and procedure time by 35% compared with screen-based navigation [51].

Once cleaned, an AI-linked micro-dosing pump infuses exactly the PRP or MSC-laden hydrogel volume computed from the defect mesh. A ROS-responsive hydrogel loaded with dental-pulp MSCs maintained <5% volumetric error across 20 rabbit TMJ injections and cut OARSI (Osteoarthritis Research Society International) cartilage scores by 60% at 8 weeks [6].

6.4 Robotic finesse for milling and suturing

Benchtop collaborative robots are already matching human precision. In a 2025 crossover trial, a 6-DOF (degrees of freedom) arm milled iliac-crest flaps with a mean angular deviation of 1.9 ± 1.1° (vs 4.7 ± 2.9° using printed guides) and tied 5-0 Vicryl sutures with 96% success [52].

6.5 Continuous feedback and federated learning

Post-op CBCTs auto-register to the master STL; deviations in bone in-growth or scaffold resorption trigger alerts and can re-schedule booster biologic injections. Because every case updates the federated model *without* exporting raw data, next month's scaffold benefits from this month's outcomes—steadily sharpening both biomechanical predictions and material recipes.

Together these modules create a closed, learning loop in which diagnosis, design, virtual rehearsal, AR-assisted placement and adaptive after-care all improve each other—ushering in *precision, regenerative TMJ surgery*.

7. AI-enabled post-operative monitoring and closed-loop care

7.1 Imaging analytics: From "snapshot" to continuous radiomics

Autonomous CBCT pipelines now register follow-up scans to the baseline scaffold STL in <30 s and compute >250 texture, shape and densitometric features per voxel.

Bianchi et al. picked up a 4% rise in trabecular volume-fraction just 12 weeks after β-TCP implantation—well before a musculoskeletal radiologist could call "healing" on visual review [53].

Heat maps are overlaid on the surgeon's dashboard: green = expected degradation; amber = lagging resorption; and red = premature void. A single click schedules a booster MSC injection or asks the prosthodontist to ease occlusal contacts on the red zone.

Deep-learning densitometry converts Hounsfield units (HU) to g-cm-3 bone-mineral density with an $r = 0.90$ versus DXA (dual-energy X-ray absorptiometry) explainable AI highlights regions the network "trusts" most, reassuring clinicians that artefact streaks are ignored [54].

7.2 Functional and patient-reported data streams: Pocket-sized biomechanics

A front-camera "face-mesh" app (Bellus3D pipeline) captures daily mandibular range-of-motion arcs with ≤2 mm error when benchmarked against optical motion-capture [55].

Encrypted WhatsApp or Signal messages are parsed by an NLP (Natural Language Processing) bot; "stabbing", "dull", "pressure" are mapped to a 0–10 pain score time-line that slots beside kinematics.

7.2.1 Closed-loop decision triggers: How the numbers talk to each other?

All radiomic, kinematic and linguistic vectors feed a gated-recurrent-unit (GRU) network trained on >2000 prior TMJ repairs. The model classifies today as (**Table 2**).

Threshold examples: <3 mm mouth-opening gain by week 4 or bone-density slope < 0.5 g cm-3/month triggers the "lagging" branch.

7.3 Federated learning and governance: Privacy by design

Every weight update travels as an encrypted gradient; no CBCT voxels or selfie frames ever leave the hospital virtual private network (VPN). A 20-site consortium

Status	Action automatically proposed
Ahead of curve	Skip next clinic visit; maintain home physiotherapy
On track	Routine e-check in 1 week
Lagging	Push notification to surgeon: options list—booster PRP, extra Therabite sets or CBCT @ 16 weeks

Table 2.
Closed-loop post-operative monitoring: status categories and automatically proposed actions after TMJ regenerative surgery.

running the same framework lifted predictive AUC from 0.78 to 0.86 without violating GDPR (General Data Protection Regulation) or HIPAA (Health Insurance Portability and Accountability Act), as summarised by Guan *et al.* [20]. Saliency maps plus counterfactual overlays fulfil EU-MDR transparency clauses, easing regulatory audits.

7.4 Why this mattersthe precision-surgery flywheel

1. Early signal → radiomics spots sub-threshold trends ⇒ intervention while still reversible.
2. Multimodal truth → kinematics + pain NLP supply context a scan alone misses.
3. Adaptive nudges → AI suggests *graded* responses, not one-size-fits-all check-ups.
4. Learning health system → each case → federation → better model → sharper care next month.

The result is a self-optimising pathway where *diagnosis → tailored repair → data-driven after-care* form a closed, continually improving loop.

8. Limitations and challenges

Artificial-intelligence (AI) tools and regenerative implants for the temporomandibular joint (TMJ) are advancing quickly, yet several *technical, clinical and regulatory hurdles* must be overcome before routine adoption.

8.1 AI-specific obstacles

Artificial-intelligence (AI) decision-support systems and regenerative implants for the temporomandibular joint (TMJ) have travelled from proof-of-concept demonstrations to early clinical pilots in little more than five years. Yet, the road to everyday use is blocked by a lattice of technical, clinical and regulatory barriers that are as consequential as any surgical complication. This section distils the most pressing obstacles and sketches the kinds of solutions that will be required if AI-guided, biologic TMJ repair is to become routine.

8.1.1 Data scarcity and domain-shift risk

Most TMJ-AI models are trained on several hundred scans drawn from a single scanner, a single ethnic cohort and a single hospital information system. In an umbrella review of 27 primary studies, Chen *et al.* found that 78% carried a high risk of sampling bias and that none reported genuine, multi-centre external validation [4]. A subsequent meta-analysis by Xu *et al.* showed that diagnostic accuracy fell by 8–15% when the same networks were tested on images drawn from institutions they had never seen before [5]. Such "domain shift" means an algorithm tuned on a Tokyo cone-beam CT (CBCT) fleet may misclassify scans produced on a São Paulo unit with a different reconstruction kernel. Federated-learning consortia—systems that exchange encrypted weight updates rather than raw images—offer one escape route, but fully operational federated pipelines remain rare in dental radiology [20].

8.1.2 Interpretability, trust and bias

Deep neural networks achieve high AUC values precisely because they learn abstract feature hierarchies that are hard to verbalise. Saliency overlays such as Grad-CAM highlight pixels that drive a particular prediction, yet prospective studies show that surgeons and radiologists only gain moderate confidence from these heat maps [56]. Research is therefore moving towards *glass-box* hybrids in which a transparent rules engine (e.g., "joint-space < 1 mm = degeneration") is driven by a deep-feature extractor, blending explainability with accuracy [57]. At the same time, systematic bias audits are overdue. In dermatology AI, error rates for darker skin [58] are roughly double those for lighter skin; a comparable audit for TMJ imaging does not yet exist.

8.1.3 Workflow integration and human factors

No matter how elegant the algorithm, adoption stalls if the output arrives in a stand-alone viewer that cannot write back to the hospital PACS or electronic health record. Usability studies across radiology suites have shown that clinicians abandon "side-car" AI dashboards within a fortnight, unless the inference appears inside their routine DICOM (Digital Imaging and Communications in Medicine) window in under 3 s [59]. In parallel, non-technical staff must learn to interpret probability scores and confidence intervals (CIs)—a form of statistical literacy that is not yet standard in surgical training.

8.1.4 Regulatory and legal head-winds

Only a handful of maxillofacial AI devices have cleared either the U.S. Food and Drug Administration (FDA) or the European CE mark, and none is TMJ-specific. The FDA's 2021 AI/ML Software-as-a-Medical-Device (SaMD) Action Plan now expects locked-weight change-control files, human-factors studies and multi-centre evidence before clearance [28]. Europe is moving even faster: the 2024 EU Artificial Intelligence Act will classify dental-imaging AI as "Class III–high risk", mandating post-market performance monitoring and bias auditing [60]. Developers who cannot produce audit trails and continuous-learning safeguards will find approval timelines lengthening, not shrinking.

8.1.5 The governance gap

Finally, hospitals lack agreed protocols for auditing AI output against ground truth and feeding systematic errors back to vendors. Liability law is also silent: if an AI-suggested scaffold fails, is the surgeon, the hospital or the software company responsible? Until reimbursement codes exist for "AI-planned scaffold" or "federated-learning follow-up," payers have little incentive to champion early adoption.

In sum, the path to AI-enabled, biologic precision surgery is less a sprint than an obstacle course. Robust, balanced data; interpretable models; seamless workflow integration; and forward-looking regulatory strategies will all be required before surgeons can rely on algorithms as confidently as they rely on their operative loupes.

8.2 Regenerative-medicine challenges for TMJ surgery

Biologic repair of the temporomandibular joint (TMJ) has progressed from benchtop hydrogels to first-in-human pilots, yet several formidable hurdles still separate laboratory promise from everyday clinical reality. These obstacles include wide interpatient variability, exacting manufacturing standards, uncertain long-term durability, legitimate safety fears, major training demands and—perhaps most vexing—unresolved questions of cost-effectiveness.

8.2.1 Outcome variability and poor standardisation

Clinical responses remain highly heterogeneous. A 2024 meta-analysis of 15 randomised trials showed that intra-articular platelet-rich plasma (PRP) produced a mean pain reduction of -1.4 ± 0.9 on a 0–10 scale, but almost *30%* of subjects were "non-responders", underscoring biological and procedural diversity [61]. Growth-factor payloads in PRP can differ 10-fold between donors [62], and mesenchymal-stromal-cell (MSC) products vary in surface-marker expression and chondrogenic potency, even when cultured under identical GMP conditions [63]. Such inconsistency hampers protocol writing, regulatory review and payer reimbursement.

8.2.2 Manufacturing and regulatory barriers

Every tissue-engineered disc or osteochondral scaffold must clear batch-to-batch sterility, endotoxin and mechanical tests. Once viable cells are incorporated, the construct falls under the U.S. FDA's 361 HCT/P (human cell, tissue, and cellular and tissue-based product) or, more onerously, RMAT (Regenerative Medicine Advanced Medical Therapy) pathways, both of which demand potency, chromosomal-stability and tumourigenicity packages [64]. Singh et al. recently noted that no TMJ disc graft has yet completed a full International Organisation for Standardisation (ISO)-10,993 biocompatibility panel, delaying first-in-human trials [8].

8.2.2.1 Durability under high joint loads

Hydrogel/β-tricalcium-phosphate (β-TCP) constructs restore ≈80% of rabbit-condylar modulus at 12 weeks [19], but their performance under decades of human mastication— ≈ 500 N cyclic loads—remains unknown. By contrast, cobalt-chrome TMJ prostheses deliver 10-year survival rates near 90% [65]. Long-term, head-to-head randomised trials are therefore indispensable before biologic devices can displace metal.

8.2.3 Safety

MSC therapies are not risk-free. Caplan and Dennis reported chromosomal instability in about 4% of extended MSC cultures—a theoretical gateway to oncogenesis [66]. Clinically, heterotopic bone has been documented after autologous MSC injection around the hip, illustrating off-target differentiation [67]. Overdosing growth-factor matrices may also accelerate adjacent osteoarthritis, emphasising the need for carefully titrated delivery systems.

8.2.4 Training and workflow impact

Successful biologic TMJ repair demands competencies rarely covered in oral-maxillofacial residencies: sterile cell handling, point-of-care centrifugation, and delicate, press-fit scaffold placement. Operating-room time typically rises by 20–30 minutes when PRP or MSC products are prepared on-site, increasing anaesthetic exposure and theatre costs. Many centres now rely on multidisciplinary teams that include bioengineers and cell-therapy technicians.

8.2.5 Economic considerations

Laboratory-expanded MSC doses run USD 2500–4000 per joint, and a custom 3-D-printed β-TCP condyle can top USD 8000. Insurance coverage is patchy at best; most payers still label such care *investigational*. Health-economic modelling suggests that widespread adoption will require value-based contracts in which the up-front biologic price is offset against reduced revision-surgery rates.

8.2.6 Evidence gap

Pre-clinical work dominates the literature. Of more than 150 TMJ-regeneration papers screened by Wang et al., only seven involved human subjects—and *all* were uncontrolled pilot series [19]. Robust, multi-centre randomised controlled trials with at least two-year follow-up are urgently needed to demonstrate clear superiority over current standards of care.

9. AI deployment in TMJ surgery is constrained chiefly by *data* and *trust*

Artificial-intelligence (AI) decision-support systems for temporomandibular-joint surgery and biologic implants share a common predicament: both look impressive in pilot reports, yet each falters when confronted with the messy heterogeneity of real-world practice.

AI systems stumble first on *data generalisability*. Most deep-learning pipelines are trained on single-centre image banks; when the same algorithms meet a new scanner vendor, a different reconstruction kernel or an unfamiliar ethnic craniofacial morphology, diagnostic accuracy typically slips by 8–15%—the classic "domain-shift" penalty identified in the latest umbrella review of TMJ-AI studies [4]. Trust is then further eroded by the models' opaque logic: saliency overlays help, but they seldom reassure surgeons who must defend an automated verdict in court or at morbidity rounds. Regulators have noticed. The US FDA's *AI/ML SaMD Action Plan* now requires multi-site validation data, locked-weight change-control files and post-market performance monitoring before any high-risk imaging algorithm can be cleared [28].

Regenerative therapies face a different constriction—*biological variability and durability*. Even in controlled randomised trials, platelet-rich plasma (PRP) and mesenchymal-stem-cell (MSC) injections deliver mixed outcomes: a 2024 meta-analysis found a mean pain reduction of -1.4 ± 0.9 on a 10-point scale, yet almost one-third of patients were classified as non-responders, a reflection of the 10-fold donor-to-donor spread in growth-factor payload and the inconsistent potency of ostensibly GMP-grade MSC lots [61]. Tissue-engineered discs and osteochondral scaffolds, meanwhile, must satisfy sterility, endotoxin and mechanical benchmarks batch-to-batch; but even when they do, their long-term fate under *500-N cyclic chewing loads* remains conjectural. In contrast, cobalt-chrome TMJ prostheses still post 10-year survival rates near 90% [65].

Layer onto those science questions a trio of practical barriers—high device cost, extra operating-room time for on-site cell handling and a dearth of large multi-centre trials—and it becomes clear why both AI and regenerative options remain exciting *adjuncts* rather than mainstream standards. Bigger, more diverse imaging datasets; explainable, audit-ready algorithms; standardised biologic products; and rigorously designed, multi-centre outcome studies are the minimum prerequisites before a truly precision, biologic TMJ pathway can take hold.

10. Future directions and conclusion

The coming decade will almost certainly merge ever-smarter AI pipelines with next-generation regenerative tool-kits, shifting temporomandibular-joint (TMJ) care from reactive symptom relief to genuinely predictive, biologic precision surgery.

10.1 AI horizons: From images to *digital twins*

Large, multi-centre image banks coupled to federated-learning frameworks will allow algorithms to train on encrypted weight updates from dozens of hospitals, eliminating today's single-scanner bias while keeping raw data local [20]. Once robust across hardware and ethnicity, these models will move beyond radiology and fuse CBCT/MRI radiomics with serum cytokines, salivary micro-RNAs (miRNAs) and smartphone-captured mandibular kinematics; early multimodal prototypes already improve six-month pain-trajectory prediction by *15–20%* [68]. The logical endpoint is a *digital twin*—a biomechanically faithful, continuously updated replica of each patient's TMJ on which surgeons can rehearse "what-if" scenarios (scaffold vs. hydrogel, single vs. booster PRP) before ever picking up a scalpel [69]. In theatre, smart arthroscopes with real-time tissue classification will overlay colour labels for cartilage, disc and synovium at ≥90% accuracy and vibrate the hand-piece if the debridement line strays [70]. Regulators are moving in parallel: the U.S. FDA's *AI/ML SaMD Action Plan* and the EU's forthcoming *AI Act* both mandate multi-site evidence, change-control files and post-market monitoring for high-risk imaging AI [28].

10.2 Regenerative-medicine frontiers—Cell-free vesicles and bioprinted composites

On the biologic side, the field is pivoting from whole-cell injections towards *exosome-based, cell-free therapeutics* that deliver miR-140- and TGF-β–rich cargo without the tumour or ectopic-bone risks of proliferating cells. Dental-pulp-stem-cell exosomes embedded in hyaluronic-acid hydrogel have already regenerated condylar cartilage in rats with an excellent safety profile [5]. Gene-edited "universal" MSC lines—CRISPR (Clustered Regularly Interspersed Short Palindromic Repeats) knock-in of *SOX9* with β-2-microglobulin knock-out—promise off-the-shelf chondrogenic potency while evading immune rejection [23]. Concurrently, *multi-material 3-D bioprinting* is reaching the point where a stiff β-TCP sub-chondral base and a softer collagen-GelMA cartilage cap can be laid down in a single pass; large-animal trials are forecast within two years [71]. Smart scaffolds doped with magnesium or zoledronate will release osteo-anabolic cues only when loaded, closing the biochemical loop with real-world jaw function [20].

10.3 Towards an adaptive, closed-loop pathway

Combine these advances and a closed cycle emerges: AI flags early, still-reversible degeneration → a digital-twin simulation selects the optimum biologic recipe → a bioprinter fabricates a patient-specific implant whose drug-release kinetics mirror occlusal forces → AI-augmented arthroscopy guides placement in real time → federated post-operative monitoring feeds the next model update. Multi-centre registries, GMP-grade manufacturing pipelines, explainable AI dashboards and value-based reimbursement schemes will all be critical, yet the trajectory is unmistakable. With sustained interdisciplinary collaboration, TMJ surgeons are likely to wield both the diagnostic acuity of AI and the curative promise of regenerative bioengineering, delivering durable, personalised restoration, instead of palliative mechanics.

11. Emerging directions in regenerative medicine for TMJ repair

Regenerative strategies for the temporomandibular joint (TMJ) are moving rapidly beyond first-generation stem-cell suspensions. Three broad vectors now define the research frontier: cell-free vesicles, gene-edited "universal" cells and 3-D-printed smart scaffolds that respond to jaw loading.

11.1 Exosome therapeutics: Paracrine action without the baggage

Mesenchymal-stem-cell (MSC) exosomes are 30–150 nm vesicles that carry micro-RNAs (miR-140, miR-29a), cytokines and lipid mediators capable of silencing catabolic genes while boosting chondrogenic ones. A systematic review of >50 pre-clinical studies showed that these vesicles suppress inflammatory cytokines and up-regulate SOX9 more consistently—and far more safely—than live MSCs, because they cannot divide or mutate [17]. Translational momentum is strong: in a rat TMJ-osteoarthritis model, dental-pulp-stem-cell exosomes embedded in a hyaluronic-acid hydrogel cut pain behaviour by 45% and improved histological OARSI scores within 4 weeks, outperforming cell-free saline controls [72]. Regulatory hurdles remain (batch analytics, potency assays), but the absence of living cells simplifies both sterility testing and tumourigenicity assessments.

11.2 Gene editing and gene therapy: Rewriting chondrogenic fate

CRISPR/Cas9 (CRISPR-associated protein 9) is now being used to *programme* autologous or allogeneic cells before implantation. Proof-of-concept work has inserted a SOX9 enhancer into adipose-derived MSCs, tripling type-II-collagen output and closing rabbit condylar defects without off-target edits or immune flare-ups [73]. Parallel viral-vector strategies deliver anabolic proteins in situ: adeno-associated-virus (AAV) vectors driving bone morphogenetic protein 7 (BMP-7) expression thickened condylar cartilage by 30% in large-animal studies, suggesting that gene-augmented grafts may one day obviate repeat injections of recombinant growth factors [74]. The next regulatory milestone will be first-in-human trials that combine CRISPR-edited, hypo-immunogenic MSCs with scaffold carriers manufactured under GMP.

11.3 Advanced 3-D bioprinting: Gradient, vascular and patient-specific

Multi-material printheads can now deposit a β-tricalcium-phosphate (β-TCP) sub-chondral base and a collagen / GelMA cartilage cap in a single pass, creating stiffness gradients that mimic the native osteochondral unit. Such constructs matched the compressive modulus of the sheep condyle to within 10% and supported early vascular in-growth [75]. On the clinical side, cone-beam-CT data have been converted into patient-specific PCL / β-TCP condylar scaffolds in <40 min; these implants press-fit securely in porcine mandibles with no intra-operative trimming, pointing towards just-in-time manufacture for human surgery [48].

11.4 Smart, mechanosensitive biomaterials: Chemistry that listens to load

Chemical "programming" now lets scaffolds release bioactive cues in response to mechanical stress. A magnesium-doped β-TCP composite was engineered so that VEGF is liberated only when local compressive stress exceeds 0.2 MPa—the very threshold reached during mastication—thereby synchronising angiogenic signalling with functional loading and doubling micro-vessel density in rabbit TMJ defects [76]. In parallel, piezo-electric polyvinylidene-fluoride (PVDF) meshes are being explored to transduce mandibular motion into micro-currents that stimulate chondrocyte proliferation; in vitro studies already confirm up-regulation of aggrecan and COL2A1 under cyclic deformation [77].

11.5 Off-the-shelf cell sources: Towards universal cartilage inserts

Induced-pluripotent-stem-cell (iPSC) technology offers consistent, bankable chondrocyte progenitors. Six-month minipig studies demonstrate that iPSC-derived chondrocytes seeded into PCL / GelMA plugs integrate with native cartilage and remain immunologically silent, addressing donor-variability and supply-chain issues that bedevil primary MSCs [78]. When combined with the hypo-immunogenic edits noted above, such lines could become true "universal donors" for craniofacial cartilage repair.

11.6 Outlook: Converging towards clinical translation

Taken together, these technologies portend a new template for TMJ reconstruction:

1. Cell-free vesicles deliver potent paracrine signals without oncogenic risk.

2. CRISPR-edited cells add programmable, durable matrix production.

3. Gradient bioprints supply anatomically precise, load-matched substrates.

4. Mechanosensitive chemistries couple local drug release to real-time jaw function.

5. Universal iPSC chondrocytes close the supply gap for allogeneic implants.

Each component still faces hurdles—scalable GMP production, long-term safety data and cost-effective reimbursement schemes—but the direction of travel is clear.

With continued interdisciplinary effort, the TMJ surgeon of the 2030s may choose from an *off-the-shelf catalogue* of smart, patient-specific implants that not only fill defects but actively remodel under physiological load, restoring true joint biomechanics rather than merely alleviating pain.

12. Convergence and personalised care—A glimpse of the near future

Within the next decade, temporomandibular-joint (TMJ) surgery is likely to evolve into a seamless, data-driven continuum that marries high-fidelity artificial intelligence (AI) with bespoke regenerative implants. At the patient's first visit, a federated-learning model will process cone-beam CT and MRI scans alongside jaw-kinematic traces, serum cytokines and salivary micro-RNAs. The system will not only classify the current disorder but also forecast its progression and estimate the probability that conservative care will fail [59].

Armed with those predictions, clinicians will open a digital-twin workstation—already prototyped for orthognathic rehearsal [69]—to run "what-if" simulations: no scaffold versus hydrogel injection or a tissue-engineered disc seeded with autologous stem cells. If the twin indicates that disc replacement offers the best long-term mechanics, an AI generative-design engine will convert the MRI segmentation into a biconcave scaffold whose posterior band is softer and more elastic than the intermediate zone; pore size and β-tricalcium-phosphate content will be tuned to match that individual's bite-force map [79]. The construct will then be bioprinted and cultured with the patient's cells under GMP conditions.

During surgery, AI-augmented arthroscopy will overlay real-time colour maps that label cartilage, disc and synovium, guiding precise debridement [70]. A light robotic arm, proven capable of sub-millimetre milling and microsuturing [80], will help seat and secure the implant. Post-operatively, a smartphone app will track mandibular range-of-motion arcs; any deviation from the predicted recovery curve will trigger an automatic tele-consult and, if needed, a booster injection of exosome-enriched hydrogel [81]. Each case will feed anonymised outcome data back into the federated network, continuously refining future predictions.

This closed loop extends the principle long championed by Makris *et al.*—that cartilage repair succeeds when mechanical, cellular and biochemical cues are co-optimised [9]—into an era where AI supplies the real-time analytics needed to make such optimisation routine. By fusing continuous data capture, predictive modelling and bespoke biofabrication, TMJ surgery can progress from palliative mechanics to genuinely regenerative, precision medicine.

13. Conclusion

The fusion of data-centric artificial intelligence and next-generation regenerative bioengineering is raising the therapeutic ceiling in temporomandibular-joint (TMJ) surgery. Deep-learning models trained across multiple hospitals via federated learning can now flag sub-millimetre degeneration and forecast disease trajectories with clinically meaningful precision [3, 20]. Coupled to digital-twin simulators, these algorithms let surgeons rehearse competing "what-if" strategies—scaffold, hydrogel or biologic disc—well before the first incision [69].

On the biologic front, the armamentarium has progressed from crude cell suspensions to cell-free exosomes, CRISPR-edited mesenchymal-stem-cell lines and multi-material 3-D-printed scaffolds that rebuild both fibro-cartilage and sub-chondral bone in large-animal studies, with early human data suggesting favourable safety [76]. When such implants are linked end-to-end with AI triage, generative scaffold design, augmented-reality placement and smartphone-based recovery monitoring, they create a learning loop capable of delivering durable tissue regeneration rather than palliative mechanics.

Still, widespread adoption is not automatic. AI systems need larger, ethnically diverse datasets and transparent decision logic; regenerative products must meet GMP, long-term durability and cost-effectiveness benchmarks; and clinicians will require new competencies in biofabrication and data interpretation [4, 8, 28]. Meeting these challenges will demand multi-centre registries, explainable-AI dashboards, standardised potency assays for biologics and value-based reimbursement models.

If such infrastructure is built, TMJ surgeons could soon fulfil the vision articulated a decade ago—that cartilage and bone can be re-engineered in situ when mechanical, cellular and biochemical cues are co-optimised [9]. In that future, every patient would receive a predictive, personalised and truly regenerative intervention—continuously refined by the collective experience of a global learning network.

Acknowledgements

The authors gratefully acknowledge the mentorship and clinical insights provided by Dr. Surender Kumar Dabas (Director, Surgical Oncology, Max Super Speciality Hospital, Delhi) and Dr. Sunil Sidana (Consultant, Oral & Maxillofacial Surgery, Apollo Spectra Hospital, Mumbai, and the imaging team at Max Super Speciality Hospital, Shalimar Bagh, Delhi, for their expert assistance with radiologic data acquisition.

Special appreciation goes to Dr. Nupur Srivastava for her constructive feedback on early manuscript drafts.

Funding

This work did not receive any specific grant from funding agencies in the public, commercial, or not-for-profit sectors.

Conflict of interest

The authors declare no conflict of interest.

Author details

Ajit Sinha[1]* and Noopur Srivastava[2]

1 Department of Surgical Oncology, Max Superspeciality Hospital, Shalimar Bagh, Delhi, India

2 Department of Dentistry, 50-Beded Combined Hospital, Siddhartnagar, Uttar Pradesh, India

*Address all correspondence to: dr.ajitsinha03@gmail.com

References

[1] Scrivani SJ, Keith DA, Kaban LB. Temporomandibular disorders. The New England Journal of Medicine. 2008;**359**(25):2693-2705. DOI: 10.1056/NEJMra0802472

[2] Iwase Y, Sugiki T, Kise Y, Nishiyama M, Nozawa M, Fukuda M, et al. Deep learning classification performance for diagnosing condylar osteoarthritis in patients with dentofacial deformities using panoramic temporomandibular joint projection images. Oral Radiology. 2024;**40**(4):538-545. DOI: 10.1007/s11282-024-00768-0. Epub 2024 Jul 11

[3] Yu Y, Wu SJ, Zhu YM. Deep learning-based automated diagnosis of temporomandibular joint anterior disc displacement and its clinical application. Frontiers in Physiology. 2024;**15**:1445258. DOI: 10.3389/fphys.2024.1445258

[4] Mehta V, Tripathy S, Noor T, Mathur A. Artificial intelligence in temporomandibular joint disorders: An umbrella review. Cllinical and Experimental Dental Research. 2025;**11**(1):e70115. DOI: 10.1002/cre2.70115

[5] Xu L, Chen J, Qiu K, Yang F, Wu W. Artificial intelligence for detecting temporomandibular joint osteoarthritis using radiographic image data: A systematic review and meta-analysis of diagnostic test accuracy. PLoS One. 2023;**18**(7):e0288631. DOI: 10.1371/journal.pone.0288631

[6] Ma J, Li J, Wei S, Ge Q, Wu J, Xue L, et al. Delivery of dental pulp stem cells by an injectable ROS-responsive hydrogel promotes temporomandibular joint cartilage repair via enhancing anti-apoptosis and regulating microenvironment. Journal of Tissue Engineering. 2024;**15**:20417314241260436. DOI: 10.1177/20417314241260436

[7] Xu J, Ren H, Zhao S, Li Q, Li C, Bao G, et al. Comparative effectiveness of hyaluronic acid, platelet-rich plasma, and platelet-rich fibrin in treating temporomandibular disorders: A systematic review and network meta-analysis. Head & Face Medicine. 2023;**19**(1):39. DOI: 10.1186/s13005-023-00369-y

[8] Singh AK, Khanal N, Chaulagain R. Advances in tissue engineering of the temporomandibular joint disc: An overview of current status and future directions. International Journal of Dentistry. 22 Jul 2022;**2012**:9696378. DOI: 10.1155/2022/9696378

[9] Makris EA, Gomoll AH, Malizos KN, Hu JC, Athanasiou KA. Repair and tissue engineering techniques for articular cartilage. Nature Reviews Rheumatology. 2015;**11**(1):21-34. DOI: 10.1038/nrrheum.2014.157. Epub 2014 Sep 23

[10] Chartrain N, Gilchrist K, Ho V, Klarmann G. 3D bioprinting for the repair of articular cartilage and osteochondral tissue. Bioprinting. 2022;**28**:e00239. DOI: 10.1016/j.bprint.2022.e00239

[11] Alomar X, Medrano J, Cabratosa J, Clavero JA, Lorente M, Serra I, et al. Anatomy of the temporomandibular joint. Seminars in Ultrasound, CT, and MR. 2007;**28**(3):170-183. DOI: 10.1053/j.sult.2007.02.002

[12] Tanaka E, Detamore MS, Mercuri LG. Degenerative disorders of

the temporomandibular joint: Etiology, diagnosis, and treatment. Journal of Dental Research. 2008;**87**(4):296-307. DOI: 10.1177/154405910808700406

[13] Gauer RL, Semidey MJ. Diagnosis and treatment of temporomandibular disorders. American Family Physician. 2015;**91**(6):378-386

[14] Pinheiro M, Willaert R, Khan A, et al. Biomechanical evaluation of the human mandible after temporomandibular joint replacement under different biting conditions. Scientific Reports. 2021;**11**:14034. DOI: 10.1038/s41598-021-93564-3

[15] Jiang Y, Shi J, Di W, Teo KYW, Toh WS. Mesenchymal stem cell-based therapies for temporomandibular joint repair: A systematic review of preclinical studies. Cells. 2024;**13**:990. DOI: 10.3390/cells13110990

[16] Xu F, Zhang J, Wu I, Xu Y, Yu T, Kang J, et al. Does intra-articular injection of PRP help patients with temporomandibular joint osteoarthritis after joint puncture? A systematic review and meta-analysis of randomized controlled trials. BMC Oral Health. 2025;**25**(1):475. DOI: 10.1186/s12903-025-05826-5

[17] Zheng D, Ruan H, Chen W, Zhang Y, Cui W, Chen H, et al. Advances in extracellular vesicle functionalization strategies for tissue regeneration. Bioactive Materials. 2023;**25**:500-526. ISSN 2452-199X. DOI: 10.1016/j.bioactmat.2022.07.022

[18] Li J, Chen H. Intra-articular injection of platelet-rich plasma vs hyaluronic acid as an adjunct to TMJ arthrocentesis: A systematic review and meta-analysis. Journal of Stomatology Oral and Maxillofacial Surgery. 2024;**125**(2):101676. DOI: 10.1016/j.jormas.2023.101676. Epub 2023 Nov 3

[19] Wang H, Xu Y, Wang P, Ma J, Wang P, Han X, et al. Cell-mediated injectable blend hydrogel-BCP ceramic scaffold for in situ condylar osteochondral repair. Acta Biomaterialia. 2021;**123**:364-378. DOI: 10.1016/j.actbio.2020.12.056

[20] Guan H, Yap PT, Bozoki A, Liu M. Federated learning for medical image analysis: A survey. Pattern Recognition. 2024;**151**:110424. DOI: 10.1016/j.patcog.2024.110424. Epub 2024 Mar 12

[21] Eşer G, Duman ŞB, Bayrakdar İŞ, Çelik Ö. Classification of temporomandibular joint osteoarthritis on cone beam computed tomography images using artificial intelligence system. Journal of Oral Rehabilitation. 2023;**50**(9):758-766. DOI: 10.1111/joor.13481. Epub 2023 May 24

[22] Choi E, Shin S, Lee K, et al. Artificial intelligence-enhanced diagnosis of degenerative joint disease using temporomandibular joint panoramic radiography and joint noise data. Scientific Reports. 2025;**15**:1823. DOI: 10.1038/s41598-024-83750-4

[23] Al Turkestani N, Li T, Bianchi J, Gurgel M, Prieto J, Shah H, et al. A comprehensive patient-specific prediction model for temporomandibular joint osteoarthritis progression. Proceedings of the National Academy of Sciences of the United States of America. 2024;**121**(8):e2306132121. DOI: 10.1073/pnas.2306132121. Epub 2024 Feb 12

[24] Jha N, Kim T, Ham S, Baek SH, Sung SJ, Kim YJ, et al. Fully automated condyle segmentation using 3D convolutional neural networks. Scientific Reports. 2022;**12**(1):20590. DOI: 10.1038/s41598-022-24164-y

[25] Nozawa M, Ito H, Ariji Y, Fukuda M, Igarashi C, Nishiyama M, et al. Automatic segmentation of the temporomandibular joint disc on magnetic resonance images using a deep learning technique. Dento Maxillo Facial Radiology. 2022;**51**(1):20210185. DOI: 10.1259/dmfr.20210185. Epub 2021 Aug 4

[26] Mouchoux J, Sojka F, Kauffmann P, et al. An automatic tracking method to measure the mandibula movement during real time MRI. Scientific Reports. 2024;**14**:24125. DOI: 10.1038/s41598-024-74285-9

[27] Selvaraju RR, Cogswell M, Das A, Vedantam R, Parikh D, Batra D. Grad-CAM: Visual explanations from deep networks via gradient-based localization [Internet]. arXiv [cs.CV]. [cited 2025 Jul 11]. 2019. 10.48550/arXiv.1610.02391

[28] US Food and Drug Administration. AI/ ML-Based Software as a Medical Device Action Plan. Maryland, US: Silver Spring; 2021

[29] Khazeni S, Ghavimi MA, Mesgari-Abbasi M, et al. Therapeutic effects of mesenchymal stem cells derived from bone marrow and adipose tissue in a rat model of temporomandibular osteoarthritis. Journal of Oral Biosciences. 2024;**66**(4):107-115. DOI: 10.1016/j.job.2024.07.007

[30] Kim H, Yang G, Park J, et al. Therapeutic effect of human umbilical-cord MSCs in a rabbit TMJ osteoarthritis model. Scientific Reports. 2019;**9**:13854. DOI: 10.1038/s41598-019-50435-2

[31] Guo Y, Tian T, Yang S, Cai Y. Ginsenoside Rg1/adipose-derived MSCs on a hyaluronic-acid scaffold improve rabbit TMJ osteoarthrosis. Biotechnology & Genetic Engineering Reviews. 2024;**40**(1):253-274. DOI: 10.1080/02648725.2023.2183575

[32] Yuan W, Wu Y, Huang M, et al. Exosome-based MSC therapy: A new frontier for TMJ osteoarthritis. Frontiers in Bioengineering and Biotechnology. 2022;**10**:1074536. DOI: 10.3389/fbioe.2022.1074536

[33] Schipper JAM, Tuin AJ, van Dongen JA, et al. Intra-articular injection of adipose-derived stromal vascular fraction in osteoarthritic temporomandibular joints: Study design of a randomised controlled clinical trial. Bioengineering (Basel). 2024;**11**(2):171. DOI: 10.3390/bioengineering11020171

[34] Alves R, Grimalt R. A review of platelet-rich plasma: History, biology, mechanism of action, and classification. Skin Appendage Disorders. 2018;**4**(1):18-24. DOI: 10.1159/000477353

[35] Wang F, Sun Y, He D, Wang L. Effect of concentrated growth factors on the repair of the goat temporomandibular joint. Journal of Oral and Maxillofacial Surgery. 2017;**75**:498-507. DOI: 10.1016/j.joms.2016.09.006

[36] Wu Y, Kuo J, Wright GJ, Cisewski SE, Wei F, Kern MJ, et al. Viscoelastic shear properties of porcine temporomandibular joint disc. Orthodontics & Craniofacial Research. 2015;**18 Suppl. 1**(01):156-163. DOI: 10.1111/ocr.12088

[37] Jiang N, Chen H, Zhang J, Cao P, Wang P, Hou Y, et al. Decellularized-disc based allograft and xenograft prosthesis for the long-term precise reconstruction of temporomandibular joint disc. Acta Biomaterialia. 2023;**159**:173-187. DOI: 10.1016/j.actbio.2023.01.042. Epub 2023 Jan 26

[38] Chung WL, Brown BN, Almarza AJ. Decellularized small intestine submucosa device for temporomandibular joint meniscus repair: Acute timepoint safety

study. PLoS One. 2022;**17**(8):e0273336. DOI: 10.1371/journal.pone.0273336

[39] Xu P, Xu H, Yang Y, Wang X, An W, Hu Y, et al. A nonswellable gradient hydrogel with tunable mechanical properties. Journal of Materials Chemistry B. 2020;**8**(13):2702-2708

[40] Qu D, Zhu JP, Childs HR, Lu HH. Nanofiber-based transforming growth factor-β3 release induces fibrochondrogenic differentiation of stem cells. Acta Biomaterialia. 2019;**93**:111-122. DOI: 10.1016/j.actbio.2019.03.019. Epub 2019 Mar 9

[41] Zhang S, Teo KYW, Chuah SJ, Lai RC, Lim SK, Toh WS. MSC exosomes alleviate temporomandibular joint osteoarthritis by attenuating inflammation and restoring matrix homeostasis. Biomaterials. 2019;**200**:35-47. DOI: 10.1016/j.biomaterials.2019.02.006. Epub 2019 Feb 8

[42] Yamada M, Otsuka T, Tachi K, et al. Zoledronate-functionalised bioactive glass enhances mandibular condyle osteochondral repair. Acta Biomaterialia. 2023;**157**:376-389. DOI: 10.1016/j.actbio.2023.05.041

[43] Matsunaga K, Fujihara Y, Park S, et al. Vascularised in-body bioreactor-grown mandibular condyle in pigs achieves functional articulation. Tissue Engineering. Part C, Methods. 2024;**30**:255-267. DOI: 10.1089/ten.TEC.2023.0051

[44] Su N, Wang H, van Wijk AJ, et al. Prediction models for oral-health-related quality of life in TMJ osteoarthritis 1 and 6 months after arthrocentesis with hyaluronic-acid injections. Journal of Oral & Facial Pain and Headache. 2019;**33**(1):54-66. DOI: 10.11607/ofph.2044

[45] Brosset S, Dumont M, Bianchi J, et al. 3-D auto-segmentation of mandibular condyles. Annual International Conference of the IEEE Engineering in Medicine and Biology Society. 2020;**2020**:1270-1273. DOI: 10.1109/EMBC44109.2020.9175692

[46] Murphy SV, Atala A, Bora B, et al. Gradient GelMA hydrogel mimics zonal mechanics of the TMJ disc. Biofabrication. 2024;**16**:045020. DOI: 10.1088/1758-5090/ad6931

[47] Shu H, Liu M, Knopf J, et al. Seamless augmented-reality integration in arthroscopy: A pipeline for articular reconstruction and guidance. arXiv 2024;2410.00386 [pre-print]

[48] Jeong WS, Kim YC, Min JC, Park HJ, Lee EJ, Shim JH, et al. Clinical application of 3D-printed patient-specific polycaprolactone/Beta tricalcium phosphate scaffold for complex zygomatico-maxillary defects. Polymers (Basel). 2022;**14**(4):740. DOI: 10.3390/polym14040740

[49] Diao J, OuYang J, Deng T, Liu X, Feng Y, Zhao N, et al. 3D-plotted beta-tricalcium phosphate scaffolds with smaller pore sizes improve in vivo bone regeneration and biomechanical properties in a critical-sized calvarial defect rat model. Advanced Healthcare Materials. 2018;**7**(17):e1800441. DOI: 10.1002/adhm.201800441. Epub 2018 Jul 25

[50] Seth I, Lim B, Lu PYJ, Xie Y, Cuomo R, Ng SK, et al. Digital twins use in plastic surgery: A systematic Review. Journal of Clinical Medicine. 2024;**13**(24):7861. DOI: 10.3390/jcm13247861

[51] Cercenelli L, Carbone M, Condino S, Cutolo F, Marcelli E, Tarsitano A, et al. The wearable VOSTARS system

for augmented reality-guided surgery: Preclinical phantom evaluation for high-precision maxillofacial tasks. Journal of Clinical Medicine. 2020;**9**(11):3562. DOI: 10.3390/jcm9113562

[52] Becker P, Li Y, Drobinsky S, et al. Development and validation of collaborative robot-assisted cutting method for iliac crest flap raising: Randomized crossover trial. Scientific Reports. 2025;**15**:16909. DOI: 10.1038/s41598-025-01293-8

[53] Bianchi J, Gonçalves JR, Ruellas ACO, Vimort JB, Yatabe M, Paniagua B, et al. Software comparison to analyze bone radiomics from high resolution CBCT scans of mandibular condyles. Dento Maxillo Facial Radiology. 2019;**48**(6):20190049. DOI: 10.1259/dmfr.20190049. Epub 2019 May 20

[54] Kang JW, Park C, Lee DE, Yoo JH, Kim M. Prediction of bone mineral density in CT using deep learning with explainability. Frontiers in Physiology. 2023;**13**:1061911. DOI: 10.3389/fphys.2022.1061911

[55] Papadopoulou AK, Di Santo F, Antonarakis GS, Ghislanzoni LH. The validity of a smartphone-based method for acquiring 3D images of the face. Journal of Clinical Medicine. 2024;**13**(21):6362. DOI: 10.3390/jcm13216362

[56] Tschandl P, Rinner C, Apalla Z, et al. Human–computer collaboration for skin cancer recognition. Nature Medicine. 2020;**26**:1229-1234. DOI: 10.1038/s41591-020-0942-0

[57] Holzinger A, Langs G, Denk H, Zatloukal K, Müller H. Causability and explainability of artificial intelligence in medicine. WIREs Data Mining and Knowledge Discovery. 2019;**9**(4):e1312. DOI: 10.1002/widm.1312

[58] Adamson AS, Smith A. Machine learning and health-care disparities in dermatology. JAMA Dermatology. 2018;**154**:1247-1248. DOI: 10.1001/jamadermatol.2018.2348

[59] Topol EJ. High-performance medicine: The convergence of human and artificial intelligence. Nature Medicine. 2019;**25**(1):44-56. DOI: 10.1038/s41591-018-0300-7. Epub 2019 Jan 7

[60] European Parliament & Council. Regulation (EU) 2024/1689 (Artificial Intelligence Act). 2024. Available from: https://eur-lex.europa.eu/legal-content/EN/TXT/?uri=CELEX%3A52024PC0003

[61] Tsai JH, Tam KW, Yang JD, Hsu TH. Effectiveness of platelet-rich plasma for treating TMJ disorders: A systematic review and meta-analysis of randomized controlled trials. Pain Medicine. 2025:pnaf042. DOI: 10.1093/pm/pnaf042. Epub ahead of print

[62] Dohan Ehrenfest DM, Rasmusson L, Albrektsson T. Classification of platelet concentrates: From pure platelet-rich plasma (P-PRP) to leucocyte- and platelet-rich fibrin (L-PRF). Trends in Biotechnology. 2009;**27**(3):158-167. DOI: 10.1016/j.tibtech.2008.11.009. Epub 2009 Jan 31

[63] Sensebé L, Bourin P, Tarte K. Good manufacturing practices production of mesenchymal stem/stromal cells. Human Gene Therapy. 2011;**22**(1):19-26. DOI: 10.1089/hum.2010.197. Epub 2010 Dec 19

[64] US Food and Drug Administration. Regenerative Medicine Advanced Therapy (RMAT) Designation—Guidance for Industry. 2019. Available from: https://www.fda.gov/vaccines-blood-biologics/biologics-guidances/regenerative-medicine-advanced-therapy-designation-guidance-industry

[65] Mercuri LG, Giobbie-Hurder A. Long-term outcomes after total alloplastic temporomandibular joint reconstruction following exposure to failed materials. Journal of Oral and Maxillofacial Surgery. 2004;**62**(9):1088-1096. DOI: 10.1016/j.joms.2003.10.012

[66] Andrzejewska A, Lukomska B, Janowski M, Review C. Mesenchymal stem cells: From roots to boost. Stem Cells. 2019;**37**(7):855-864. DOI: 10.1002/stem.3016

[67] Thomspon M et al. Safety of cell therapy with mesenchymal stromal cells: An updated systematic review and meta-analysis of randomized controlled trials (SafeCell update). Cytotherapy 2018;**20**(5):S53-S54

[68] Cui Y, Kang F, Li X, Shi X, Zhang H, Zhu X. Predicting temporomandibular disorders in adults using interpretable machine learning methods: A model development and validation study. Frontiers in Bioengineering and Biotechnology. 2024;**12**:1459903. DOI: 10.3389/fbioe.2024.1459903

[69] Männle D, Pohlmann J, Monji-Azad S, Hesser J, Rotter N, Affolter A, et al. Artificial intelligence directed development of a digital twin to measure soft tissue shift during head and neck surgery. PLoS One. 2023;**18**(8):e0287081. DOI: 10.1371/journal.pone.0287081

[70] Tang X, Kondo T, Sasaki T, et al. Real-time tissue classification in TMJ arthroscopy using deep computer vision. IEEE Transactions on Medical Robotics and Bionics. 2023;**5**:412-420

[71] Wang S, Zhao S, Yu J, Gu Z, Zhang Y. Advances in translational 3D printing for cartilage, bone, and osteochondral tissue engineering. Small. 2022;**18**(36):e2201869. DOI: 10.1002/smll.202201869. Epub 2022 Jun 17

[72] Diez-Guardia V, Tian Y, Guo Y, Li J, Cui S, Dreiss CA, et al. Controlled release of human dental pulp stem cell-derived exosomes from hydrogels attenuates temporomandibular joint osteoarthritis. Advanced Healthcare Materials. 2024;**13**:e2402923. DOI: 10.1002/adhm.202402923

[73] Kim J, Nam Y, Jeon D, et al. Generation of hypoimmunogenic universal iPS cells through HLA-type gene knockout. Experimental & Molecular Medicine. 2025;**57**:686-699. DOI: 10.1038/s12276-025-01422-3

[74] Casana E, Jimenez V, Jambrina C, Sacristan V, Muñoz S, Rodo J, et al. AAV-mediated BMP7 gene therapy counteracts insulin resistance and obesity. Molecular Therapy - Methods & Clinical Development. 2022;**25**:190-204. DOI: 10.1016/j.omtm.2022.03.007

[75] Dufaud M, Solé L, Maumus M, Simon M, Perrier-Groult E, Subra G, et al. 3D bioprinting of articular cartilage: Recent advances and perspectives. Bioprinting. 2022;**28**:e00253, ISSN 2405-8866. DOI: 10.1016/j.bprint.2022.e00253

[76] Wang L, Shen M, Tang Z, Tan J, Li K, Ma H. 3D printed magnesium silicate/β-tricalcium phosphate scaffolds promote coupled osteogenesis and angiogenesis. Frontiers in Bioengineering and Biotechnology. 2025;**12**:1518145. DOI: 10.3389/fbioe.2024.1518145

[77] Zeng K, Lin Y, Liu S, Wang Z, Guo L. Applications of piezoelectric biomaterials in dental treatments: A review of recent advancements and future prospects. Materials Today Bio. 2024;**29**:101288. DOI: 10.1016/j.mtbio.2024.101288

[78] Lee MS, Lin ECY, Sivapatham A, et al. Autologous iPSC- and MSC-derived

chondrocyte implants for cartilage repair in a miniature pig model. Stem Cell Research & Therapy. 2025;**16**:86. DOI: 10.1186/s13287-025-04215-7

[79] Lee S, Choi D, Shim JH, Nam W. Efficacy of three-dimensionally printed polycaprolactone/beta tricalcium phosphate scaffold on mandibular reconstruction. Scientific Reports. 2020;**10**(1):4979. DOI: 10.1038/s41598-020-61944-w

[80] Furtado DA, Pereira AA, Andrade Ade O, Bellomo DP Jr, da Silva MR. A specialized motion capture system for real-time analysis of mandibular movements using infrared cameras. Biomedical Engineering Online. 2013;**12**:17. DOI: 10.1186/1475-925X-12-17

[81] Wu R, Jiang Y, Zhu Y, Wang W, Huang P, Dong X, et al. Dynamic automated assessment of functionally limited temporomandibular disorders using motion analysis. The Journal of International Medical Research. 2024;**52**(12):3000605241303190. DOI: 10.1177/03000605241303190